Chronic Disorders in Children and Adolescents

Mark L. Goldstein · Stephen Morewitz

Chronic Disorders in Children and Adolescents

Springer

Mark L. Goldstein
Sheridan Rd., Suite 215 1893
60035 Highland Park
Chicago, IL
USA
mlglmr@aol.com

Stephen Morewitz
Noe Street 695
94114 San Francisco
CA, USA
morewitz@earthlink.net

ISBN 978-1-4899-9852-1 ISBN 978-1-4419-9764-7 (eBook)
DOI 10.1007/978-1-4419-9764-7
Springer New York Dordrecht Heidelberg London

Printed on acid-free paper

Springer is part of Springer Science+Business Media (www.springer.com)

Acknowledgments

Steve would like to thank Mrs. Myra Kalkin Morewitz and Dr. Harry A. Morewitz for their advice and support. He would like to thank Ms. Vandana Ganatra for her research assistance.

Mark would like to thank his wife, Lisa, for her support, understanding, encouragement, and love. He would also like to thank his children, Ashley and Jonathan, who provide healthy role models.

We would also like to thank Bill Tucker, Public Health Editor at Springer, who has been supportive, as well as thorough and thoughtful.

Contents

About the Authors

Dr. Mark L. Goldstein is a licensed clinical psychologist, who specializes in the diagnosis and treatment of children, adolescents, and families. He also has served as an expert witness in over 1,100 forensic cases and consults to suburban school systems in the Chicago area. Dr. Goldstein was previously an associate professor at the Illinois School of Professional Psychology and served as an adjunct professor at the University of Illinois College of Medicine, Roosevelt University, Forest Institute of Professional Psychology, and the Chicago School of Professional Psychology. He has presented numerous papers at national and international conferences and has published a number of articles, book chapters, and the book, *Aging and Chronic Disorders* (Springer, 2007, with Dr. Stephen Morewitz).

Dr. Stephen Morewitz is a lecturer in the Department of Nursing and Health Sciences at California State University, East Bay, and is president of the consulting firm, Stephen Morewitz, Ph.D., & Associates, Buffalo Grove, IL, San Francisco, and Tarzana, CA. Dr. Morewitz was a professor and research dean at the California School of Podiatric Medicine, CA. He has been on the faculty or staffs of Michael Reese Hospital and Medical Center, University of Illinois at Chicago, College of Medicine and School of Public Health, DePaul University, and Argonne National Laboratory, Division of Biological and Medical Research. Dr. Morewitz is the author of more than 100 publications, including the award-winning book, *Domestic Violence and Maternal and Child Health* (New York: Kluwer Academic/Plenum Publishers, 2004), *Chronic Diseases and Health Care* (New York, Springer Science+Business Media, Inc., 2006), *Aging and Chronic Disorders* (New York, Springer, 2007) with Mark L. Goldstein, the award-winning book, *Stalking and Violence* (New York: Kluwer Academic/Plenum Publishers, 2003), and *Death Threats and Violence* (New York: Springer Science+Business Media, L.L.C., 2008).

Chapter 1
Epidemiology, Health Services Utilization, and Costs

Health-care access, utilization, quality, and expenditures have changed for children and youth in recent decades. In the USA, Simpson et al. (2004) used the 1996–2001 Medical Expenditure Panel Survey and the Nationwide Inpatient Sample (1995–2000) from the Healthcare Cost and Utilization project, and the National Medical Expenditure Survey (1987) to evaluate trends in insurance coverage, health-care utilization, perceived quality of care, and costs for children and youth. The authors discovered that since 1987, health care for children and youth has changed substantially, especially between 1987 and 1996. Their results showed that insurance coverage has improved, care has shifted from hospital to ambulatory settings, hospital use has declined, and the costs related to the care of children and youth as a percentage of the total health-care costs have declined.

Although hospital use has declined, hospital costs remain substantial, especially for freestanding children's hospitals. Higher health-care costs are associated with children's hospitals compared to other health-care settings. A variety of factors contribute to these higher health-care costs. Using data from the Healthcare Cost and Utilization Project Kids' Inpatient Database 2000, Merenstein et al. (2005) discovered that freestanding children's hospitals offered health care to children who were more likely to be at higher risk for health-care problems, have more co-diagnoses, come from minority backgrounds, and be enrolled in Medicaid than non-children's hospitals. Children's hospitals did not differ in median length of stay with non-children's hospitals. However, the investigators showed that children's hospitals had higher total costs than non-children's hospitals. Children's hospitals had a median cost of admission that was $1,294 more per hospitalization than non-children's hospitals.

National policies, such as the State Children's Health Insurance Program (SCHIP), have been developed to improve children's access to health care. Researchers have shown that children and adolescents who participate in SCHIP improve their access to care. For example, Klein et al. (2007) showed that adolescents in New York's SCHIP were more likely to report a usual source of care than before entering into the program.

Nevertheless, many children and youth have difficulty accessing health-care services in the USA and in other countries. According to Fry-Johnson et al. (2005), almost 8½ million children were uninsured in the USA The authors noted that

M.L. Goldstein, S. Morewitz, *Chronic Disorders in Children and Adolescents*,
DOI 10.1007/978-1-4419-9764-7_1, © Springer Science+Business Media, LLC 2011

Medicaid and the SCHIP have not accomplished expected results since more than 70% of uninsured children are eligible for either of these public programs. Moreover, families of uninsured children are confronted with non-financial barriers to health care such as not having continuous care provided by a primary care professional and insufficient visit time.

Researchers find that low-income families have problems with insurance coverage, health-care utilization, and quality of care for their children. Simpson et al. (2005) discovered that children from low-income families were more likely than children from middle–high-income families to be uninsured or have public insurance and less likely to be privately insured. Children from low-income families were less likely to have had a medical office visit or a dental office visit than children from middle–high-income families for office-based visits, less likely to have prescribed medications, or have used hospital outpatient services. However, children from low-income families were more likely than children from middle–high-income families to use emergency departments. Children from low-income families were more likely than children from middle–high-income families to have their parents report major difficulty in obtaining health care and obtaining a referral to a specialist.

The following analysis examines the epidemiology, health utilization, and costs of selected diseases in childhood and adolescence.

Genetic and Chromosomal Disorders

Researchers are recognizing the increasing role of genetics in childhood diseases (McCandless et al., 2004). However, experts have not documented the full impact of genetics on pediatric conditions. About 4,000 genetic disorders are currently known and more are being discovered. Genetic disorders and congenital abnormalities occur in approximately 2–5% of all live births.

Prevalent genetic syndromes include chromosomal rearrangements, Down syndrome, DiGeorge syndrome, fragile X syndrome, Marfan syndrome, neurofibromatosis, Turner syndrome, and Williams syndrome.

According to Emery and Rimoin (1990), genetic disorder constitutes up to 30% of pediatric hospitalizations, and in developed countries, they are responsible for about 30% of childhood deaths (Emery and Rimoin, 1990). Based on a sample of 5,747 consecutive admissions to Rainbow Babies and Children's Hospital in 1996, McCandless et al. (2004) discovered that 34% had clearly genetic underlying conditions. These genetic disorders made up 50% or more than $31 million of the total hospital charges. Patients with a genetic underlying disorder had an average length of hospital stay that was 40% longer than for patients without an underlying genetic disease.

Cerebral Palsy

The incidence of cerebral palsy (CP) is about 1.5–2 cases per 1,000 live births in the USA and other countries. CP is the most common cause of severe childhood disability.

In a Danish study, Kruse et al. (2009) evaluated the lifetime costs of CP using the Danish Cerebral Palsy Register, which comprises the eastern area of the nation and has approximately 50% of the persons with CP. The investigators divided the lifetime costs associated with the condition into health-care costs, productivity costs, and social costs. Based on a sample of 2,367 persons with CP who were born between 1930 and 2000, the authors demonstrated that for men, the lifetime costs of the disease were approximately 860,000 €, while for women, the lifetime costs were approximately 800,000 €. Social care costs, especially during childhood, accounted for the largest percentage of the costs. The authors performed a sensitivity analysis, which showed that changes in social care costs had a small impact on total lifetime costs. In contrast, reducing the discount rate of social care costs from 5 to 3% significantly raised total lifetime costs.

Using a sample of caregivers of 319 CP patients in specialty hospitals in five cities in 2004, Wang et al. (2008) assessed the economic burden of CP in China. They showed that the average lifetime costs associated with a new CP patient was US $67,044 in 2003. The life span total economic costs related to all new patients with CP in 2003 were US $2–4 billion. The researchers found that indirect costs (productivity) accounted for 93% of total economic costs and direct health-care and developmental costs made up 3–4% each. Loss of productivity, lower life expectancy, increased dependence, progressive loss in motor physical function, and continuous use of rehabilitation services account for the high costs associated with CP.

Autism Spectrum Disorders

Autism spectrum, also called autism spectrum disorders (ASD) or autism spectrum conditions (ASC), refers to a range of behavioral problems that involve impairment in social interactions and communication, severely restricted interests, and repetitive behaviors.

The prevalence of autism ranges from 0.7 to 72.6 per 10,000 (Fombonne, 2009). Other reports estimate a prevalence of 1–2 per 1,000 for autism and almost 6 per 1,000 for ASD. These data may underestimate ASD's true prevalence because of measurement difficulties. The majority of individuals with ASD are classified as PDD-NOS. Asperger's is about 0.3 per 1,000 and the remaining ASD types are much rarer. In the 1990s and early 200s, the number of reported cases of autism increased dramatically. Alterations in diagnostic practices, referral patterns, availability of services, age at diagnosis, and public awareness may have led to these increases in prevalence, although unknown environmental risk factors cannot be disregarded.

An estimated 0.5–10% of individuals with ASD show unusual abilities, ranging from splinter skills, such as the memorization of trivia, to the extraordinarily rare talents of prodigious autistic savants.

Based on a literature review, McCarthy (2007) demonstrated that children with ASD and intellectual disability have a high rate of comorbid conditions, such as attention-deficit/hyperactivity disorder (ADHD), mood disorders, catatonia, and repetitive behaviors, compared to children without ASD. Children and adolescents with ASD have high rates of mental health services, which increase the costs of health-care expenditures.

Knapp et al. (2009) examined the economic costs of ASD in the UK using data on prevalence, intellectual disability level, residence, annual costs of services and support, and opportunity costs of lost productivity. The authors estimated that £2.7 billion were spent annually to support children with ASD. Twenty-five billion pounds were spent each year to support ASD adults. After discounting for a person with ASD and intellectual disability, the estimated lifetime cost was £1.23 million, while for an individual with ASD without intellectual disability the lifetime cost was estimated to be £0.80 million.

ADHD

ADHD is one of the most prevalent chronic disorders in childhood and negative effects continue into adolescence and adulthood (Leibson and Long, 2003). Disease burden is substantial for afflicted persons, their families, and society as a whole. Investigations reveal that direct medical costs for young people with ADHD are about twice those for young persons without the disorder. Cross-sectional research indicate that ADHD-related incremental costs are greatest for mental health services and medication costs and are highest for young people who have comorbid psychiatric disorders and for youth being treated with stimulants.

Based on a literature review, Pelham et al. (2007) analyzed the costs of ADHD in childhood and adolescence. They reviewed 13 investigations, 2 of which were longitudinal studies of children with ADHD who were followed into adolescence. The investigators examined ADHD treatment costs and other medical care costs and several studies analyzed the costs related to education (special education and disciplinary costs), parental work loss, and juvenile justice. The authors estimated the annual cost of illness of the disorder in children and adolescents to be $14,576 per person in $2005, with a range between $12,005 and $17,458 per person. Using a prevalence rate of 5%, they estimated conservatively that the annual societal cost of illness to be $45.2 billion, with a range between $36 billion and $52.4 billion.

Burd et al. (2003), based on data from the North Dakota Department of Health, estimated that the annual cost of care for children with ADHD in North Dakota was $5.1 million, which was 5.6% of all health-care costs for children. They showed that 1.9% of total health expenditure for children was attributable to the disorder. The researchers estimate that in the USA the cost of care attributable to the condition would be $2.15 billion per year.

Using an administrative database from a national Fortune 100 manufacturer, Swensen et al. (2003) estimated the direct and indirect costs of treating children with ADHD and their families. They demonstrated that the annual average direct cost for a patient with ADHD was $1,574 compared to $541 for matched controls. The annual average payment (direct combined with indirect cost) per family member was $2,728 for non-ADHD family members of ADHD patients, compared to $1,440 for family members of matched controls. The investigators conclude that the disorder imposes substantial medical care costs and productivity loss for patients and family members.

Based on the 1996 Medical Expenditure Panel Survey, Chan et al. (2002) compared the costs of treating children with ADHD with the costs of treating children with asthma and the general pediatric population. The investigators discovered that children with ADHD had higher average total health-care costs ($1,151) than children with asthma ($1,091) and the general pediatric population ($712). After controlling for age, sex, and other variables, the excess total costs were $479 for children with ADHD and $437 for children with asthma. The researchers conclude that the costs of treating children with ADHD is similar to the costs for treating children with asthma and is substantially greater than the costs of providing care to the general pediatric population. They note that since ADHD-associated services take place in school and mental health organizations, the data in this study probably underestimate the costs of treating children with this condition.

Leibson et al. (2006) assessed whether the use of stimulants reduced emergency department use and medical cost among young people with ADHD. They discovered that treatment with stimulants was related to less emergency room (ER) use, but higher total medical costs.

Children and adolescents with ADHD and comorbid conditions can have higher use of services, resulting in increased expenditures. Jones and Foster (2009) examined service use, including mental health, school services, and juvenile justice system, and the costs of treating young people, aged 12–17, diagnosed with ADHD and comorbid conduct disorder (CD). They discovered that over a 6-year period, the public costs of caring for young people with ADHD were on average more than $40,000 per child, which were more than twice the expenditures for youth without this condition. Treatment costs for young people with ADHD and comorbid CD were twice as much as the treatment costs for youth with ADHD by itself.

Researchers have evaluated health services utilization and costs associated with treating preschoolers with ADHD. Marks et al. (2009) assessed the use of speech and language therapy, occupational therapy, physical therapy, and special education programs by 3- and 4-year-old children with ADHD compared to a control group. They discovered that preschool children with the disorder had a greater probability of using individual and multiple services compared with their peers. Higher use of services resulted in higher costs for each individual service except physical therapy services.

In other countries, the costs of treating ADHD are substantial. Internationally, drug spending for patients with the condition has increased during the last decade. Schlander (2007) predicts more than a sixfold increase in ADHD drug expenditures for children and adolescents over the decade from 2002 to 2012 using the framework of the National Health Service in the UK and the Gesetzliche Krankenversicherung in Germany.

Psychiatric/Behavioral and Emotional Disorders

Various studies have examined the epidemiology of psychiatric/behavioral and emotional problems in children and adolescents (Mehler-Wex and Kolch, 2008; Lavigne et al., 2009; Keenan et al., 2004).

Depression in children and adolescents has prevalence rates up to 8.9% (Mehler-Wex and Kolch, 2008). Other studies report that 3–5% of children and adolescents have major depression (Bhatia and Bhatia, 2007). Approximately 2% of children of school age and 5–8% of adolescents have depression (Jellinek and Synder, 1998; Birmaher et al., 1998). In successive generations, depression seems to be increasing in prevalence and the onset of the disorder is occurring at younger ages (Klerman et al., 1985; Gershon et al., 1987).

In their literature review, Mehler-Wex and Kolch (2008) discovered that children have a high rate of spontaneous remissions (33%). In addition, they discovered that 80% of cases of depression in childhood and adolescence persisted into adulthood.

Using a sample of 794 4-year-old children selected from schools and pediatric settings, Lavigne et al. (2009) discovered that the most prevalent psychiatric disorders were oppositional defiant disorder (ODD) and ADHD. In less than 1% of the sample, generalized anxiety disorder (GAD) and depressive disorders were found. ADHD-inattentive type was more prevalent among boys than girls. The researchers found no gender differences for GAD, major depressive disorder (MDD), dysthymia, separation anxiety disorder, or ODD. The authors did not discover any racial or ethnic differences in major depressive disorder. The preschoolers had a comorbidity rate of 6.4%. About 3% of the children with a psychiatric diagnosis had been treated in a mental health setting.

Using a community sample of 2,451 girls, aged 5–8 years old, from the Pittsburgh Girls Study, Keenan et al. (2004) showed that less than 1% of the girls had five or more symptoms of an MDD, according to the caregiver reports.

Based on a survey with the Aquitaine Sentinelle Network, Mathet et al. (2003) showed that more than 1 child out of 10 under 13 years had a depressive disorder and the prevalence of depressive disorders in an adolescent sub-group was 5%. In 6% of the children, an MDD occurred, in 4%, dysthymia was present, and in 1%, maladjustment with depressive mood occurred. The researchers discovered that all of the depressive disorders were moderate in nature. In about 50% of the depressed adolescents, atypical depression was present. The young people were diagnosed with other conditions, including anxiety disorders, obsessive–compulsive disorder, and panic disorder. The authors discovered that disruptive disorders were much less prevalent in this sample. Fifty percent of the young people with psychiatric disorders had psychiatric comorbid disorders, especially anxiety disorders. The authors estimated that 70% of the diagnoses of depression were not made during the visits to the general practitioners. The authors recommend training general practitioners to enhance their screening of depressive disorders in young people.

Researchers have studied the increased rates of bipolar disorder (BD) among children and adolescents in certain countries. Using data from the National Hospital Discharge Survey, Blader and Carlson (2007) found that the population-adjusted rates of hospital discharges of children with BD as a primary diagnosis increased in a linear fashion between 1996 and 2004. In 1996, the rate was 1.3 per 10,000 US children and increased to 7.3 per 10,000 US children in 2004. Among adolescents, hospital discharges associated with BD increased fourfold during this period. The investigators discovered that hospitalization associated with BD were more prevalent among female adolescents, while male children were more at risk than female children. Diagnoses for BD in children tended not to specify a prevailing mood state. The authors conclude that the higher rates of BD-related hospital admissions may be due to clinicians' greater recognition of affective dysfunction in children and adolescents or upcoding to more severe problems for reimbursement or administrative purposes.

Holtmann et al. (2010), based on registry data from the German Federal Health Monitoring System, reported that between 2000 and 2007, hospital admissions for BD among German children and adolescents increased to 68.5%, from 1.13 to 1.91 per 100,000. Children under 15 years of age had a non-significant decline, while adolescents, aged 15–19, had the largest relative increase in BD-associated hospitalizations. In their study, hospital admissions for depressive disorders increased by 219.6% and by 111.3% for hyperkinetic disorders. CD-related hospitalizations increased by 18.1%, which was less than the overall increase for all mental disorders. Psychotic disorders were the only diagnostic category to decline significantly (−11.8%) in children and adolescents. In 2000, BD-related hospital admissions constituted only 0.22% of all hospital admissions for mental disorders and 0.27% in 2007. The investigators suggested that the increased rates of BD-associated hospital admissions may be the result of increased clinicians' recognition of mood dysfunction in children and adolescents and re-considering the diagnosis of psychotic problems in young people.

Evans-Lacko et al. (2009), based on a national sample of young people, aged 6–18 years of age, discovered that children and adolescents with BD had a higher rate of comorbid medical conditions than those with other psychiatric disorders. Thirty-six percent of young people with BD suffered from two or more chronic health problems, compared with 8% of young persons with other psychiatric disorders. Youth with BD were more likely to have heart, gastrointestinal/hepatic, neurological, musculoskeletal, female reproduction, and respiratory problems than those with other psychiatric diagnoses. Young people with BD suffered more toxic effects and adverse events than youth with other psychiatric problems. The authors suggest that various factors may explain why young people with BD have higher medical comorbidity, including more side effects from medications, unhealthy lifestyles, worse access to health care, low socioeconomic status, and biologic susceptibility.

Researchers are evaluating the cost-effectiveness of treatments for adolescent depression. Domino et al. (2009), using data from the Treatment of Adolescents with Depression Study (TADS), evaluated the cost-effectiveness of fluoxetine by itself, cognitive behavior therapy (CBT) alone, or both fluoxetine and CBT in treating major depression in adolescents, aged 12–18. The investigators discovered that CBT was the most expensive treatment (mean $1,787 for CBT by itself). Combination therapy was likely to be more cost-effective than fluoxetine by itself at 36 weeks.

The costs of treating children with a CD and other behavioral problems can be substantial especially since multiple agencies often incur costs. The costs of treating a person with CD by the age of 28 were about 10 times higher than for individuals with no problems (Dretzke et al., 2005). Using public sector expenditure data during a 7-year period from mental health, medical care, school, and juvenile justice settings, Foster and Jones (2005) discovered that additional public costs per child associated with CD was more than $70,000 over a 7-year period. In another report, Jones et al. (2002) note that preventing one high-risk child from having bad outcomes may yield net savings to society of almost $2 million as well as enhance the life of that child and her/his family.

Treating children with behavioral disorders who also have emotional disorders may be associated with even higher expenditures. Using data from the 1996 Medical Expenditure Panel Survey, researchers discovered that among children with behavioral disorders, those with emotional disorders were associated with significantly more total costs than children with disruptive disorders (Guevara et al., 2003).

Mental health utilization and expenditures are substantial in foster care settings. Based on analysis of Medicaid claim and eligibility records in southwestern Pennsylvania, Harman et al. (2000) showed that children in foster care are more likely to have mental health problems and use more mental health and general health care than children in the Aid to Families with Dependent Children. Foster care children had service utilization and costs similar to children with disabilities.

Medicaid reimburses behavioral health services for school-aged children. An investigation by Mandell et al. (2008) demonstrated that in Philadelphia, PA, 21% of the children receiving special education used Medicaid-reimbursed behavioral health care and 15% of the other Medicaid-enrolled children used Medicaid-reimbursed behavioral health care. Forty percent of the total expenditures ($197.8 million) for Medicaid-reimbursed behavioral health care were spent on 5,728 special education children and 60% was spent on 15,092 children. The authors conclude that children in special education receive a disproportionate amount of the Medicaid-reimbursed behavioral health services, and the Deficit Reduction Act may jeopardize the financing of these services.

Eating Disorders

Eating disorders (EDs) are prevalent among adolescents (Cozzi and Ostuzzi, 2007). Among females, the lifetime prevalence of anorexia nervosa (AN) is about 0.5% (American Psychiatric Association, Diagnostic and Statistical Manual of Mental Disorders, 4th Edit., Text Revision). Clinicians are more likely to see persons who are sub-threshold for the condition, such as those who have an ED that is not otherwise specified. Compared to females, the prevalence of AN among males is about one-tenth of the rate. In recent decades, the incidence of AN seems to have increased.

Among women, the lifetime prevalence of bulimia nervosa (BN) is about 1–3% (American Psychiatric Association, Diagnostic and Statistical Manual of Mental

Disorders, 4th Edit., Text Revision). Among males, the prevalence is about one-tenth of that in females.

Studies of the prevalence of EDs among adolescents vary. In Spain, Olesti Baiges et al. (2008) showed that AN occurred in 0.9% of the adolescent girls, aged 12–21 years old. BN occurred in 2.9% and other EDs occurred in 5.3% of the adolescent girls studied. In another investigation in Spain, Rodriguez-Cano et al. (2005) discovered that the prevalence of EDs in adolescents (500 males and 576 females) was 3.71%. AN occurred in 0.1%, BN in 0.75%, and ED not otherwise specified occurred in 2.88%. In their investigation, the rate of false negatives was 2.6% of the control group, indicating that up to the present, the prevalence of EDs in Spanish adolescents may be underestimated.

Researchers have studied the health service use and costs associated with EDs. Simon et al. (2005) reviewed 2 cost-of-illness investigations from the UK and Germany, 1 burden-of-disease report from Australia, and 14 other publications and pertinent data from Denmark, the Netherlands, Austria, the UK, and the USA. The health-care cost of AN in the UK was estimated to be £4.2 million in 1990. In 1998, the health service cost of AN in Germany was estimated to be 65 million € and 10 million € for BN. In Australia, researchers estimated the health services' costs of EDs to be AUS $22 million for the period 1993–1994.

Simon et al. (2005) discovered that other investigations have mainly emphasized inpatient health services and have generated a range of cost estimates for the treatment of EDs. They found few studies of non-health-care costs related to EDs.

Based on a sample of 123 adult HMO patients, Lynch et al. (2010) evaluated the cost-effectiveness of cognitive behavior therapy-guided self-help treatment (CBT-GSH) for recurrent binge eating (BE). The investigators discovered that compared to usual care, CBT-GSH produced 25.2 more BE-free days and had lower total societal costs of $427 over a 1-year period after treatment. The researchers found that the lower costs were due to the reduction in usual care treatment services by patients in the CBT-GSH group.

Obesity

In North America and around the world, overweight and obesity in childhood is epidemic and is increasing at a disturbing rate (Ogden et al., 2010; Van Cleave et al., 2010; Anderson and Whitaker, 2009; Centers for Disease Control and Prevention, 2007; National Center for Health Statistics, 2007; Baker et al., 2007; Deckelbaum and Williams, 2001; Troiano and Flegal, 1998). Worldwide, more than 22 million children under 5 years of age are overweight. Around the world, including developing countries where western lifestyles and nutritional patterns are being adopted, doubling rates are occurring.

In the last two to three decades in the USA, the number of overweight children and adolescents has increased significantly. Using the 2007–2008 National Health and Nutrition Examination Survey (NHANES), Ogden et al. (2010) discovered that 9.5% of infants and toddlers were at or above the 95th percentile of the weight for recumbent length growth charts. Almost 17% of children and adolescents, aged 2–19 years, were at or above the 95th percentile of the BMI for age growth charts, and almost 32% were at or above the 85th percentile of BMI for age.

Researchers have examined the prevalence of obesity in different racial and ethnic groups. Based on the Early Childhood Longitudinal Study, Anderson and Whitaker (2009) revealed that among preschool children, American Indian/Native Alaskans had the highest prevalence of obesity (BMI at or above the 95th percentile for age of the sex-specific Centers for Disease Control and Prevention growth charts) (31.2%). They had twice the rate of obesity compared to non-Hispanic whites (15.9%). Twenty-two percent of Hispanic and 20.8% of non-Hispanic black preschoolers were obese.

Earlier data from the 1999 to 2002 NHANES revealed that about 16% of children and adolescents aged 16–19 were overweight. This prevalence is a 45% increase in the percentage of overweight children and adolescents in this age group, reported for the period 1988–1994. The results of two NHANES surveys for the periods 1976–1980 and 2003–2004 showed that the prevalence of overweight has increased for different age groups. For children, aged 2–5 years, the prevalence increased from 5 to 13.9%. The prevalence increased from 6.5 to 18.8% for children, aged 6–11 years, and 5–17.4% for young persons, aged 12–19 years. In 2004, about 9 million children in the USA were regarded as obese (Institute of Medicine, 2005).

Obesity during childhood and adolescence is related to risk factors for later health problems and with the early onset of these problems. Based on a literature review of the prevalence rates associated with impaired glucose tolerance, hyperinsulinemia, type 2 diabetes mellitus (DM), cardiovascular risk factors, and other conditions among obese children, Lobstein and Jackson-Leach (2006) estimate that over 20,000 in the European Union have type 2 DM and 400,000 have impaired glucose tolerance. The authors estimate that over a million obese children are likely to have a range of cardiovascular disease indicators such as hypertension, elevated blood cholesterol levels, and three or more risk factors for the metabolic syndrome. In addition, they estimate that over 1.4 million children may be in the early phases of liver disease.

In the USA, Van Cleave et al. (2010) used the National Longitudinal Survey of Youth–Child Cohort (1988–2006) of three cohorts of children and youth to analyze the dynamics of obesity and chronic health conditions (defined as obesity, asthma, other physical conditions, and behavioral/learning problems) in these samples. The authors discovered that between 1988 and 2006, the prevalence of chronic disorders increased among children and youth. In cohort 1, the end-study prevalence of any chronic problem was 12.8% in 1994. In 2000, the prevalence was 25.1% for cohort 2, and the prevalence was 26.5% for cohort 3 in 2006. The three cohorts experienced a significant amount of turnover in chronic health problems during the study period. In all cohorts, 7.4% had a chronic health problem at the start of the investigation that lasted to the end of the study. A little more than 9% of participants had chronic disorders at the beginning of the study that was resolved within 6 years, and 13.4% developed new chronic disorders during the study. Male, Hispanic, and African-American youth had higher rates of chronic health problems.

Trasande and Chatterjee (2009) analyzed the impact of obesity on health service utilization and costs in childhood. Using data on 6- to 19-year-olds in the 2002–2005 Medical Expenditure Panel Survey, they discovered that obese children had $194 higher outpatient expenditures than normal/underweight children. Obese children also had $114 higher prescription drug expenditures and $12 higher ER expenditures than normal/underweight children. The authors estimate that high BMI during childhood is related to $14.1 billion in additional expenditures for prescription drugs, ER, and outpatient visits per year.

Similar trends are found when analyzing health-care use in specific health-care organizations. Based on an Israeli sample of 363 obese children and 382 matched controls, Hering et al. (2009) demonstrated that obese children had more clinic visits, more hospitalizations, had longer hospital stays, and had higher medication use than the matched controls.

In a study of obesity and type 2 DM among children in Germany, Wolfenstetter (2006) showed that the mean annual direct costs of obesity were 44 million € during 2003. Rehabilitation costs were 36.4 million €, hospitalization 3.6 million €, and 3.9 million € for special medical care programs. The average costs per treated obese were 3,484 €.

Childhood obesity has an impact on employers. Based on an investigation of one large employer, Sepulveda et al. (2010) discovered that for an obese child, the average per capita health claims' costs were $2,907 in 2008 and were $10,780 for a child with type 2 DM. For children with type 2 DM, the average claims were higher than the average claims for adults with the condition ($8,844).

Children with obesity-associated health problems who have been diagnosed with psychiatric conditions may use more health services than those without psychiatric diagnoses. Using a sample of 13,688 young people with type 2 DM, metabolic syndrome, dyslipidemia, or obesity, Janicke et al. (2009) discovered that having any type of a psychiatric diagnosis was linked to increased use of health services. They also found that children with both an externalizing and internalizing psychiatric conditions used health services more than those with only one of these disorders.

In US adults, the cost of obesity-related health care is estimated to be $100 billion per year (Wang, 2001; Connolly et al., 2002).

Diabetes Mellitus

Insulin-dependent diabetes mellitus (IDDM) is one of the most prevalent chronic disorders in children (LaPorte et al., 1995). About 13,171 children develop IDDM annually. There are about 17 new cases of IDDM per 100,000 children per year, compared to about 12 new cases of cancer and about 2 new cases of juvenile rheumatoid arthritis. The number of children who acquire IDDM each year is about 14 times the number of children who develop AIDS (Libman et al., 1993).

Studies of different geographical areas in the USA showed that there are racial and ethnic differences in the incidence of IDDM in children (LaPorte et al., 1995). For example, in the Philadelphia, PA, area, Hispanic and white children had the highest incidence (15.2 per 100,000 children and 13.3 per 100,000 children, respectively), followed by African-American children with 11.0 per 100,000 children. LaPorte et al. (1995) note that Hispanic children had the highest incidence in Philadelphia, but these data are based on only a few studies.

Research on IDDM incidence by gender in Allegheny County, PA, revealed that white children had a slight increased incidence in males (LaPorte et al., 1995). Non-white children had a slight increased incidence in females. The results revealed that age at onset tended to peak at puberty. Girls had an earlier pubertal peak incidence than boys, and girls tended to experience the pubertal peak 1 year earlier than boys. Data from a number of registries in the USA and other countries have revealed a similar pattern. Few infants acquire IDDM in the first year of life.

In children, temporal trends in IDDM have been identified (LaPorte et al., 1995). IDDM incidence has spiked over time, which are indicative of epidemics of the disease. For instance, in the US Virgin Islands, the incidence of the disease in children rose substantially in the mid-1980 period (Tull et al., 1991). Barbados and other regions of the Caribbean showed a similar epidemic pattern (Jordan et al., 1994). In Birmingham, AL, in 1983, IDDM incidence increased significantly (Wagenknecht et al., 1991). This substantial increase occurred at the same time as a coxsackievirus infection.

According to worldwide incidence data, there may have been a pandemic of IDDM in the USA and in a large percentage of other nations throughout the world (Dokheel, 1993; Diabetes Epidemiology Research International Group, 1990). These findings indicate that globally IDDM incidence is on the rise and that the epidemics may explain the total increase.

In children, studies in the USA have shown that the prevalence of IDDM varies from 0.6 per 1,000 to 2.5 per 1,000 (LaPorte et al., 1995). Most estimates are about 1.7 per 1,000. Based on these data, about 123,032 persons, aged 19 years or younger, in the USA have IDDM.

The economic impact of childhood IDDM is substantial. The cost through the age of 40 years is nearly $40,000 per patient (Songer et al., 1988). These costs can be high because children afflicted with the disorder have a high risk of developing major complications.

Wolfenstetter (2006) discovered that the mean annual direct costs of hospitalization and rehabilitation for children with type 2 DM were 1.4 million € during 2003. The mean costs per treated obese child with type 2 DM were 8,539 €.

Based on a literature, Icks et al. (2007) reported that hospitalization due to poor metabolic control, education, and acute complications account for the substantial costs of treating children with type 1 DM. The authors conclude that hospitalization contributes significantly to the costs of treating children and adolescents with type 1 DM. They suggest that home interventions may be more cost-effective than traditional treatment models. However, additional investigations are warranted.

Juvenile Asthma

In the USA, from 1980 to the late 1990s, asthma period prevalence among children, aged 0–17 years, more than doubled (Akinbami, 2006). In 1980, asthma period prevalence was 3.6% and at the peak of the trend in 1995, it was 7.5%. The prevalence of asthma remains at historically high rates. In 2005, 8.9% or 6.5 million children, aged 0–17 years, currently had asthma. In this same year, 5.2% or 3.8 million children suffered at least one asthma attack in the previous 12 months. In 2005, almost two of every three children who currently have asthma had at least one attack in the previous 12 months.

In 2005, 12.7% or 9 million children, aged 0–17 years, had been diagnosed with asthma at some point in their life (Akinbami, 2006). Seventy percent or 6.5 million of these children currently have asthma.

Asthma prevalence increases with age (Akinbami, 2006). For the period, 2004–2005, current asthma prevalence was 6.2% for children, aged 0–4 years, 9.3% for children, aged 5–10 years, and 10.0% for children aged 11–17 years.

Asthma prevalence varies by gender, with boys having higher current asthma prevalence than girls (Akinbami, 2006). For 2004–2005, boys, aged 0–4 years, had a current asthma prevalence of 7.4%, compared to 5.0%. In the 5-to 10-year age group, boys had a current asthma prevalence of 11.1%, while girls had a rate of 7.4%. In the 11 to 17-year age group, boys had a current asthma prevalence of 11.1%, while girls had a rate of 8.8%.

Racial disparities in childhood asthma prevalence are substantial (Akinbami, 2006). Compared to whites, African-American children have about 60% higher asthma prevalence for the period 2004–2005. During this period, Native American or Alaska Native children had about 25% higher asthma prevalence than white children. The lowest prevalence rates occurred among Asian children. Puerto Rican children had the highest asthma prevalence of all groups (19.2%), when taking into account both race and ethnicity. Their rate was 140% higher than that of children of non-Hispanic white origin. In contrast, Mexican children had the lowest asthma prevalence rate (6.4%).

Significant morbidity and disability is associated with the condition (Akinbami, 2006). In 2003, children, ages 0–17 years, with at least one asthma attack (4 million) in the past 12 months missed about 12.8 million school days because of their disorder.

Among children, asthma deaths are rare but potentially avoidable (Akinbami, 2006). A number of factors increase a child's risk of dying from asthma. If children have severe, uncontrolled asthma, have suffered an almost fatal asthma attack, and have a history of repeated ER visits, hospitalizations, or intubation for asthma, they are at increased risk of dying from asthma (McFadden and Warren, 1997).

Asthma deaths among children have declined recently after a rising trend during the period 1980–1996. There were 2.5 deaths due to asthma per 1,000,000 children, aged 0–17 years, in 2004. The proportional impact of asthma deaths in the 2003–2004 period is highest for non-Hispanic children, followed by Hispanic and white children.

Although overall asthma death rates have declined since 1999, death rates for African-American children have remained fairly flat (Akinbami, 2006). As a result, since 1999, the racial disparity in asthma death rates has increased. A number of factors may explain why asthma death rates among African-American children remain high relative to white children. African-American children and their families may experience more severe disease, more environmental hazards, such as pollution and poverty, delays in receiving the latest asthma treatments, a lack of asthma education, and more problems in adopting asthma control strategies.

According to Center for Disease Control and Prevention (CDC), asthma accounts for 14 million lost days of school missed annually; this problem is compounded by an estimated $1 billion in lost productivity for their working parents. In the USA, asthma-related health-care costs approximately $10.7 billion in 1994, including a direct health-care cost of $6.1 billion. Indirect costs, such as lost work days, amounted to $4.6 billion. Furthermore, asthma affects the academic performance of the children in the school and other social and leisure pursuits (Weiss et al., 2000) (http://www.urbancollaborative.org/asthma.asp#impact).

Asthma creates a substantial burden on afflicted children and their families. The disorder can impair playing, learning, and sleep, may require complex and expensive treatment, and produces both direct medical costs and indirect costs, such as missed school days and work days (Akinbami, 2006).

Physician offices are the sites of a majority of non-urgent asthma-related ambulatory visits. In 2004, children had 6.5 million visits or 89 visits to physician offices per 1,000 children for asthma care. That same year, there were 0.5 million visits to hospital outpatient departments or 6 visits to hospital outpatient department per 1,000 children for asthma treatment. Of all ambulatory visits among children in the 0–17 age group, a little over 2.5% were related to asthma.

Ambulatory care for asthma has continued to increase since 2000 despite the plateau in childhood asthma prevalence (Akinbami, 2006). Various factors may account for this increase in ambulatory care utilization. Children may be suffering greater disease severity. Increased utilization is also related to improved asthma control because of greater awareness of the public and health-care professionals. Increased ambulatory care use has occurred during a period in which the total rate of ambulatory care for children did not rise (Hing et al., 2006).

At ERs, children are often treated for asthma attacks or exacerbations (Akinbami, 2006). Asthma-related ER visits may indicate that the child has severe asthma or that the disease is out of control. ER visits for asthma also may reflect inadequate access to specialist care or inappropriate use of emergency services (Shields et al., 2004; Halfon et al., 1996). Frequent ER visits and hospitalizations are associated with an increased risk for fatal asthma attacks (McFadden and Warren, 1997).

Implementing environmental control strategies, minimizing exposure to allergens and irritants, taking medication, and effective patient and health-care professional education can minimize poor outcomes (Akinbami, 2006; National Heart, Lung, and Blood Institute, 1997). However, children and their families can face significant difficulties in undertaking these often complex primary and secondary intervention activities. In fact, children who are seen in the ER for asthma continue to experience symptoms and impairment in daily activities despite receiving emergency medical services (Lenhardt et al., 2006).

Data on ER visits for children with asthmatic attacks provide a crude description of the burden of severe and out-of-control disease on children, families, and the health-care system. In the USA, between 1992 and the late 1990s, the rate of ER visits for asthma increased. After 1999, the rate reached a plateau and has remained fairly flat through 2004 (Akinbami, 2006). In 2004, 103 visits per 10,000 children or a total of 750,000 ER visits were for asthma. Of all ER visits in 2004, asthma-associated ER visits accounted for 2.8% of the visits among children, aged 0–17 years.

Children with severe exacerbation of their asthma often require hospitalization for treatment and increased monitoring of their condition (Akinbami, 2006). Hospitalization entails substantial costs to the families of the children and to the health-care system. Previous hospitalization for asthma, prior intubation for asthma, and severe symptoms increase the risk of hospitalization (Pollack et al., 2002).

Hospitalizations can be mostly prevented if patients, families, and health-care providers receive effective education about the disorder and have access to quality health care (Homer et al., 1996; Akinbami, 2006). However, some hospitalizations may not be avoided, especially in very young children who have respiratory infections.

An analysis of hospitalization trends can reveal the extent to which primary and secondary prevention strategies are effective in controlling the burden of the disease (Akinbami, 2006). For children, aged 0–17 years, asthma-related hospitalization rates increased from 1980 through the mid-1990s. This trend paralleled the asthma prevalence rates, although the increased rates are due in part to improvements in the diagnosis of the condition (Akinbami, 2006; Akinbami and Schoendorf, 2002). The asthma-related hospitalization rates among children have reached a plateau at historically high rates since the late 1990s.

There were 27 asthma-associated hospitalizations per 10,000 children or 198,000 hospitalizations in 2004 (Akinbami, 2006). Three percent of all hospitalizations among children were for asthma.

Hospitalization rates for asthma have remained fairly level at a time when the overall hospitalization rate among children has decreased (DeFrances and Podgornik, 2006). Children who are hospitalized in recent years may have more severe exacerbations relative to prior years.

Asthma-associated health-care utilization generally decreases throughout childhood and adolescence, with the highest use among very young children (Akinbami, 2006). Infants and toddlers frequently experience wheezing because their small airways are more susceptible to airflow obstruction and they have a high rate of respiratory infections. Clinicians have difficulty diagnosing asthma in this population because many conditions can cause wheezing in infants and toddlers. In addition, very young children who experience wheezing during respiratory infections tend to have temporary symptoms (Reed, 2006; Martinez et al., 1995; Wright, 2002; Eggleston et al., 2005). Health-care providers are hesitant to diagnose a child with these symptoms as having a chronic disease. Nevertheless, in infants and toddlers, respiratory distress can quickly become life-threatening and necessitate immediate assessment. As a result of the above factors, utilization of ERs and hospitalizations is high in this population.

In the school-age population, allergies and atopic sensitization are important determinants of wheezing and replace respiratory infections as the primary causes of asthma attacks (Reed, 2006; Wright, 2002).

Juvenile Arthritis

Juvenile arthritis (JA) refers to any form of arthritis or an arthritis-related condition that develops in children or teenagers who are less than 18 years of age (Lawrence et al., 1998; Arthritis Foundation Website). Approximately 294,000 children under the age of 18 are affected by pediatric arthritis and rheumatologic conditions (Sacks et al., 2007).

Juvenile idiopathic arthritis (JIA), also known as juvenile rheumatoid arthritis (JRA), or juvenile chronic arthritis (JCA), is the most common form of arthritis in children and is a chronic inflammatory disease of the joints (Cassidy and Petty, 1995; Janz et al., 1993). Although JIA is often a mild condition that causes few problems over time, it can be more problematic and cause joint and tissue damage in some children, leading to more severe complications.

JIA affects between 60,000 and 200,000 children and adolescents in the USA (Cassidy and Petty, 1995; Erlandson, 1989). Approximately 5% of children diagnosed with JIA have recurrent episodes of arthritis as adults and about 10% begin adulthood with severe functional disabilities (Robinson, 1998). Of children diagnosed with JIA, 60–80% do not suffer permanent joint damage (Milota et al., 1991). Death occurs in 2–4% of children with JIA worldwide. In the USA, the majority of deaths are associated with a type of JIA known as systemic JIA; in many cases, infections were contributing causes as well (Cassidy and Petty, 1995).

Ambulatory care visits for pediatric arthritis and rheumatologic conditions averaged 827,000 annually (Sacks et al., 2007). In addition to obtaining allopathic care, children with JA use complementary and alternative medicine (CAM). A cohort study of 182 patients with JIA who went to outpatient clinics were studied for 1 year (April et al., 2009). Based on parents' reports, the investigators discovered that 36.4% of the sample used at least one form of CAM over the 1-year period. The authors discovered that 72% of the parents who had obtained CAM for their children indicated that CAM was at least somewhat helpful.

Arthritis and related conditions such as JA cost the US economy nearly $128 billion per year in medical care and indirect expenses, including lost wages and productivity (MMWR, 2007).

In Germany, Minden et al. (2009) evaluated the economic burden of JIA based on a sample of 369 outpatients with the condition. They estimated that the average total cost of JIA per patient per year was 4, 663 €. Patients with seropositive polyarthritis and systemic arthritis had the highest costs (7,876 €) and patients with persistent oligoarthritis had the lowest costs (2,904 €). Health-care expenditures made up 89% of the total costs, and medications contributed to almost 50% of the health-care expenditures. Families paid a substantial part of the health-care costs; their average out-of-pocket costs were 223 €, and their average indirect costs associated with time away from work were 270 € per year per family. Disease activity and pain, duration of the disorder, uveitis, and time period from onset of symptoms to having the first pediatric rheumatologist visit were associated with increased costs. However, the investigators showed that functional status was the only factor that predicted changes in the patient total costs.

In the UK, data from the Childhood Arthritis Prospective Study evaluated JIA patient-based costs during the first year after diagnosis (Thornton et al., 2008). Based on 297 children who had a 12-month follow-up visit, the researchers discovered that the average annual total cost per child was £1,649. Appointments with pediatric rheumatologists comprised the largest part of health-care costs. Children with enthesitis-associated, systemic JIA or persistent oligoarthritis had the highest average total costs.

HIV and AIDS

Although the majority of people living with HIV are still adults, children under 15 account for one in six AIDS-related deaths and one in seven new infections. As we enter the third decade of the epidemic, a child under 15 dies of an AIDS-associated illness every minute of every day, and a young person aged 15–24 contracts HIV every 15 s. Every day, over 6,000 young people aged 15–24 are newly infected with HIV; there are almost 1,800 new pediatric infections and 1,400 children under 15 die of AIDS-related illness (CDC, HIV/AIDS Surveillance Report, 2006. Vol. 18).

Globally, 15 million children have lost at least one parent to HIV/AIDS. By 2010, approximately 18 million children in sub-Saharan Africa alone will have lost at least one parent to AIDS (CDC, HIV/AIDS Surveillance Report, 2006. Vol. 18).

Most children living with HIV, around 9 out of 10, live in Sub-Saharan Africa, the region of the world where AIDS has taken its greatest toll. Large numbers of children with HIV also live in the Caribbean, Latin America, and South/Southeast Asia. Around 90% of all children living with HIV acquired the infection from their mothers during pregnancy, birth, or breastfeeding. Many countries that had previously seen child-survival rates rise, as a result of improved healthcare, are now seeing these rates fall again. In Botswana and Zimbabwe, for instance, child mortality rates have nearly doubled since 1990 (Hunter and Williamson, 2000).

The first case of AIDS was reported in the USA in 1981, but the disease may have existed unrecognized for many years before that time. HIV infection leading to AIDS has been a major cause of illness and death among children, teens, and young adults worldwide. AIDS has been the sixth leading cause of death in the USA among 15- to 24-year-olds since 1991 (UNAIDS, *AIDS Epidemic Update*, December 2003).

More than 700,000 cases of AIDS have been reported in the USA since 1981, and as many as 900,000 Americans may be infected with HIV. The epidemic is growing most rapidly among minority populations and is a leading killer of African-American males. According to the CDC, AIDS affects nearly seven times more African-Americans than whites and three times more Hispanics than whites (CDC HIV/AIDS Surveillance Report, Vol. 12, 2000).

Because every child today is growing up in a world where AIDS is a devastating reality, some people say that every child is affected by the epidemic, whether they are infected or not. Other researchers study children who are orphaned by AIDS or those who are HIV positive. Children are affected by HIV in many ways, and their families and friends also are adversely affected as a result of the epidemic (Brown et al., 2000).

The aging of the population with HIV and innovations in antiretroviral therapy for children may have produced changes in health services utilization among HIV-infected children. Rutstein et al. (2005), based on a study of four HIV primary pediatric and specialty care sites in different geographical regions, found that between 2000 and 2001, hospitalization rates decreased significantly from 39.2 to 25.3% admissions per 100 patients. Factors associated with increased hospitalizations were high immunosuppression, 2 years of age and younger, and AIDS. In their investigation, average outpatient visits did not change between 2000 and 2001. Patients who had greater outpatient utilization were those children who were 2 years and younger, those who were on highly active antiretroviral treatment, those who had AIDS, and those on Medicaid. Patients who had higher HIV-1 RNA had more outpatient visits than those with less disease progression.

Investigations reveal that in resource-poor settings, highly active antiretroviral treatments can be administered effectively and safely to children (Klein et al., 2004). However, pediatric HIV care is difficult to implement in resource-poor countries. In resource-limited countries, prevention of mother-to-child transmission (PMTCT) services are difficult to implement because of a lack of health-care infrastructure, a scarcity of health-care personnel, and competing health-care priorities (Paintsil and Andiman, 2009).

In South Africa, Meyers et al. (2007) note that too few infants and children are being diagnosed early, and cotrimoxazole prophylaxis coverage is insufficient. The authors report that health-care practitioners are not adequately trained and facilities are inadequate.

Another study in South Africa evaluated socioeconomic conditions and follow-up rates of HIV-exposed infants (Jones et al., 2005). Based on cross-sectional data from 176, the investigators demonstrated that poverty, geographical relocation, and the inability of fathers to support their children reduce the ability of families to adhere to a PMTCT program.

Ginsburg et al. (2007) evaluated PMTCT services in 18 resource-limited countries and discovered that PMTCT services are integrated into maternal-child health services. However, they discovered that adult and pediatric care frequently operates without adequate coordination with PMTCT services.

Using medical visit and hospitalization data from the HIV Research Network and other data sources, Schackman et al. (2006) showed that the discounted lifetime cost of HIV care in the USA is $385,200 and undiscounted cost is $618,900 per person with a projected life expectancy of 24.2 years. Antiretroviral medications account for 73% of the costs, inpatient care 13%, 9% outpatient care, and 5% other HIV-associated drugs and laboratory costs. The investigators conclude that antiretroviral treatment has enhanced survival and have increased the lifetime cost of HIV medical care in the USA.

According to UNAIDS (2007), an estimated $10 billion is spent for HIV/AIDS prevention, care, and support in low- and middle-income countries. UNAIDS (2007) estimate that $42 billion in 2010 is needed to increase HIV/AIDS prevention, care, and support in these countries in order to achieve universal access. For fiscal year 2009, the US President's budget request for HIV/AIDS funding for HIV/AIDs prevention, care, and research in low-and middle-income countries was $5.9 billion (Kaiser Family Foundation, 2008).

Cancer and Leukemia

Nearly 30% of USA population is under the age of 20. In the USA in 2007, approximately 10,400 children under age 15 were diagnosed with cancer and about 1,545 children were died from the disease (American Cancer Society, 2007).

Although this makes cancer the leading cause of death by disease among USA in children 1–14 years of age, cancer is still relatively rare in this age group. On average, one to two children develop the disease each year for every 10,000 children in the USA (Ries et al., 2004).

Over the past 20 years, the incidence of children diagnosed with all forms of invasive cancer has increased from 11.5 cases per 100,000 children in 1975 to 14.8 per 100,000 children in 2004. During this same time, however, death rates declined dramatically and 5-year survival rates increased for most childhood cancers. For example, the 5-year survival rates for all childhood cancers combined increased from 58.1% in 1975–1977 to 79.6% in 1996–2003 (Ries et al., 2004).

Lymphomas account for 10% of all childhood cancers (National Children's Cancer Foundation, 1997). Lymphoma, a cancer of the lymph nodes, has two types: non-Hodgkin's lymphoma (NHL) and Hodgkin's lymphoma (HL). NHL and HL are cancers that start in lymph tissues, such as the tonsils, lymph nodes, and thymus. These cancers may spread to bone marrow and other organs, which can cause different symptoms depending on where it is growing. They also can cause fever, sweats, weakness, and swollen lymph nodes in the neck, armpit, or groin.

NHL is most common in pre-adolescents and adolescents. The most common symptoms of NHL are enlarged lymph nodes, difficulty breathing because of enlarged lymph nodes in the chest, an abdominal tumor from enlarged lymph nodes, fevers, weight loss, and lethargy. This cancer tends to metastasize to other areas rapidly, most commonly to the bones, CNS, and the bone marrow. Due to the link between the lymph node system and the immune system, Horowitz and Pizzo (1990) predict that the incidence of NHL may increase as the number of children with the AIDS virus increases.

HL "differs from NHL in that it usually demonstrates a slower onset and an orderly progression, involving contiguous lymph node areas" (Granowetter, 1994). The peak incidence of HL occurs in late adolescence, early adulthood, and middle age (Majhail et al., 2007).

Armstrong et al. (2010) evaluated late mortality among 5-year survivors of childhood cancer and found that 30 years from diagnosis, the overall cumulative mortality was 18.1%.

Below is a discussion of different pediatric cancers:

Leukemia (30% of All Pediatric Cancers)

Childhood leukemias are cancers of the hematopoietic system. In a majority of cases, they produce a malignant change in lymphoid progenitor cells. Less commonly, they cause changes in myeloid progenitor cells (Smith et al., 1996). About 3,250 children are diagnosed annually with leukemia. Two major types of leukemia are ALL and acute non-lymphocytic leukemia. One report found that ALL made up almost three-fourths of all leukemias, while the acute non-lymphocytic type comprised 19% (Smith et al., 1996). The symptoms of leukemia may include bone and joint pain, weakness, bleeding, and fever (American Cancer Society, 2007).

The incidence of ALL has varied with age. Smith et al. (1996) found a sharp peak in the incidence of ALL among young children, aged 2–3 years. The incidence was more than 80 per million for this age group. For children, aged 8–10 years, the rate decreases to 20 per million. The incidence of ALL is about 4 times greater than that for infants and is almost 10 times greater than that for 19-year-olds.

Racial differences have been shown in the incidence of leukemia. One report revealed that white children had a much higher incidence than African-American children for the period 1986–1995 (Smith et al., 1996). This investigation demonstrated that white children aged 0–14 years had a leukemia incidence rate of 45.6 per million compared to 27.8 per million for African-American children. This racial disparity is most evident when analyzing rates of leukemia by single year of age. White children in the 2- to 3-year age group had a three times higher incidence compared to African-American children.

Brain and Other Nervous System (22.3%)

These cancers in their early stages may produce headaches, nausea, vomiting, blurred or double vision, dizziness, and problems in walking or handling objects.

Neuroblastoma (7.3%)

Neuroblastoma is a cancer of the sympathetic nervous system. Neuroblastoma can appear at any body site but usually develops as a swelling in the abdomen.

Wilms' tumor (5.6%)

Wilm's tumor is a kidney tumor which causes a swelling or lump in the abdomen.

Non-Hodgkin Lymphoma (4.5%) and Hodgkin Lymphoma (3.5%)

NHL and HL have an impact on lymph nodes but may spread to bone marrow and other organs. They may produce swelling of lymph nodes in the neck, armpit, or groin and cause weakness and fever.

Rhabdomyosarcoma (3.1%)

Rhabdomyosarcoma, a soft-tissue sarcoma, develops in the head and neck, genitourinary area, trunk, and extremities, causing pain and/or a mass or swelling.

Retinoblastoma (2.8%)

Retinoblastoma is an eye tumor that usually afflicts children younger than 4 years of age.

Osteosarcoma (2.4%)

Osteosarcoma is a bone tumor. The disorder frequently does not cause any initial pain or symptoms until local swelling appears.

Ewing sarcoma (1.4%)

Ewing sarcoma is another cancer type that often develops in bone.

In 2007, about 1,545 deaths from pediatric cancer are expected to occur among children in the 0- to 14-year age group (American Cancer Society, 2007). About one-third of these deaths are due to leukemia. Since 1975, the mortality rates for pediatric cancers have declined by 48%. New and improved treatments are responsible for these decreased mortality rates.

Relative survival varies by cancer type. For infants, relative survival is very good for patients with neuroblastoma, Wilms' tumor, and retinoblastoma. Relative survival is fairly good for leukemia patients. Children with ALL have experienced significant improvement in survival since the early 1970s and overall survival is now about 80% (Smith et al., 1996). Age at diagnosis affects survival rates for children with ALL. Children older than 1 year of age and less than 10 years of age have the most favorable outcomes. Improvements in therapies have led to improved survival in children with ALL. Children with other types of cancer do not have a fairly good survival rate.

Cancer-Related Pediatric Health-Care Utilization and Costs

Hospitalizations of children with cancer are common, are associated with significant costs in the short term, and have predictable patterns of resource utilization (Rosenman et al., 2005). Children with cancer tend to have longer hospital hospitalizations than adults with cancer (Hendrickson and Rimar, 2009). Children with cancer also tend to have longer, more frequent, and more costly hospital admissions than hospitalized children with other conditions. Those with leukemia and central nervous system tumors in childhood often require hospitalization.

Researchers have identified disparities in access to pediatric cancer treatment. For example, Mukherjee et al. (2009) discovered racial and socioeconomic disparities in access to high-volume neurooncological care. Based on an analysis of 4,421 patients, the authors found that Hispanic ethnicity and each 1% increase in foreign residents per county were associated with worse access to care. Factors related to greater access to high-volume neurooncological care were higher county neurosurgeon density and higher county home value.

Investigators have studied other patterns of pediatric cancer care utilization and costs. Using a retrospective cohort investigation of 195 consecutively diagnosed children with cancer at a children's hospital, Rosenman et al. (2005) evaluated hospital resource utilization during 3 years after diagnosis. Of the 165 diagnoses, 65 (39%) were lymphoid malignancy, 51 (31%) solid tumors, 36 (22%) with central nervous system tumors, and 13 (8%) myeloid leukemia. They found that 62 patients (38%) were treated in the pediatric intensive care unit (PICU) at least one time and 22 patients (13%) had stem cell transplantation. Sixty-five patients (39%) participated in clinical trials. At the end of the 3-year period, 139 patients (84%) were alive.

In their study, Rosenman et al. (2005) discovered that cumulative hospital charges for the 3-year period were $16 million, with almost $100,000 spent per hospitalized child. Fifty percent of these hospital charges were incurred during the children's first 4.5 months after diagnosis. Fifty percent of the hospital charges were attributed to only 12.7% of the patients, who were more likely to be diagnosed with myeloid leukemia, to have had stem cell transplantation, and to have been treated in the PICU. The researchers found that stem cell transplantation, use of the PICU, and death within 3 years of diagnosis were independent predictors of hospital charges. Tumor type, stem cell transplantation, and death within 3 years were predictors of PICU utilization. In regard to tumor type, myeloid leukemia and central nervous system tumors positively predicted PICU utilization, whereas lymphoid malignancy and solid tumors were negative predictors of PICU use.

ALL is the most prevalent and curable malignant childhood disease (Liu et al., 2009). Based on 45 newly diagnosed children with ALL in Shanghai, China, from May 2005 to June 2006, Liu et al. (2009) found that the average total clinic expense per patient was $3,695. The average total inpatient expense per patient was $7,300 although there was substantial individual variability in expenses. Medicine accounted for 40.5% of the costs, while laboratory tests made up 21.5% of the costs. During the treatment period, patients remained at home were treated at the clinic for more than 90% of the time. Costs tended to be higher for patients with higher risk levels and severe complications. Low- and medium-risk groups had 30-month event-free survival of 94.14 and 82.81%, respectively.

Researchers have assessed resource utilization and cost of episodes of febrile neutropenia in children with acute leukemias and lymphomas. Based on an analysis of 51 episodes of febrile neutropenia in hospitalized children with leukemia and lymphoma in Sao Paulo, Brazil, Costa et al. (2003) found that median cost per treated episode was $2,660. Sixty-two percent of the total treatment costs were attributed to hospitalization costs, while 23% of the treatment costs were associated with antibacterials. Patients who had documented infections had a higher median direct cost than patients who had fever of unknown origin.

Raisch et al. (2003) compared the home care-based treatment of chemotherapy-induced febrile neutropenia with hospital-based treatment for the condition. Based on an analysis of 144 episodes of chemotherapy-induced febrile neutropenia, they showed that the median charge per febrile neutropenia episode was significantly greater in the hospital ($9,392) than in home care ($5,893). They concluded that home care-based treatment had lower median total charges than hospital-based treatment with no differences in patient care outcomes.

References

Akinbami, L.J. (2006). The state of childhood asthma, United States, 1980–2005 (Advance data from Vital Health Statistics; No. 381). Hyattsville, MD: National Center for Health Statistics.

Akinbami, L.J., Schoendorf, K.C. (2002). Trends in childhood asthma: prevalence, health care utilization, and mortality. Pediatrics, 110 (2 Pt 1), 315–322.

American Cancer Society (2007). Cancer facts and figures. Atlanta, GA: American Cancer Society. Retrieved Feb. 21, 2010, from: http://www.cancer.org/downloads/STT/CAFF2007PWSecured.pdf duplicate document.

Anderson, S.E., Whitaker, R.C. (2009). Prevalence of obesity among U.S. preschool children in different racial and ethnic groups. Arch Pediatr Adolesc Med, 163 (4), 344–348.

April, K.T., Feldman, D.E., Zunzunegui, M.V. et al. (2009). Longitudinal analysis of complementary and alternative health care use in children with juvenile idiopathic arthritis. Complement Ther Med, 17 (4), 208–215.

Armstrong, G.T., Pan, Z., Ness, K.N. et al. (2010). Temporal trends in cause-specific late mortality among 5-year survivors of childhood cancer. J Clin Oncol, 28 (7), 1224–1231.

Baker, J.L., Olsen, L.W., Sorensen, T.I. (2007). Childhood body-mass index and the risk of coronary heart disease in adulthood. N Engl J Med, 357 (23), 2329–2337.

Bhatia, S.K., Bhatia, S.C. (2007). Childhood and adolescent depression. Am Fam Physician, 75 (1), 73–80.

Birmaher, B., Brent, D.A., Benson, R.S. (1998, November). Summary of the practice parameters for the assessment and treatment of children and adolescents with depressive disorders. Amer Acad Child Adol Psychiatry, 37 (11), 1234–1238.

Blader, J.C., Carlson, G.A. (2007). Increased rates of bipolar disorder diagnoses among U.S. child, adolescent, and adult inpatients, 1996–2004. Biol Psychiatry, 62 (2), 107–114.

Brown, L.K., Lourie, K.J., Pao, M. (2000). Children and adolescents living with HIV and AIDS: a review. J Child Psychol Psychiatry, 41 (1), 81–96.

Burd, L., Klug, M.G., Coumbe, M.J. et al. (2003). Children and adolescents with attention deficit-hyperactivity disorder: 1. prevalence and cost of care. J Child Neurol, 18 (8), 555–561.

Cassidy, J., Petty, R. (1995). Textbook of pediatric rheumatology (3rd ed.). Philadelphia, PA: W.B. Saunders.

CDC (2000). HIV/AIDS surveillance report, Vol. 12. Atlanta, GA: CDC.

CDC (2006). HIV/AIDS surveillance report, Vol. 18. Atlanta, GA: CDC.

Centers for Disease Control and Prevention (2007, June 28). HIV/AIDS and African Americans. Retrieved March 3, 2010 from: http://www.cdc.gov/hiv/topics/aa/

Chan, E., Zhan, C., Homer, C.J. (2002). Health care use and costs for children with attention-deficit/hyperactivity disorder: national estimates from the Medical Expenditure Panel Survey. Arch Pediatr Adolesc Med, 156 (5), 504–511.

Connolly, J., Gargiula, L., Reeve, D. (2002). Selections from current literature treatment issues in childhood obesity. Fam Pract, 19 (3), 304–309.

Costa, V.C., Ferra, M.B., Petrilli, A.S. et al. (2003). Resource utilization and cost of episodes of febrile neutropenia in children with acute leukemias and lymphomas. Support Care Cancer, 11 (6), 356–361.

Cozzi, F., Ostuzzi, R. (2007). Relational competence and eating disorders. Eat Weight Disord, 12 (2), 101–107.

Deckelbaum, R.J., Williams, C.L. (2001). Childhood obesity: the health issue. Obes Res, 9 (Suppl 4), 239S–243S.

DeFrances, C.J., Podgornik, M.N. (2006, May 4). 2004 National hospital discharge survey. Adv Data, 371, 1–19.

Diabetes Epidemiology Research International Group (1990). Secular trends in incidence of childhood IDDM in 10 countries. Diabetes, 39, 858–864.

Dokheel, T.M. (1993). An epidemic of childhood diabetes in the United States? Evidence from Allegheny County, PA. Diabetes Care, 16, 1606–1611.

Domino, M.E., Foster, E.M., Vitiello, B. et al. (2009). Relative cost-effectiveness of treatments for adolescent depression: 36-week results from the TADS randomized trial. J Am Acad Child Adolesc Psychiatry, 48 (7), 711–720.

Dretzke, J., Frew, E., Davenport, C. et al. (2005). The effectiveness and cost-effectiveness of parent training/education programmes for the treatment of conduct disorder, including oppositional defiant disorder, in children. Health Technol Assess, 9 (50), iii, ix–x, 1–233.

Eggleston, P.A., Diette, G., Lipsett, M. et al. (2005, October). Lessons learned for the study of childhood asthma from the Centers for Children's Environmental Health and Disease Prevention Research. Environ Health Perspect, 113 (10), 1430–1436.

Emery, A.E.H., Rimoin, D.L. (1990). Principles and practice of medical genetics (2nd ed.), Vols. 1 & 2. Edinburgh, UK: Churchill Livingstone.

Erlandson, D. (1989). Juvenile rheumatoid arthritis. In M. Logigian & J. Ward (Eds.), Pediatric rehabilitation: a team approach for therapists. Boston: Little Brown and Co.

Evans-Lacko, S.E., Zeber, J.E., Gonzalez, J.M. et al. (2009). Medical comorbidity among youth diagnosed with bipolar disorder in the United States. J Clin Psychiatry, 70 (10), 1461–1466.

Fombonne, E. (2009). Epidemiology of pervasive developmental disorders. Pediatr Res, 65 (6), 591–598.

Foster, E.M., Jones, D.E. (2005). The high costs of aggression: public expenditures resulting from conduct disorder. Am J Public Health, 95 (10), 1767–1772.

Fry-Johnson, Y.W., Daniels, E.C., Levine, R. et al. (2005). Being uninsured: impact on children's healthcare and health. Curr Opin Pediatr, 17 (6), 753–758.

Gershon, E.S., Hamovit, J.H., Guroff, J.J. et al. (1987, April). Birth-cohort changes in manic and depressive disorders in relatives of bipolar and schizoaffective patients. Arch Gen Psychiatry, 44 (4), 314–319.

Ginsburg, A.S., Hoblitzelle, C.W., Sripipatana, T.L. et al. (2007). Provision of care following prevention of mother-to-child HIV transmission services in resource-limited settings. AIDS, 21 (18), 2529–2532.

Granowetter, L. (1994). Pediatric oncology: a medical overview. In D.J. Bearison, R.K. Mulhern (Eds.), Pediatric psychooncology: psychological perspectives on children with cancer. New York, NY: Oxford University Press, pp. 9–34.

Guevara, J.P., Mandell, D.S., Rostain, A.L. (2003). National estimates of health services expenditures for children with behavioral disorders: an analysis of the medical expenditure panel survey. Pediatrics, 112 (6 Pt 1), e440.

Halfon, N., Newacheck, P.W., Wood, D.L. et al. (1996). Routine emergency department use for sick care by children in the United States. Pediatrics, 98 (1), 28–34.

Harman, J.S., Childs, G.E., Kelleher, K.J. (2000). Mental health care utilization and expenditures by children in foster care. Arch Pediatr Adolesc Med, 154 (11), 1114–1117.

Hendrickson, K.C., Rimar, J. (2009). Patterns of hospital resource utilization of children with leukemia and CNS tumors: a comparison of children who survive an those who die within 3 years of diagnosis. Nurs Econ, 27 (1), 35–44.

Hering, E., Pritdker, I., Gonchar, L. et al. (2009). Obesity in children is associated with increased health care use. Clin Pediatr (Phila), 48 (8), 812–818.

Hing, E., Cherry, D.K., Woodwell, D.A. (2006). National ambulatory medical care survey: 2004 (Advance data from Vital Health Statistics; No. 374). Hyattsville, MD: National Center for Health Statistics.

Holtmann, M., Duketis, E., Poustka, L. et al. (2010). Bipolar disorder in children and adolescent in Germany: national trends in the rates of inpatients, 2000–2007. Bipolar Disord, 12 (2), 155–163.

Homer, C.J., Szilagyi, P., Rodewald, L. et al. (1996). Does quality of care affect rates of hospitalization for childhood asthma? Pediatrics, 98 (1), 18–23.

Horowitz, M.E., Pizzo, P.A. (1990). Cancer in the child infected with human immunodeficiency virus. J Pediatr, 116, 730–731.

Hunter, S., Williamson, J. (2000). Children on the brink: executive summary. Washington, DC: USAID.

Icks, A., Holl, R.W., Giani, G. (2007). Economics in pediatric type 1 diabetes – results from recently published studies. Exp Clin Endocrinol Diabetes, 115 (7), 448–454.

Institute of Medicine (2005). Childhood obesity in the United States, facts and figures, fact sheet, September 2004. Drawn from: Preventing childhood obesity: Health in the balance. Retrieved on Feb. 20, 2010 from: http://www.iom.edu/~/media/Files/Report20Files/2004/Preventing-Childhood-Obesity-Health-in-the-Balance/FINALfactsandfigures2.ashx.

Janicke, D.M., Harman, J.S., Kelleher, K.J. et al. (2009). The association of psychiatric diagnoses, health service use, and expenditures in children with obesity-relate health conditions. J Pediatr Psychol, 34 (1), 79–88.

Janz, J., Harrison, J., Caldwell, T. (1993). Children with special health needs in school: developing and individualized educational program and an individualized health care plan. Paper presented at the Annual Convention of the Council for Exceptional Children, San Antonio, TX.

Jellinek, M.S., Synder, J.B. (1998, August). Depression and suicide in children and adolescents. Pediatr Rev, 19 (8), 255–264.

Jones, D., Dodge, K.A., Foster, E.M. et al. (2002). Early identification of children at risk for costly mental health service use. Prev Sci, 3 (4), 247–256.

Jones, D.E., Foster, E.M. (2009). Service use patterns for adolescents with ADHD and comorbid conduct disorder. J Behav Health Serv Res, 36 (4), 436–449.

Jones, S.A., Sherman, G.G., Varga, C.A. (2005). Exploring socio-economic conditions and poor follow-up rates of HIV-exposed infants in Johannesburg, South Africa. AIDS Care, 17 (4), 466–470.

Jordan, O.W., Lipton, R.B., Stupnicka, E. et al. (1994). Incidence of type I diabetes in people under 30 years of age in Barbados, West Indies, 1982–1991. Diab Care, 17, 428–431.

Kaiser Family Foundation (2008, April). U.S. federal funding HIV/AIDS: the FY 2009 budget request.
Keenan, K., Hipwell, A., Duax, J. et al. (2004). Phenomenology of depression in young girls. J Am Acad Child Adolesc Psychiatry, 43 (9), 1098–1106.
Klein, M.W., Matusa, R.F., Copaciu, L. et al. (2004). Comprehensive pediatric human immunodeficiency virus care and treatment in Constanta, Romania: implementation of a program of highly antiretroviral therapy in a resource-poor setting. Pediatr Infect Dis J, 23 (8), 695–700.
Klein, J.D., Shone, L.P., Szilagyi, P.G. et al. (2007). Impact of the State Children's Health Insurance Program on adolescents in New York. Pediatrics, 119 (4), e885–e892.
Klerman, G.L., Lavori, P.W., Rice, J. et al. (1985, July). Birth-cohort trends in rates of major depressive disorder among relatives of patients with affective disorder. Arch Gen Psychiatry, 42 (7), 689–693.
Knapp, M., Romeo, R., Beecham, J. (2009). Economic cost of autism in the U.K. Autism, 13 (3), 317–336.
Kruse, M., Michelsen, S.I., Flachs, E.M. et al. (2009). Lifetime costs of cerebral palsy. Dev Med Child Neurol, 51 (8), 622–628.
LaPorte, R.E., Matsushima, M., Chang, Y-F. (1995). Prevalence and incidence of insulin-dependent diabetes. In R. Aubert, Diabetes in America. Bethesda, MD: National Institute of Health, National Institute of Diabetes, and Digestive and Kidney Diseases, National Diabetes Data Group, NIH Publication No. 95–1468.
Lavigne, J.V., Lebailly, S.A., Hopkins, J. et al. (2009). The prevalence of ADHD, ODD, depression, and anxiety in a community sample of 4-year-olds. J Clin Child Adolesc Psychol, 38 (3), 315–328.
Lawrence, R.C., Helmick, C.G., Arnett, F.C. et al. (1998). Estimates of the prevalence of arthritis and selected musculoskeletal disorders in the United States. Arthritis Rheum, 41 (5), 778–799.
Leibson, C.L., Barbaresi, W.J., Ransom, J. et al. (2006). Emergency department use and costs for youth with attention-deficit/hyperactivity disorder: associations with stimulant treatment. Ambul Pediatr, 6 (1), 45–53.
Leibson, C.L., Long, K.H. (2003). Economic implications of attention-deficit hyperactivity disorder for healthcare systems. Pharmacoeconomics, 21 (17), 1239–1262.
Lenhardt, R.O., Catrambone, C.D., McDermott, M.F. et al. (2006). Improving pediatric asthma care through surveillance: the Illinois Emergency Department Asthma Collaborative. Pediatrics, 117 (4 Pt, 2), S96–S105.
Libman, I., Songer, T., LaPorte, R. (1993). How many people in the U.S. have IDDM? Diab Care, 16, 841.
Liu, Y., Chen, J., Tang, J. et al. (2009). Cost of childhood acute lymphoblastic leukemia care in Shanghai, China. Pediatr Blood Cancer, 53 (4), 557–562.
Lobstein, T., Jackson-Leach, R. (2006). Estimated burden of paediatric obesity and co-morbidities in Europe. Part 2. Numbers of children with indicators of obesity-related disease. Int J Pediatr Oes, 1 (1), 33–41.
Lynch, F.L., Striegel-Moore, R.H., Dickerson, J.F. et al. (2010, June). Cost-effectiveness of guided self-help treatment for recurrent binge eating. J Consult Clin Psychol, 78 (3), 322–333.
Majhail, N.S., Ness, K.K., Burns, L.J. et al. (2007). Late effects in survivors of Hodgkin and non-Hodgkin lymphoma treated with autologous hematopoietic cell transplantation: A report from the Bone Marrow Transplant Survivor Study. Biol Blood Marrow, 13 (10), 1153–1159.
Mandell, D.S., Machefsky, A., Rubin, D. et al. (2008). Medicaid's role in financing health care for children with behavioral health care needs in the special education system: implications of the Deficit Reduction Act. J School Health, 78 (10), 532–538.
Marks, D.J., Mlodnicka, A., Bernstein, M. et al. (2009). Profiles of service utilization and the resultant economic impact in preschoolers with attention deficit/hyperactivity disorder. J Pediatr Psychol, 34 (6), 681–889.
Martinez, F.D., Wright, A.L., Taussig, L.M. et al. (1995, January 19). Asthma and wheezing in the first six years of life. The Group Health Medical Associates. New Engl J Med, 332 (3), 133–138.

Mathet, F., Martin-Guehl, C., Maurice-Tison, S. et al. (2003). Prevalence of depressive disorders in children and adolescents attending primary care. A survey with the Aquitaine Sentinelle Network. Encephale, 29 (5), 391–400.

McCandless, S.E., Brunger, J.W., Cassidy, S.B. (2004). The burden of genetic disease in inpatient care in a children's hospital. Am J Hum Genet, 74 (1), 121–127.

McCarthy, J. (2007). Children with autism spectrum disorders and intellectual disability. Curr Opin Psychiatry, 20 (5), 472–476.

McFadden, E.R., Jr., Warren, E.L. (1997). Observations on asthma mortality. Ann Intern Med, 127 (2), 142–147.

Mehler-Wex, C., Kolch, M. (2008). Depression in children and adolescents. Dtsch Arztebl Int, 105 (9), 149–155.

Merenstein, D., Egleston, B., Diener-West, M. (2005). Lengths of stay and costs associated with children's hospitals. Pediatrics, 115 (4), 839–844.

Meyers, T., Moultrie, H., Naidoo, K. et al. (2007). Challenges to pediatric HIV care and treatment in South Africa. J Infect Dis, 196 (Suppl 3), S474–S481.

Milota, C., Goldberg, M., Goldberg, P. et al. (1991). Count me in: resource manual on disabilities. Minneapolis, MN: PACER Center Inc. Retrieved February 27, 2010 from: http://www.eric.ed.gov/ERICDocs/data/ericdocs2sql/content_storage_01/0000019b/80/3/98/8a.pdf.

Minden, K., Niewerth, M., Listig, J. et al. (2009). The economic burden of juvenile idiopathic arthritis-results from the German paediatric rheumatologic database. Clin Exp Rheumatol, 27 (5), 863–869.

MMWR (2007). National and state medical expenditures and lost earnings attributable to arthritis and other rheumatic conditions–United States, 2003. MMWR Morb Mortal Wkly Rep, 56 (1), 4–7. Retrieved February 27, 2010 from: http://www.ncbi.nlm.nih.gov/pubmed/17218935?itool=EntrezSystem2.PEntrez.Pubmed.Pubmed_ResultsPanel.Pubmed_RVDocSum&ordinalpos=1.

Mukherjee, D., Kosztowski, T., Zaidi, H.A. et al. (2009, October). Disparities in access to pediatric neurooncological surgery in the United States. Pediatrics, 124 (4), e688–696.

National Center for Health Statistics (2007). Health & Stats, Prevalence of overweight among children and adolescents: United States, 1999–2002. Hyattsville, MD: U.S. DHHS, CDC, National Center for Health Statistics. Retrieved February 27, 2010 from: http://www.cdc.gov/nchs/data/hestat/overwght99.htm.

National Children's Cancer Foundation (1997). Facts about childhood cancer. National Children's Cancer Foundation.

National Heart, Lung, and Blood Institute. (1997). Managing asthma long term in children 0–4 years and 5–11 years of age. Expert panel report: guidelines for the diagnosis and management of asthma. Bethesda, MD: National Heart, Lung, and Blood Institute (rev. Aug. 2007), pp. 281–325.

Ogden, C.L., Carroll, M.D., Curtin, L.R. et al. (2010). Prevalence of high body mass index in U.S. children and adolescents, 2007–2008. J Am Med Assoc, 303 (3), 242–249.

Olesti Baiges, M., Pinol Moreso, J.L., Martin Vergara, N. et al. (2008). Prevalence of anorexia nervosa, bulimia nervosa and other eating disorders in adolescent girls in Reus, Spain. An Pediatr (Barc), 68 (1), 18–23.

Paintsil, E., Andiman, W.A. (2009). Update on successes and challenges regarding mother-to-child transmission of HIV. Curr Opin Pediatr, 21 (1), 94–101.

Pelham, W.E., Foster, E.M., Robb, J.A. (2007). The economic impact of attention-deficit/hyperactivity disorder in children and adolescents. Ambul Pediatr, 7 (1 Suppl), 121–131.

Pollack, C.V., Jr., Pollack, E.S., Baren, J.M. et al. (2002). A prospective multicenter study of patient factors associated with hospital admission from the emergency department among children with acute asthma. Arch Pediatr Adolesc Med, 156 (9), 934–940.

Reed, C.E. (2006, September). The natural history of asthma. J Allergy Clin Immunol, 118 (3), 543–548.

Raisch, D.W., Holdsworth, M.T., Winter, S.S. et al. (2003). Economic comparison of home-care-based versus hospital-based treatment of chemotherapy-induced febrile neutropenia in children. Value Health, 6 (2), 158–166.

Ries, L.A.G., Melbert, D., Krapcho, M. et al. (2004). SEER cancer statistics review, 1975–2004. Bethesda, MD: National Cancer Institute. Retrieved June 19, 2008, from http://seer.cancer.gov/csr/1975_2004.

Robinson, E.L. (1998). Arthritis (juvenile rheumatoid). In LeAdelle Phelps (Ed.), Health related disorders in children and adolescents: a guidebook for understanding and educating. Washington, DC: American Psychological Association, pp. 62–67.

Rodriguez-Cano, T., Beato-Fernandez, L., Belmonte-Llario, A. (2005). New contributions to the prevalence of eating disorders in Spanish adolescents: detection of false negatives. Eur Psychiatry, 20 (2), 173–178.

Rosenman, M.B., Vik, T., Hui, S.L. et al. (2005). Hospital resource utilization in childhood cancer. J Pediatr Hematol Oncol, 27 (6), 295–300.

Rutstein, R.M., Gebo, K.A., Siberry, G.K. et al. (2005). Hospital and outpatient health services utilization among HIV-infected children in care, 2000–2001. Med Care, 43 (9 Suppl), III31–9.

Sacks, J., Helmick, C., Yao-Hua, L. et al. (2007). Prevalence of and annual ambulatory health care visits for pediatric arthritis and other rheumatologic conditions in the US in 2001–2004. Arthritis Rheum, 57, 1439–1445.

Schackman, B.R., Gebo, K.A., Walensky, R.P. et al. (2006). The lifetime cost of current human immunodeficiency virus care in the United States. Med Care, 44 (11), 990–997.

Schlander, M. (2007). Impact of attention-deficit/hyperactivity disorder (ADHD) on prescription drug spending for children and adolescents: increasing relevance of health economic evidence. Child Adolesc Psychiatry Ment Health, 1 (1), 13.

Sepulveda, M.J., Tait, F., Zimmerman, E. et al. (2010). Impact of childhood obesity on employers. Health Aff (Millwood), 29 (3), 513–521.

Shields, A.E., Comstock, C., Weiss, K.B. (2004). Variations in asthma care by race/ethnicity among children enrolled in a state Medicaid program. Pediatrics, 113 (3 Pt 1), 496–504.

Simon, J., Schmidt, U., Pilling, S. (2005). The health service use and cost of eating disorders. Psychol Med, 35 (11), 1543–1551.

Simpson, L., Owens, P.L., Zodet, M.W. et al. (2005). Health care for children and youth in the United States: annual report on patterns of coverage, utilization, quality, and expenditures. Ambul Pediatr, 5 (1), 6–44.

Simpson, L., Zodet, M.W., Chevarley, F.M. et al. (2004). Health care for children and youth in the United States: 2002 report on trends in access, utilization, quality, and expenditures. Ambul Pediatr, 4 (2), 131–153.

Smith, M., Arthur, D., Camitta, B. et al. (1996). Uniform approach to risk classification and treatment assignment for children with acute lymphoblastic leukemia. J Clin Oncol, 14 (1), 18–24.

Songer, T.J., LaPorte, R.E., Dorman, J.S. (1988). The individual costs of insulin-dependent diabetes mellitus (IDDM) expected through age 40. Diabetes Res Clin Pract Suppl, 1–5, S354.

Swensen, A.R., Birnbaum, H.G., Secnik, K. et al. (2003). Attention-deficit/hyperactivity disorder: increased costs for patients and their families. J Am Acad Child Adolesc Psychiatry, 42 (12), 1415–1423.

Thornton, J., Lunt, M., Ashcroft, D.M. et al. (2008). Costing juvenile idiopathic arthritis: examining patient-based costs during the first year after diagnosis. Rheumatology (Oxford), 47 (7), 985–990.

Trasande, L., Chatterjee, S. (2009). The impact of obesity on health service utilization and costs in childhood. Obesity (Silver Spring), 17 (9), 1749–1754.

Troiano, R., Flegal, K. (1998). Overweight children and adolescents: description, epidemiology, and demographics. Pediatrics, 101 (3 Supp), 497–504.

Tull, E.S., Roseman, J.M., Christian, C.L.E. (1991). Epidemiology of childhood IDDM in U.S. Virgin Islands from 1979 to 1988. Diab Care, 14 (7), 558–564.

UNAIDS (2007, September). Financial resources required to achieve universal access to HIV prevention, treatment, care, and support.
Van Cleave, J., Gortmaker, S.L., Perrin, J.M. (2010). Dynamics of obesity and chronic health conditions among children and youth. J Am Med Assoc, 303 (7), 623–630.
Wagenknecht, L.E., Roseman, J.M., Herman, W.H. (1991). Increased incidence of insulin-dependent diabetes mellitus following an epidemic of coxsackievirus B5. Ann J Epidemiol, 133, 1024–1031.
Wang, Y. (2001). Cross-national comparison of childhood obesity: the epidemic and the relationship between obesity and socioeconomic status. Int J Epidemiol, 30, 1129–1136.
Wang, B., Chen, Y., Zhang, J. et al. (2008). A preliminary study into the economic burden of cerebral palsy in China. Health Pol, 87 (2), 223–234.
Weiss, K.B., Sullivan, S.D., Lyttle, C.S. (2000, September). Trends in the cost of illness for asthma in the United States, 1985–1994. J Allergy Clin Immunol, 106 (3), 493–499.
Wolfenstetter, S.B. (2006). Juvenile obesity and comorbidity type 2 diabetes mellitus (T2 DM) in Germany; development and cost-of-illness analysis. Gesundheitswesen, 68 (10), 600–612.
Wright, A.L. (2002, February). Epidemiology of asthma and recurrent wheeze in childhood. Clin Rev Allergy Immunol, 22 (1), 33–44.

Chapter 2
Chromosomal Abnormalities

Numerous chromosomal and genetic disorders exist, and several volumes would be needed to delineate each of them. For the purposes of this chapter, the authors have chosen to focus largely on several chromosomal disorders, mainly the trisomies. Other common genetic disorders will be briefly referenced and sources will be provided for those interested in understanding these disorders in greater detail.

About 1 in 150 babies is born with a chromosomal abnormality (American College of Obstetricians and Gynecologists, 2001, 2005; Carey, 2003). These disorders are caused by errors in the number or structure of chromosomes, which usually result from an error that occurred when an egg or sperm cell was developing. Babies may be born with too few or too many chromosomes. In some instances, a piece of a chromosome may be missing or the chromosomes may be rearranged. However, it is still unknown why these errors occur. Nonetheless, these errors can cause a variety of birth defects ranging from mild to severe.

Many children with a chromosomal abnormality have mental and/or physical birth defects, ranging from mild to severe. In addition, some chromosomal abnormalities result in miscarriage or stillbirth. Research indicates that nothing that a parent does or does not do during pregnancy can cause a chromosomal abnormality.

A common type of chromosomal abnormality is a trisomy, where there are three copies, instead of two, of a specific chromosome. In most instances, an embryo with the wrong number of chromosomes does not survive and a miscarriage results, often during the first trimester. In fact, 75% of first trisemester miscarriages are caused by chromosomal abnormalities in the embryo (American College of Obstetricians and Gynecologists, 2005).

Other errors can also occur, usually prior to fertilization. Alteration in the structure of one or more chromosomes can result. Chromosomes may be deleted, misplaced, inverted, duplicated, or exchanged with part of another chromosome. These structural rearrangements have no effect at times if all of the chromosome is present, but is just rearranged. However, an increased risk of miscarriage or birth defects exists nevertheless.

Errors in cell division may also occur after fertilization, resulting in mosaicism, a condition in which an individual has cells with different genetic makeups. The severity of the condition is dependent primarily on the percentage of abnormal cells. As result, some people are only mildly affected while others are profoundly impacted.

M.L. Goldstein, S. Morewitz, *Chronic Disorders in Children and Adolescents*,
DOI 10.1007/978-1-4419-9764-7_2, © Springer Science+Business Media, LLC 2011

Down syndrome (DS) is one of the most common chromosomal abnormalities, affecting approximately 1 in 800 babies (American College of Obstetricians and Gynecologists, 2005; National Down Syndrome Society, 2006). Significantly, the risk of DS and other trisomies increases with the mother's age. According to the American College of Obstetricians and Gynecologists (2005), a woman's risk of having a baby with DS is 1 in 1,000 at age 30, 1 in 400 at age 35, and 1 in 100 at age 40.

In addition to mother's age, other parental characteristics may be associated with an increased risk of certain congenital malformations in offspring. Research suggests that parental occupation and Hispanic ethnicity may increase the risk of some birth defects. A case–control investigation of babies born in Texas from 1996 through 2000 revealed that maternal occupation as a cook or nurse was related to an increased risk of oral clefts and neural tube defects among births to Hispanic women, but not among births to non-Hispanic White mothers (Brender et al., 2008). Hispanic fathers who were electricians had a greater risk of having babies with chromosomal abnormalities, particularly trisomy 18. These associations did not occur among the babies of non-Hispanic White fathers.

Maternal smoking and other behaviors may increase the risk of chromosomal abnormalities. For example, in their investigation of the effects of maternal smoking on prenatal screening for DS and trisomy 18 in the first trimester of pregnancy, Miron et al. (2008) demonstrated that maternal smoking was associated with an increase in average risk and rates of trisomy 18, but not an increase in the average risk and rates of DS.

Babies can also be born with an extra chromosome 13 or 18, both trisomies which are significantly more severe than DS. Carey (2003) reported that about 1 in 10,000 babies are born with trisomy 13 (Patau syndrome). SOFT (2006) reported that 1 in 6,000 babies are born with trisomy 18 (Edwards syndrome).

As a result of new technology, some uncommon chromosomal abnormalities have been identified. In some of these cases, the abnormalities are so rare that only a few children may be impacted. Some of the uncommon abnormalities include deletion, in which a small section of a chromosome is missing and microdeletion, in which a single gene or minute amount of material is missing. In addition, a translocation occurs, in which a section of a chromosome is attached to another chromosome, or an inversion takes place, in which a section of a chromosome is inserted upside down. Furthermore, duplication occurs, resulting in extra genetic material, or a ring chromosome develops, where material is deleted at each end of a chromosome and the new ends then join to form a ring.

Some of these abnormalities, particularly inversions and translocations, may not impact a child's health if no genetic material is missing or duplicated. However, deletions, even small deletions, often result in severe complications. Prader–Willi syndrome, Cri-du-chat syndrome, Wolf–Hirschhorn syndrome, and 22q11 deletion syndrome are well-known examples.

Typically, the risk of parents having another child with a chromosomal abnormality is low. Carey reported that parents with a child with DS had a 1% risk of having another DS baby, if the mother is younger than 35 years of age. Those mothers over 35 have a risk similar to others of their age. Nonetheless, there are exceptions.

Early diagnosis and intervention are essential. Genetic counseling is often recommended and supportive counseling for the parents is usually helpful, particularly group support. In some cases, early education intervention, particularly with non-fatal disorders like DS or Klinefelter syndrome, is vital. Furthermore, expert medical care is necessary.

Down Syndrome (DS)

Down syndrome (DS) is a chromosomal condition related to chromosome 21. The extra number 21 chromosome interrupts the normal course of development, causing the characteristic clinical features. However, some individuals have an extra chromosome 21 in only some of their cells, resulting in mosaic Down syndrome (MDS). In addition, a small number of people with DS have the syndrome because part of chromosome 21 translocated to another chromosome, either before or at the time of conception. As a result, these individuals have two copies of chromosome 21 and additional material from chromosome 21 attached to another chromosome.

DS is typically not inherited. MDS is also not inherited, but is the result of random error during cell division, resulting in some cells having an extra copy of the chromosome. Translocation DS may be inherited.

DS affects 1 in 800 to 1 in 1,000 live born infants (National Human Genome Research Institute, 2008). Individuals with DS have learning problems, mental retardation, poor muscle tone in infancy, as well as a characteristic facial feature. They also have an increased risk for having heart defects. Approximately 40–60% of those born with DS have a heart defect (Drew, 1990).

Those with DS also have more digestive problems, including gastroesophageal reflux or celiac disease. Some infants with DS have problems with swallowing or they can experience bowel blockage. Some also have hypothyroidism.

DS children often have frequent colds as well as sinus and ear infections. Others experience sucking problems during infancy, as a result of poor muscle tone. Sucking problems create difficulty with breast feeding initially. Furthermore, some infants have eye problems, most notably strabismus and cataracts.

Intellectually, DS children may function from a low-normal to a mentally handicapped range. Wisniewski et al. (1996) found varying degrees of cognitive and other neurological dysfunction in DS children. Furthermore, Anderson (1998) and Nadel (1996) have also commented extensively on the wide range of intellectual functioning.

Researchers have evaluated language comprehension in children with DS and other disorders. Price et al. (2007) compared the receptive vocabulary, grammatical morphology, and syntax skills of DS boys with those of boys with fragile X syndrome (FXS) (who were also classified as having autism, autism spectrum disorder, or no autism) and typically developing (TD) boys. The DS boys performed lower in language comprehension than the FXS boys without autism and TD boys. DS boys and FXS boys varied in receptive language performance, indicating unique language patterns for each disorder. The investigators recommend targeting language comprehension in assessing and treating these groups.

Ferrier et al. (1991) investigated the conversational skills of persons with FXS, compared to two matched groups of individuals with autism and DS. The researchers found that the FXS group relied on more eliciting forms in conversation than the DS group. The FXS group also used partial self-repetition more frequently than both the DS and autism groups. The DS group exhibits more speech dysfluencies than the autism group, but no more than the FXS group. Compared to the other groups, the autism group used more inappropriate phrases.

Research on the phonological accuracy and speech intelligibility has shown differences based on the type of disorder. Based on a sample of boys with FXS with autism spectrum disorder (ASD), FXS only, DS, and typically developing (TD) boys, Barnes et al. (2009) discovered that DS boys had lower scores on phonological accuracy and the occurrence of phonological processes than all other groups of boys. DS boys also relied on fewer intelligible words than did boys in the TD group. The investigators concluded that DS boys exhibited more extensive delays in all phonological indicators than boys in the FXS and TD groups.

Wright, Lewis, and Collis (2006) found that object search and play behaviors of children with DS rely more heavily on imitation than is the case for typically developing children. In another investigation, Landry et al. (1994) related that DS children initiated fewer exchanges in less structured situations than normal peers, but were more likely to increase compliance with directive requests.

Cicchetti (1991) expressed concern about the biologically based risk factors on early self-development, particularly self-concept, in children with DS. Dykens et al. (2007) examined the self-perceptions, thoughts, hopes, and inner lives of children with DS and Prader–Willi syndrome (PWS). Positive and negative self-appraisal was found to be related to syndrome status or maladaptive behavior. Hodapp et al. (1997) reported that the amount of the child's maladaptive behavior is highly correlated with parental stress and that the parents of DS children generally report lower levels of stress, related to the degree to which the child is reinforcing and acceptable to the child. Finally, Ghosh et al. (2008) indicated that ASD manifests as a distinct behavioral phenomenon in DS, and DS children with ASD display more restricted repetitive and stereotyped patterns of behavior, interests, and activities.

Prader–Willi Syndrome (PWS)

First reported in 1956, the Prader–Willi syndrome (PWS) occurs when there is a paternal deletion on chromosome 15, a maternal uniparental disomy, or an imprinting defect. According to the Prader–Willi Association (2008), every case of PWS is the result of the baby failing to receive active genes from a specific section of the father's chromosome 15. Approximately 70% of all cases are the result of paternal deletion or microdeletion. Usually a deletion occurs for no known reason and there is less than a 1% chance of reoccurrence. About 25% of all cases are the result of maternal uniparental trisomy, where the developing embryo begins with three copies of chromosome 15 and one of the copies is "lost," the chromosome 15 from the father. The result is the same as deletion, even though there are two complete copies of the mother's chromosome 15. Finally, less than 5% of all cases results from an imprinting defect. In these instances, the PWS genes on the father's chromosome are present but do not work because the imprinting process is faulty.

PWS occurs equally in both genders and all races and has a prevalence of 1 in 12,000–15,000. The major characteristics include hypotonia, hypogonadism, hyperphagia, cognitive impairment, and problematic behaviors. The major medical concern is morbid obesity, due to a tendency to impulsively overeat. Morbid obesity is worsened by decreased energy expenditure and reduced physical activity (Whitman et al., 2002).

PWS first appeared in the medical literature when endocrinologists Prader, Labhart, and Willi reported an unusual pattern of abnormalities, including diminished fetal activity, profound poor muscle tone, feeding problems in infancy, underdeveloped sex organs, short stature and retarded bone age, small hands and feet, delayed developmental milestones, characteristic faces, cognitive impairment, onset of gross obesity in early childhood due to insatiable hunger, and a tendency to develop diabetes mellitus (DM) in adolescence and adulthood when weight was not controlled. Butler and Thompson (2000), Cassidy and Schwartz (1998), and Cassidy and Schwartz (2009) have offered an expanded understanding of the syndrome.

Obesity and the concomitant development of DM have been of most concern for individuals with PWS. Dudley et al. (2008) conducted a cross-cultural comparison of body mass index and PWS. They discovered that obesity was similar for children with PWS in the USA, France, and Germany, but that French adults with PWS had significantly higher rates of obesity than adults in the USA or Germany.

Persons with PWS are at increased risk of experiencing emotional, behavioral, and cognitive problems (Whitman et al., 2002). Researchers have identified similar difficulties related to short stature among non-PWS individuals with growth hormone (GH) deficiency and idiopathic short stature. Moreover, normal adults with GH deficiency have reported a lower quality of life (QOL) and psychosocial problems.

During adolescence and adulthood, individuals with PWS develop psychiatric conditions, including acute cycloid psychosis, and obsessive–compulsive, bipolar, and pervasive developmental disorders (Descheemaeker et al., 2002). Persons with PWS may exhibit literal mindedness, inflexibility, and impaired social cognition (Whittington et al., 2004).

Growth hormone replacement therapy (GHRT) has produced positive changes in PWS children's physical measures. In an investigation of adults with PWS, Hoybye et al. (2005) discovered that when GHRT was discontinued, the individuals exhibited impairments in both physical and social status and overall functioning.

GHRT has shown significant positive psychosocial and behavioral effects in non-PWS individuals (Whitman et al., 2002). In non-PWS populations, GHRT has enhanced alertness, physical activity, endurance, and extroversion. This therapy has also reduced irritability and a person's tendency to worry. These outcomes have improved relationships and reduced conflicts.

Based on a 2-year investigation, Whitman et al. (2002) discovered that GHRT significantly reduced symptoms of depression and did not result in a deterioration of behaviors during the treatment. The authors recommend using GHRT to treat PWS.

Bertella et al. (2007) assessed the QOL of those diagnosed with PWS who underwent growth hormone treatment. Results suggested that those with PWS had significant improvement with regard to both psychological and physical well-being.

Angelman Syndrome (AS)

When a deletion of chromosome 15 is found on the mother's chromosome 15, the result is a syndrome different from PWS, known as Angelman syndrome (AS). AS appears to occur spontaneously for unknown reasons, as a result of deletion or disruption of a certain gene or genes on the long arm of chromosome 15 (15q11–q13). The syndrome was first identified by Angelman (1950), who described some children in his pediatric practice as having flat heads, jerky movements, protruding tongues, and having bouts of laughter (Angelman Syndrome Foundation, 2005; National Organization for Rare Disorders, 2003). The disease was initially referred to as the "happy puppet syndrome."

AS is clinically characterized by severe mental retardation, lack of speech, EEG abnormalities, ataxia and stiff, atactic gait (Brouwer et al., 1990; Moncia et al., 1994; Robb et al., 1989). Other symptoms identified with AS include developmental delay, absence or near absence of speech, prolonged episodes of inappropriate laughter, characteristic facial features and episodes of seizures (Clayton-Smith and Laan, 2003; Garcia-Ramirez et al., 2008; Turchetti et al., 2006). Abnormalities of the head and face are typical, including microcephaly, deeply set eyes, macrostomia, maxillary hypoplasia, mandibular prognathism, and widely spaced teeth.

Infants with AS appear normal at birth, but often have feeding problems in the first few months of life. In addition, abnormal sleep patterns are typical. Furthermore, by early childhood, severe developmental delays are evident. Those with AS may also exhibit ataxia, resulting in a stiff manner of walking, with jerky arm movements and a characteristic positioning of the arms with flexion of the elbows and wrists.

Seizures often begin between 2 and 3 years of age. Although affected individuals may be unable to speak, many eventually learn to communicate through other means, particularly sign language. Others have adequate receptive language in order to respond to simple commands. The prevalence of autistic disorder is still debated (Pelc, Cheron, and Dan, 2008). Furthermore, Walz and Baranek (2006) confirmed a high degree and variety of sensory processing abnormalities in individuals with AS.

Although behavior problems have been documented in children with AS, researchers know little about their developmental course and outcome (Summers et al., 1995). Drawing on a review of case reports and parent responses to a survey, Summers et al. (1995) discovered that both male and female children of all ages exhibited behavior problems, including language impairments, excessive laughter, hyperactive behavior, short attention span, eating and sleeping difficulties, aggressive behaviors, and non-compliance. Moreover, the AS children mouthed objects, had tantrums, and engaged in repetitive and stereotyped behavior. The authors recommend that clinicians identify and treat severe behavior disorders in AS children to enhance their social functioning.

Those with AS tend to have normal life spans and generally do not show developmental regression with age.

Patau Syndrome (PS)

Patau syndrome (PS), also known as trisomy 13, is a congenital disorder associated with the presence of an extra copy of chromosome 13 or a translocation of a portion of chromosome 13 (Patau et al., 1960). First identified by Dr. Klaus Patau, in 1960, the condition is also called Bartholin–Patau syndrome, named in part for Thomas Bartholin, a French physician, who described an infant with the syndrome in 1656.

The incidence of PS is approximately 1 per 12,000 live births (Baty et al., 1994b; Baty et al., 1994a; Delatycki and Garder, 1997).

Seventy-five to eighty percent of cases are caused by a trisomy, whether a full or partial trisomy. In the latter, physical symptoms tend to be less severe. In the remaining cases, there is an inherited translocation of chromosome 13. PS occurs in approximately 1 in 8,000–12,000 live births. Miscarriages frequently occur, while in other instances, stillbirths occur. As is typical with other trisomies, the risk of PS increases with the mother's age, particularly if she is over 30. Gender, racial, or ethnic differences do not occur among individuals with PS.

According to Beers and Berkow (2004) and Best and Stallworth (2002), severity and symptoms vary from individual to individual, but are most severe when there is full trisomy 13. Holoprosencephaly and microcephaly usually occur. In addition, myelomeningocele may exist, where the spinal cord protrudes through a defect in the vertebrae of the spinal column. In addition, incomplete development of the optic and olfactory nerves usually accompany brain defects. The eyes may be unusually small or one eye may be missing. At times, the eyes are set close together or even fused into a single structure.

PS also results in individuals being born either partially or totally deaf. Many also have recurring ear infections. Furthermore, facial features appear flattened; the ears are malformed and low-set; and a cleft palate, cleft lip, or both are common. In addition, those with PS may have extra toes or fingers, permanently closed fingers, noticeably prominent heels, missing ribs, and loose folds of skin at the back of the neck.

Genital malformations are typical in those with PS, including ambiguous genitalia in males, an abnormally formed uterus in females, undescended testicles, and an abnormally developed scrotum.

In nearly all cases, the infant has respiratory problems and heart defects, including holes between the chambers of the heart, holes in the valves of the lungs and the heart, and malformed ducts that result in abnormal direction of blood flow and misplacement of the heart in the right side of the chest. Frequently, cysts develop in the kidneys and/or gastrointestinal system.

After the first month after birth, infants with PS are likely to experience feeding problems; reflux disease; constipation; high blood pressure; low muscle tone; ear, eye, and urinary tract infections; light sensitivity; irritability; scoliosis; and slow growth rate.

With partial PS of the distal segment, there is evidence of a distinctive facial appearance, with a short upturned nose, a longer than usual area between the upper lip and nose, and bushy eyebrows. Tumors on the forehead are also typical. With partial PS of the proximal segment, there may be a variety of facial features, including a receding jaw, large nose, and a short upper lip. Although partial PS results in severe mental retardation, these individuals typically live far beyond those with full PS.

Approximately 45% of PS babies die within 1 month after birth. As many as 70% die within the first 6 months. Survival into adulthood is very rare. However, Nanjiani, Hossain, and Mahgoub (2007) described a 51-year-old woman with PS.

Duarte et al. (2004) reported on a PS patient who had a long survival. They examined a 28-month-old girl who at birth was cyanotic, icteric, spastic, and who cried weakly. She had polydactyly in the left hand, congenital club foot and convex soles, and ocular hypertelorism. The girl also had a low nasal bridge, many hemangiomas throughout her body, cardiomegaly, and perimembranous interventricular communication. However, the patient did not have a cleft lip or palate. She had neuropsychomotor development retardation at birth, but had improved after physiotherapy and recreational treatments.

Edwards Syndrome (ES)

Edwards syndrome (ES) is another chromosomal disorder, specifically the result of an extra copy of chromosome 18. Also known as trisomy 18, ES affects approximately 1 in 3,000 live births and is the second most common trisomy. Data from the Support Organization for Trisomy 18, 13 and Related Disorders (SOFT) indicates that approximately 75–80% of newborns impacted by ES are female. As with other trisomies, as a woman becomes older, she has a greater risk of having a child with ES. Very rarely, a translocation may occur, resulting in a partial trisomy. As a result, the individual may have fewer and less pronounced symptoms.

Physical symptoms include clenched hands with index fingers overlapping other fingers, crossed legs, a hole, split, or cleft in the iris, low set and malformed ears, small jaw, small head, separation between the two sides of the rectus abdominis muscle, unusual shaped chest, underdeveloped fingernails, undescended testicles, and hernia. Abnormalities in the lungs, diaphragm, heart, and blood vessel formations are also common. In addition, the kidneys may be malformed. Furthermore, the baby may have clubbed feet and either webbed or fused toes. Low birth weight is typical. Severe mental deficiency is expected as well.

In the most comprehensive study of trisomy 18, Naguib et al. (1999) evaluated 118 children diagnosed with ES. They reported that the majority of children died before the second week of life and that congenital heart and gastrointestinal abnormalities were the most prevalent medical issues. The investigators also reported that maternal age was associated with ES.

Double trisomy is rare. Tennakoon et al. (2008) reported on a male neonate with double trisomy (48XYY, +18), who was born to a 28-year-old gravida three, parity one mother at 35 weeks of gestation. The baby exhibited clinical characteristics of ES. The male neonate did not have a family history of DM and had not been exposed to chemicals. Discrepancy between genders may explain why the Y-chromosome is rarely involved in ES.

Cri du Chat Syndrome (CdCS)

Cri du chat syndrome (CdCS), also known as 5-p syndrome and cat cry syndrome, is a relatively rare genetic disorder caused by the deletion of the p arm of chromosome 5. The cause is unknown. Most cases are not inherited. The deletion usually occurs as a random event. Individuals with CdCS typically have no history of the condition in their family. About 10% inherit the chromosome with a deleted segment from an unaffected parent who has a balanced translocation.

Mainardi (2006) reported that the incidence ranges from 1 in 15,000 to 1 in 50,000 live births. Distinctive features of CdCS include small head, broad nasal bridge, weak muscle tone, widely spaced eyes, and low birth weight. A high-pitched, cat-like cry is the most prominent clinical feature in the newborn and is typically diagnostic for the disorder. The high-pitched, cat-like cry has been localized to chromosome 5p15.3.

Symptoms vary from one individual to the next (Fang et al., 2008). The variability is usually related to different sizes and locations of deletions in chromosome 5p. Nonetheless, common clinical symptoms include a high-pitched "cat-like" cry, delayed development, difficulty with language, and mental retardation. Approximately 50% of the children with this syndrome learn sufficient verbal skills to communicate (National Human Genome Research Institute, 2008). Some individuals with CdCS learn to use short sentences, while others are restricted to a few basic words or gestures or sign language.

Using the Aberrant Behavior Checklist in a study of 146 persons with CdCS, Dykens and Clarke (1997) showed that hyperactivity was the most important and prevalent problem. In addition, individuals with the disorder exhibited aggressive behaviors, tantrums, stereotypic behaviors, and self-destructive behaviors. In persons with lower levels of adaptive and cognitive functioning and those who have been in medication trials, these difficulties were more evident. Symptoms of autism and social withdrawal were more common in those with translocations instead of deletions.

Clarke and Boer (1998) studied problem behaviors associated with CdCS, Prader–Willi, and Smith–Magenis. Using the Aberrant Behavior Checklist, the authors found that CdCS and the other two chromosome deletion disorders were related to more ratings of problem behaviors among individuals with these three chromosome deletion disorders than those in comparison groups.

Individuals with CdCS may engage in repetitive behavior. Moss et al. (2009) compared the prevalence and nature of repetitive behavior in genetic syndromes and found persons with this disorder exhibited unique patterns of repetitive behavior.

Researchers have investigated the behavioral aspects of CdCS during early childhood. Sarimski (2003) evaluated the early play behavior in children, aged 2–7, with the disorder and showed that these children were easily distracted and had a low rate of object-directed activities compared to two control groups. The author concluded that a low level of object-directed behaviors in young children may be early signs of hyperactivity, being easily distracted, and stereotypic behaviors, which are typical of the behavioral phenotype of older persons with CdCS.

Based on an investigation of a three-generation family with 5p terminal deletion (5p15.2-pter), Fang et al. (2008) discovered that mental symptoms varied within the family although the family members shared deletions of the same size. Two female family members with the condition showed moderate mental retardation and psychotic symptoms, such as persecution delusions, auditory hallucinations, self-talking, and self-laughing. In contrast, the other three male family members with the disorder did not exhibit any psychotic behaviors but did show evidence of mild to moderate mental retardation. The investigators suggest that other factors besides the size and location of 5p deletions may influence the development of mental symptoms in persons with this disorder.

Researchers have looked at factors that cause variability in mental retardation and related symptoms in persons with CdCS. Semaphorin F (SEMAF) and delta-catenin (CTNND2) are two genes that have been mapped to the "critical regions" (Cerrutti, 2006). These two genes may be involved in cerebral development and their deletion may cause mental retardation in individuals with CdCS. Phenotypic alterations in CsCS may result from the deletion of the telomerase reverse transcriptase (hTERT) gene, which is localized to 5p15.33.

Based on a report of a family of four who have a deletion slightly distal (6p15.3) to the critical region, Cornish et al. (1999) discovered that this family had only minimal cognitive impairment, indicating that persons who have deletions that only delete the distal critical region have milder intellectual disability and a much better prognosis than persons with the typical CdCS phenotype who can have profound learning impairment.

Most people with CdCS have normal life expectancies. Furthermore, individuals with this disorder are usually happy and friendly and appear to enjoy social interaction. However, those with severe behavioral problems can cause significant stress for their families.

Those with CdCS may also experience delays in walking, feeding problems, and scoliosis. A small percentage is born with serious organ defects and other life-threatening medical problems. Chang et al. (2007) reported that the most common heart condition was atrial septal defect, followed by ventricular septal defect. They also reported that 21% had hearing impairments and that 34% suffered from airway problems.

Wolf–Hirschhorn Syndrome (WHS)

Wolf–Hirschhorn syndrome (WHS) is the result of a genetic error on chromosome 4. However, recent research (Bergemann, Cole, and Hirschhorn 2005; Zollino et al., 2008) suggests that the deletion alone is insufficient for the full development of the disorder and that the deletion of linked genes contributes to both the severity of core characteristics and the presence of additional syndrome problems. In 87% of WHS cases, the individuals do not have a family history of the disorder. The condition is caused by partial loss of material from the distal portion of the short arm of chromosome 4 (4p16.3) and is considered a contiguous gene syndrome. First described by Hirschorn and Cooper (1961) and Hirschhorn (2008), WHS affects females more frequently than males. Battaglia, Fillippi, and Carey (2008) indicated that there is a female predilection of 2:1. The disorder is estimated to occur in 1 in 20,000 to 1 in 50,000 births.

WSS causes malformations in most parts of the body due to the genetic error. Symptoms include distinctive facial features, including prominent forehead, wide set eyes, and broad beaked nose; all these features have been collectively described as "Greek warrior helmet" features. According to Heljic et al. (2004) other common characteristics include growth retardation, mental retardation, and midline fusion defects (cleft lip or palate and cardiac septal defects). Less commonly reported problems are skeletal abnormalities, coloboma iris, dysplastic kidneys, and agenesis of corpus callosum.

Based on an analysis of 80 WHS patients, Zollino et al. (2008) defined three different types of the WHS phenotype that generally were associated with the degree of the 4p deletion. One category consisted of a small deletion that did not exceed 3.5 Mb. This category is frequently correlated with a mild phenotype in which the individual does not have substantial malformations. The second and most frequent type consists of large deletions, with an average of 5–18 MB. These deletions produce the recognizable WHS phenotype. A very large deletion of more than 22–25 MB produces the third category. This third type represents the most severe phenotype and is not defined as typical WHS.

Recently, Fisch et al. (2008) investigated the cognitive-behavioral features of children, aged 4–17 years, with WHS. They found diverse cognitive-behavioral profiles. The investigators discovered that cognitive deficits in these children ranged from mild to severe. In terms of adaptive behavior, females showed slightly higher scores than males. The children showed relative strengths in verbal and quantitative reasoning as well as in socialization. Seven of the 12 children exhibited attention-deficit hyperactivity disorder. One child had symptoms suggestive of mild autism.

Seizures have also been reported as found in 50% of those with WHS (Chen, 2003). However, Battaglia et al. (2008) reported that 93% had a seizure disorder. In addition, low muscle tone; poor muscle development; short stature; malformations of hands and feet, chest, and spine; as well as malformations or underdevelopment of urinary and genital organs have been cited.

Children with WHS frequently have sleeping problems. Extinction of these sleeping disorders may be effective if they have been influenced and positively reinforced by their parents' responses. One case study of a 6-year-old girl with WHS showed that extinction of sleeping problems was effective and was maintained during follow-up (Curfs et al., 1999).

Several factors predict prognosis of WHS children (Zollino et al., 2008). The degree of the deletion, the development of complex chromosome abnormalities, and the severity of seizures affect a person's prognosis.

Velocardiofacial Syndrome (VCFS)

Velocardiofacial syndrome (VCFS), also known as 22q11.2 syndrome, Phelan–McDermid syndrome, DiGeorge sequence, conotruncal anomaly face syndrome, CATCH 22, Sedlackova syndrome, autosomal dominant Optiz G/BBB syndrome, or Cayler Cardiofacial syndrome, is a chromosome microdeletion syndrome caused by microdeletion on chromosome 22. VCFS can result from simple deletion, translocation, ring chromosome, and less common structural changes affecting the long arm of chromosome 22, specifically the region containing the SHANK3 gene. VCFS is one of the most common genetic disorders and manifests in a variety of symptoms in multiple systems (Shprintzen, 2008; Hay, 2007). The disorder occurs with equal frequency in males and females and is underdiagnosed due to lack of clinical recognition and/or insufficient laboratory testing (Phelan, 2008). The condition affects about 1 in 2,000 to 1 in 4,000 newborns, although a number of researchers have argued that the incidence is higher (Phelan, 2008; Shprintzen, 2008).

The name, velocardiofacial syndrome, comes from the Latin words, velum, meaning palate, cardia, meaning heart, and facies, having to do with the heart. However, not all of these identifying features are necessarily evident in those with VCFS. According to Shprintzen (2008), VCFS has an expansive phenotype with more than 180 clinical features that involve essentially every organ and system. The author added that the syndrome has drawn much attention because a number of psychiatric illnesses, including attention deficit disorder, schizophrenia, and bipolar disorder, have phenotypic features similar to VCFS.

Symptoms of VCFS include cleft palate usually of the soft palate, heart problems, eye problems, feeding problems, middle ear infections, immune system problems, weak muscles, low calcium, scoliosis, tapered fingers, bony abnormalities in the neck or upper back, and distinctive facial features (elongated faces, almond-shaped eyes, long eyelashes, full cheeks, wide or bulbous nose, and unusual ears).

A report of a child with VCFS and deletion of 4q34.2 to 4qter revealed that a distal 4q deletion can produce a phenotype similar to VCFS when a 22q deletion is not identified (Tsai et al., 1999). The authors recommend searching for other karyotype abnormalities when a VCFS-like phenotype is evident and a 22q deletion has not been found.

In an investigation of VCFS phenotype and deletion of 22q11.2 in Hungarian children, Morava et al. (2000) suggest that many children with VCFS may have different etiologies other than deletion of 22q11.2 even though the VCFS phenotype seems to be prevalent among Hungarian children.

Hercher and Bruenner (2008) evaluated patients with the disorder and found that there is a 25–30% risk of developing schizophrenia for those diagnosed with VCFS. They also postulated that there is an increased risk for other psychiatric illnesses, including bipolar disorder and schizoaffective disorder as well.

A longitudinal evaluation of adolescents with VCFS by Gothelf et al. (2007) revealed that sub-acute psychotic symptoms interacted with both the catechol *O*-methyltransferase (COMT) genotype and with baseline symptoms of anxiety or depression to predict 61% of the variability in psychosis severity during the follow-up period. The investigators conclude that treating VCFS children with sub-acute signs of psychosis and internalizing conditions, particularly anxiety, can reduce their risk of acquiring psychotic disorders in adolescence.

Gothelf et al. (1997) examined VCFS manifestations and microdeletions in schizophrenic patients and found documented hemizygosity of 22q11 in 3 out of 15 patients. They recommend that psychiatrists become more aware of the signs of VCFS in psychiatric patients so that further molecular studies can be conducted. They recommend screening suspected patients with a single marker such as D22S941 and examine further only those patients who have a single electrophoretic band.

Based on a sample of 326 patients in a Japanese psychiatric hospital, Sugama et al. (1999) identified 12 patients with minor facial dysmorphia. Chromosomal analysis with fluorescent in situ hybridization (FISH) was conducted in six patients who most likely had VCFS based on additional assessment. One of these patients, a 41-year-old woman, had chromosome 22q11.2 deletion. She was schizophrenic but had no substantial dysmorphia, such as cleft palate and cardiovascular anomalies. The authors suggest that psychiatric symptoms in VCFS can develop without major developmental abnormalities. Schizophrenic patients may have subtle aspects of VCFS, but go unrecognized in routine medical examinations.

Using a sample of patients with VCFS, Papolos et al. (1996) showed a strong relationship between VCFS and early-onset bipolar disorder. Their findings indicate that the microdeletion on chromosome 22q11 may be a risk factor for early-onset bipolar disorder.

About 65% of these children have a nonverbal learning disability, resulting in learning problems. When tested cognitively, they are found to have verbal IQ scores 10 points or greater than their performance IQ scores (National Human Genome Research Institute). Children with VCFS tend to have relative strength in reading, spelling, and rote memorization and relative weakness in math and abstract reasoning (De Smedt et al., 2003). Developmental delays are also very common.

Drawing on a sample of children and adolescents with VCFS, Oskarsdottir et al. (2005) demonstrated that children with this syndrome have various neurological, motor, and cognitive difficulties. Although the number and severity of their impairments vary, the combination of disabilities in these children leads to a low level of participation in activities.

Using a sample of 25 children, aged 6–12 years, with VCFS and 25 matched controls, De Smedt et al. (2009) showed that children with VCFS scored more poorly on number comparison but not on number reading. Children with VCFS performed worse on large addition and subtraction problems compared to controls. Their ability to perform backup strategies in addition and subtraction was worse than controls. However, children with VCFS preserved retrieval of arithmetic facts.

Individuals with deletion 22q13.3 syndrome may also display delay in language development (Benitez, 2009) and autistic-like behavior (Phelan, 2008). They often have problems with communication and social interaction.

In a longitudinal investigation of four children with VCFS, Scherer et al. (1999) showed that young children with the disorder have receptive-expressive language disability from the beginning of language acquisition. In addition, the children exhibited severely delayed speech and expressive language development beyond that predicted by their other developmental or receptive language performance. They had severely limited speech sound inventories and early vocabulary development, compared to children with cleft lip and palate and children with isolated cleft palate.

Based on an analysis of VCFS children of borderline or normal intelligence, De Smedt et al. (2003) discovered that the early academic achievement of VCFS children compared on average with their age-related peers. However, at an early age, individual children with VCFS showed wide variability in the domain of counting skills and mathematics and some already exhibited distinct learning impairments.

In a report comparing children with VCFS to those with cleft palate or velopharyngeal dysfunction (VPD), Baylis et al. (2008) demonstrated that the VCFS group had lower articulation functioning and nonverbal measures of intelligence than those with cleft palate or VPD. Speech perception did not vary significantly among the three groups. Articulation skills were associated with nonverbal intelligence and level of velopharyngeal dysfunction.

Researchers have demonstrated that younger children with VCFS exhibit more speech disability than older children with the syndrome or children with some of the phenotypic aspects of VCFS but who do not have the condition (D'Antonio et al., 2001). Younger children with VCFS exhibit smaller consonant inventories, more developmental mistakes, worse articulation disorder, and more glottal stop use. The investigators suggest that children with VCFS have speech production which is not only different from normal but also may be specific to the disorder itself.

Velopharyngeal insufficiency (VPI) occurs in about 70% of patients with VCFS because of cleft palate (Ysunza et al., 2009). VPI is much more prevalent because of abnormalities related to VCFS, including platybasia, hypotrophy of adenoid, enlarged tonsils, hypotonia, and abnormal pharyngeal muscles.

Based on an evaluation of 29 patients who had velopharyngeal surgery for correcting VPI, Ysunza et al. (2009) showed that tailor-made pharyngeal flaps were the strategy for treating VPI in VCFS patients. After undergoing a pharyngeal flap operation 17 (85%) patients developed normal nasal resonance or mild hypernasality. Four patients continued to have severe hypernasality after the procedure. No surgical complications occurred.

Widdershoven et al. (2008) examined the outcome of surgical correction of VPI in patients with VCFS and a control group consisting of patients without VCSF who had a palatal lengthening surgery. The control group improved their speech hypernasality more than the VCFS group. Acoustic nasometry outcomes did not vary between the VCFS and control groups. The researchers concluded that using palatal lengthening to treat VPI in children with VCFS is safe and efficacious. However, mechanical improvement is not associated with gains in speech for children with VCFS.

Musculoskeletal problems, such as scoliosis, can occur among children with VCFS. Morava et al. (2002) evaluated 20 patients for scoliosis and connective tissue problems who were consecutively diagnosed with VCFS and 22q11.2 deletion. They discovered that three of these children had substantial scoliosis and connective tissue problems. Two of these patients were thought to have possible Marfan syndrome and were referred to a genetics evaluation. The investigators recommend that scoliosis should be viewed as a prevalent condition in VCFS patients. In addition, they suggest that 22q11.2 deletion be a possible diagnosis in patients with unexplained scoliosis and developmental delay.

Turner Syndrome (TS)

Turner syndrome (TS) is a chromosomal disorder related to the x chromosome. In TS, the syndrome happens when one of the two x chromosomes normally found in women is missing or incomplete. TS alters development in females only and occurs in 1 in 2,500 female babies. However, the syndrome is much more common among miscarriages and stillbirths. Researchers have yet to determine which genes on the x chromosome are responsible for most signs and symptoms of TS. However, researchers have identified one gene, SHOX, which is important for bone growth and development. Missing one copy of this gene likely causes short stature and skeletal abnormalities. The condition is usually not inherited in families.

Females with this disorder tend to be shorter than average and are typically unable to conceive a child due to the absence of ovarian function even though the vagina and womb are totally normal. Other common symptoms include a webbed neck with folds of skin from the tops of shoulders to the sides of the neck, puffiness or swelling of hands and feet, skeletal abnormalities, and low hairline in the back and low-set ears. In addition, there is increased risk of heart defects and kidney problems. Furthermore, there is increased risk for high blood pressure, DM, osteoporosis, thyroid problems, and cataracts.

Other symptoms include an especially wide neck, arms that turn slightly out at the elbow, scoliosis, minor eye problems, a broad chest with widely spaced nipples, and a heart murmur, sometimes associated with narrowing of the aorta.

In early childhood, those with TS may have frequent middle ear infections, which can lead to hearing loss in some cases. During the age of puberty, girls do not begin to menstruate or develop breasts without hormone treatment at this time.

Children with TS are typically of normal intelligence and have good verbal skills as well as reading ability. However, some girls have difficulty with mathematics, memory functioning, and fine motor skills.

As with other abnormalities of sex chromosomes, TS has been associated with a greater incidence of neuropsychiatric disorders. Wustmann and Preuss (2009) reviewed existing reports on TS and psychosis, while Roser and Kawohl (2008) reported that TS occurs approximately threefold more frequently in female schizophrenics than compared to the general population. Finally, Marco and Skuse (2006) cited a link between the x chromosome and autism and evaluated the incidence of autism with TS and Klinefelter syndrome.

Growth hormone injections may be beneficial for some girls with TS, resulting in an increase in adult height by a few inches. Estrogen replacement therapy is often begun at the time of normal puberty, around 12 years of age, to facilitate breast development. Later, estrogen and progesterone are utilized to begin menstruation, in order to keep the womb healthy. Rubin (2008) cited the need for exogenous estrogen therapy to be initiated in coordination with the final phase of growth hormone therapy. Estrogen may also be helpful in preventing osteoporosis. Assisted reproduction techniques may assist some women with TS to become pregnant.

Klinefelter Syndrome (KS)

Klinefelter syndrome (KS), also known as an xxy male, is a condition that occurs in men as a result of an extra x chromosome. Occasionally some of the cells only have an extra chromosome, resulting in an xy/xxy mosaic. These latter individuals may have enough normally functioning cells to allow them to father children, although infertility is the most typical symptom in KS. The syndrome is found in 1 of 500–1,000 newborn males (National Institute of Child Health and Human Development, 2006). Woman who have pregnancies after age 35 have a slightly increased chance of having a child with KS.

Although the syndrome's cause is common, the symptoms and characteristics that may result from having the extra chromosome is not common. In fact, many individuals never know that they have an additional chromosome.

Men with KS may have small, firm testes, a small penis, enlarged breasts, sparse facial, body and armpit hair, tall stature, long legs, and a short trunk. In addition, they are more likely than other boys to be overweight and tend to be taller than their fathers and male siblings.

KS has also been associated with an increased risk of breast cancer, extra-gonadal germ cell tumor, lung disease, osteoporosis, and varicose veins. Furthermore, those with KS also have an increased risk for autoimmune disorders, including Sjogren's syndrome and rheumatoid arthritis (Mazzocco & Ross, 2007).

Recent research has focused on hormonal and speratogenic testicular failure in those with KS. Although infertility has been cited as a primary problem, Paduch et al. (2008) found that over 50% of men with KS had sperm, and therefore were not sterile. However, recent evidence suggests that children with KS are born with spermatogonia and lose large numbers of germ cells during puberty. There has also been some evidence that those with KS have diminished sexual drive (Hunter, 1969), but hormone treatment has been effective in reducing this issue.

Although not mentally retarded, children with KS are often diagnosed with learning disabilities. Most have some degree of language impairment and exhibit problems with learning to read and write (Graham et al., 1988). In addition, they frequently have delayed speech development. The majority have some problem with language throughout their lives. Ross et al. (2008) assessed the neuropsychological functioning of children with KS and found that specific language, academic, attentional, and motor abilities were impaired. In the language domain, there was a relative deficit in higher linguistic competence, although vocabulary and meaningful language understanding abilities were generally intact. Deficits in the ability to sustain attention without impulsivity were also evident. Furthermore, children with KS demonstrated an array of motor problems, particularly in strength and running speed.

xxy boys are usually well behaved in the classroom. They tend to be shy, quiet and want to please. When confronted with frustration academically, they tend to withdraw and daydream. Teachers sometimes fail to recognize the language problem and may dismiss them as lazy. As a result, they may fall further behind in school, and may eventually be held back. The risk of school failure and concomitant decreased self-esteem is prevalent. As a result, early identification is essential, with appropriate educational intervention.

The development of psychiatric problems has been widely discussed in the literature. For example, Polani (1969) reported that three times as many male schizophrenic patients had KS, as compared to the general population. Stuart, King, and Pai (2007) reported that autism spectrum disorders are heterogeneous with KS. However, Kessler and Moos (1973) indicated that there were no typical behavioral characteristics associated with a specific chromosomal disorder, including KS.

Developmental Disabilities (DD)

Frequently people with chromosomal abnormalities and other conditions, such as cerebral palsy and mental retardation, have developmental disabilities (DD). DD is synonymous with the terms learning disability (LD), intellectual disability (ID), and cognitive disability in certain countries.

DDs are usually classified as severe, profound, moderate, or mild, based on the individual's assessed need for supports, which may be permanent. Many social, environmental, and physical factors cause DDs, although a definite cause for a person may never be determined. Abnormalities of chromosomes and genes, brain injury, extreme prematurity, child abuse, poor diet, and growth problems are common factors causing DDs.

Between 1 and 2% of the population in most western countries acquire DDs, although statistics are flawed in this area. About 1.4% of the worldwide proportion of people is thought to have DDs (Secretary of State, UK, for Health, March 2001). DDs are twice as common in males as in females. In areas of poverty and deprivation, the prevalence of mild DDs is thought to be higher, and among people of certain ethnicities, it is also higher.

Many people with DDs suffer from various physical health problems. Individuals with DDs have inheritable disorders such as DS. However, other major contributing factors are lack of access to health services and a lack of awareness by health-care professionals. Persons who have severe communication problems have a difficult time expressing their health needs and might not recognize their own health problems without adequate support and education. They may also suffer from sensory problems, vision and hearing problems, obesity, and poor dental health. Individuals with DDs have a life expectancy that is about 20 years below average, although with innovations in adaptive and medical technologies, they are living longer and healthier lives. Freeman–Sheldon syndrome and other specific diagnoses do not affect life expectancy.

Persons with DDs are more likely to have mental health problems and psychiatric disorders than those in the general population. Traumatic events, such as abuse, bullying, and harassment, social restrictions due to low socioeconomic status (SES), biological factors, such as brain injury and alcohol abuse, and developmental factors, such as a lack of understanding of social norms, are some of the factors that produce a high incidence rate of dual diagnoses in these individuals. The difficulties that health professionals have in diagnosing mental health problems and inappropriate treatment can worsen the mental health problems of persons with DDs.

People with DDs frequently suffer abuse, including physical abuse, neglect, sexual abuse, emotional or psychological abuse, financial abuse, legal or civil abuse, systemic abuse, and passive neglect. Their low SES, low self-advocacy skills, communication deficits, and lack of understanding of social norms increase their risk of abuse.

Peer abuse is a significant, if misunderstood, problem. In addition, persons with DDs have rates of crime that are also disproportionately high, and the criminal justice systems in many countries are not equipped to meet the needs of people with DDs as both offenders and victims of crime.

Some persons with DDs engage in challenging behavior, including self-injurious behavior, aggressive behavior, inappropriate sexual behavior, behavior directed at property, and stereotyped behaviors, such as repetitive rocking. A number of factors may cause these challenging behaviors in persons with DDs, including biological, social, e.g., boredom, the insensitivity of staff and services to the individual's wishes and needs, environmental, such as noise and lighting, and psychological factors, such as feeling excluded and lonely. Challenging behavior is often learned and rewarded. However, persons with DDs are often able to learn new, positive behaviors to achieve the same aims. The challenging behavior of individuals with DDs is frequently a reaction to the challenging environments that service professionals create for people with these conditions.

Family Well-Being and Social Functioning

Families who have children with chromosomal abnormalities and associated DDs can experience a significant amount of stress, decreased QOL, and impaired social functioning. Unfortunately, families have needs during the time of clinical assessments, but their needs are often neglected because of the child-centered focus of the clinical evaluations (Head and Abbeduto, 2007).

Researchers have investigated the families of children with chromosomal abnormalities and related disabilities to determine which factors increase the risk of family stress and impairment. A family system approach is useful for analyzing how the well-being of family members can influence children with DDs (Head and Abbeduto, 2007). A family systems model can be employed to evaluate how child, parent, and family factors may affect the adjustment of children with chromosomal abnormalities and their siblings and parents. In addition, the belief systems of families with chromosomal abnormalities can influence the well-being and social functioning of the affected child and other family members.

Based on an investigation of siblings and parents of children with a disability, Giallo and Gavidia-Payne (2006) demonstrated that the level of risk for families and their degree of resilience correlated better with sibling adjustment than the sibling's own stress and coping resources. The authors conclude that family and parental factors may affect sibling adjustment more than sibling resources and coping experiences, and interventions for siblings should incorporate these findings.

Sibling adjustment is often a life-long process. A sample of 54 siblings from two linked longitudinal investigations was used to assess sibling relationship for adults who have a brother or sister with ASD or DS (Orsmond and Seltzer, 2007). The results indicated that siblings of DS adults had more contact with their brother or sister compared to siblings of ASD adults. Moreover, compared to the siblings of ASD adults, the siblings of DS adults indicated that they had higher levels of positive emotion in their relationship, felt more optimistic about the future for their brother or sister, and were less likely to note that their interactions with their parents had been altered. Siblings of DS adults had better sibling relations if the sibling had lower educational attainment, did not have children, lived in closer proximity to the brother or sister with DS, when the sibling relied on more problem-focused coping strategies, was less pessimistic about the future of the brother or sister, and when her/his life had been substantially affected by living with a brother or sister with DS.

Another investigation by Wang et al. (2007) demonstrated that DS children had better social adjustment than a mental age-matched group. However, the DS children had worse social adjustment than an age-matched group. They concluded that various factors, such as cognitive development, family factors, and newborn history, predict social adjustment of children with this disorder.

In a study of families of children with CdCS, Hodapp (2008) showed that the child's degree of maladaptive behavior was the best indicator of family stress. The investigators also found that parents and the affected child's siblings disagreed on the degree of interpersonal concerns among siblings. The siblings reported fewer interpersonal concerns compared to their parents who indicated that the siblings felt like they were being ignored and misunderstood.

In a longitudinal investigation of children with DS, Hauser-Cram et al. (2001) showed that the children's type of disability was the best predictor of changes in maternal, but not paternal child-associated stress. The disability type of the children was also correlated with parent-associated stress. In addition to disability type, the children's behavior problems and mastery motivation and other indicators of self-regulation and the mother–child interaction predicted parent well-being.

Families who have a child with a chromosomal abnormality often experience major life changes because of the consequences of coping with the child's DDs. Using the results of focus groups, King et al. (2006) discovered through alterations in their views of the world, values, and priorities, parents of children with DS or autism can acquire a sense of coherence and control. Parents achieve coherence and control by changing the ways in which they view their child, their own role as parents, and the family's role. Although families suffer the loss of goals and aspirations, they nevertheless cope with their child's disability by altering their perceptions about life and disability and come to see the positive role of their children in the family.

The Health-Care Experiences of Families

Researchers have analyzed the ways in which clinicians can improve the health-care experiences of families who are given the diagnosis of chromosomal abnormality and related DDs. Drawing on an outpatient, tertiary-based model for parents of children with a newly diagnosed visual impairment and/or ophthalmic condition, Rahi et al. (2004) suggest that the most important needs are for information, particularly about education and social services, and emotional support from professionals, social networks (both formal and informal), and support groups. Multidisciplinary teams can coordinate health, educational, and social services for newly diagnosed children and their families.

Various factors can increase the satisfaction of families who receive a prenatal diagnosis of a chromosomal disorder. In an investigation of parent-reported experiences after receiving the prenatal diagnosis of ES, Walker et al. (2008) identified several aspects of health care that affect satisfaction with health care. Provider empathy, continuity of care, communication, valuing the fetus, and participation in clinical decisions can affect parents' satisfaction. The authors conclude that training, education, or team-based strategies can potentially modify these aspects of health care and improve parents' satisfaction with their health-care experiences.

Maternal serum screening (MSS) can be effective in prenatal detection of fetal chromosome abnormalities (Hu, 2007). However, not all pregnant patients are offered MSS. A cross-sectional mailed survey of family physicians in Newfoundland and Labrador discovered more than 50% of the family physicians provided MSS to all of their pregnant patients (Cavanagh and Mathews, 2006). Another third of the family physicians surveyed offered it to some of their pregnant patients. In their study, the family physicians' practice characteristics were not associated with their attitudes toward MSS or knowledge about it. Other factors besides physician practice characteristics should be considered in developing interventions to expand the use of MSS.

Understanding women's decision to get MSS can help health-care providers expand their use of MSS. Using qualitative interviews with pregnant women, Park and Mathews (2009) demonstrated that women are more likely to put greater emphasis on information obtained from informal sources (e.g., family, friends, and the Internet) than clinicians and researchers who are more likely to rely on information obtained through rigorous, peer-review research.

Improving families' health-care experiences also can be enhanced through the use of genetic ultrasound. For example, investigations have found that second-trimester genetic sonography may be useful for identifying fetuses at risk for DS (DeVore, 2003). For high-risk women, genetic sonography is an alternative to universal amniocentesis. Genetic sonography reduces the loss rate of normal fetuses, which are subjected to amniocentesis because of risk factors related to advanced maternal age or abnormal maternal serum screening.

Drawing on Monte Carlo modeling, Benn and Egan (2008) reported that multistep screening protocols should be used to maximize the advantages of both MSS and ultrasound and minimize the amount of testing provided.

School Programs for Children with Chromosomal Abnormalities

Educational training can be beneficial for children with chromosomal abnormalities. However, many families do not have access to or participate in these training programs. Even if their children do attend these special education programs, they may not receive the appropriate interventions. In addition, more research is needed to determine the effectiveness of special education programs in improving the functioning of children and adolescents with chromosomal abnormalities.

An investigation by Jaruratanasirikul et al. (2004) evaluated a school program for DS children in southern Thailand. Among these children, congenital heart disease and gastrointestinal anomalies were prevalent. The mortality rate of these children was 13.2%. The authors discovered that a majority of the DS children (65.6%) participated in an early intervention program. However, only 38.9% received a speech intervention program. Family income predicted school attendance. Researchers are still following only 67.9% of the DS children aged over 5 years.

Researchers are examining the evolution of behavioral and psychiatric symptoms of children with chromosomal abnormalities from their primary school education to adulthood. Descheemaeker et al. (2002) analyzed the changes in behavioral and psychiatric symptoms among children, adolescents, and adults with PWS. They discovered that PWS individuals who were regarded as active and extrovert toddlers and who exhibited autistic symptoms in primary school later had psychotic episodes. These PWS individuals had moderate to severe mental retardation. In contrast, PWS persons who were considered passive and introverted as toddlers and exhibited less impaired behavior during their primary school education later had an unstable mood disorder. These PWS individuals' intellectual functioning was in the normal to borderline range.

Children with chromosomal abnormalities may have difficulty achieving their full intellectual potential in school. A variety of factors may contribute to their academic underachievement. Whittington et al. (2004) analyzed the school performance of a group of children with PWS and a comparison group of children with LD. They discovered that both groups of children had lower levels of achievement than would have been expected based on their IQ scores. Some children with PWS, however, did function as expected in at least one academic domain. Among PWS children, academic underachievement in different domains was positively associated with the amount of time spent in special school.

The authors suggest that children with PWS may be placed in special education programs in large part because of their behavioral difficulties or physical impairments or based on expectations about their disorder (Whittington et al., 2004). PWS children's impaired social behaviors may in fact cover up their true academic abilities. Interventions should take into account their behavioral problems and poor socialization skills, which may be masking their true intellectual ability.

Case Study

The following case study describes a girl with PWS. Janis is a 12-year-old Caucasian female, born to upper-middle-class parents. She has one older brother, 16 years old. She exhibited feeding problems in infancy and very poor muscle tone. The pediatrician showed no concern when the parents first expressed concern. When she was approximately 2.5 years, she began to eat excessively and exhibited pica, for example, eating dirt from plants in the home. The parents then went to a pediatrician affiliated with a children's hospital and Janis was subsequently evaluated by a geneticist and diagnosed with PWS.

She was initially sent to an early childhood education program, but her behavior was so disruptive to the other children that Janis was referred to another program for children with severe emotional and behavioral problems. At home, her behavior was also a problem, including impulsive eating and other impulsive behavior. Janis would periodically ruin her older sibling's clothes, electronics, and school work.

Eventually, a lock had to be placed on each room as well as the refrigerator, pantry, and cabinets.

Her parents had increasing conflict as Janis became older. Eventually, the child's father threatened divorce unless Janis was institutionalized. When Janis began to smear feces in the house, the mother agreed to placement. Janis has been placed in a private facility since 10 years old and goes home on weekends for visits. She has adjusted well to the private placement.

Janis's parents have also worked with a behavior therapist, in order to learn skills in helping ameliorate their daughter's behavior when she is home. The focus has been on replicating the approach utilized at the group home. Low doses of risperdal have also been utilized to control impulsive behavior.

References

Anderson, M. (1998). Mental retardation, general intelligence and modularity. Learn Indiv Differ, 10 (3), 159–178.

Angelman, S. (1950). The syndrome of obstruction of inferior vena cara in childhood. Br Med J, 2 (4682), 752–755.

Angelman Syndrome Foundation. (2005). Retrieved from http://www.angelman.org

American College of Obstetricians and Gynecologists. (2001). Prenatal diagnosis of fetal chromosomal abnormalities. ACOG Prac Bull, 27, 12.

American College of Obstetricians and Gynecologists. (2005). Your pregnancy and birth (4th ed.). Washington, DC: ACOG.

Barnes, E., Roberts, J., Long, S.H. et al. (2009). Phonological accuracy and intelligibility in connected speech of boys with fragile X syndrome or Down syndrome. J Speech Lang Hear Res, 52 (4), 1048–1061.

Battaglia, A., Fillippi, T., Carey, J.C. (2008). Update on the clinical features and natural history of Wolf-Hirshchorn syndrome. Am J Med Genet C Semin Med Genet, 148, 246–251.

Baty, B.J., Brent, L., Cary, J.C. et al. (1994a). Natural history of trisomy 18 and trisomy 13: growth, physical assessment, medical histories, survival and recurrence rate. Am J Med Genet, 49, 175–187.

Baty, B.J., Jorde, L.B., Blackburn, B.L. (1994b). Natural history of trisomy 18 and trisomy 13: psychomotor development. Am J Med Genet, 49 (2), 189–194.

Baylis, A.L., Munson, B., Moller, K.T. (2008). Factors affecting articulation skills in children with velocardiofacial syndrome and children with cleft palate or velopharyngeal dysfunction: a preliminary report. Cleft Palate Craniofac J, 45 (2), 193–207.

Beers, M.H., Berkow, R. (2004). Congenital anomalies. In the Merck manual of diagnosis and therapy. Whitehouse, NJ: Merck Research Laboratories.

Benitez, A. (2009). Genes, cognition, and language: some notes regarding velocardiofacial syndrome. Neurologia, Jan-Feb; 24 (1), 50–58.

Benn, P.A., Egan, J.F. (2008). Expected performance of second trimester maternal serum testing followed by a 'genetic sonogram' in screening of fetal Down syndrome. Prenat Diagn, 28 (3), 230–235.

Bergemann, A.D., Cole, F., Hirschhorn, K. (2005). The etiology of Wolf-Hirschhorn syndrome. Trends Genet, 21 (3), 188–195.

Bertella, L., Mori, I., Grugni, G. et al. (2007). Quality of life and psychological well-being in GH-treated, adult PWS patients: a longitudinal study. J Intell Disabil Res, 51 (4), 302–311.

Best, R.G., Stallworth, J. (2002). Patau syndrome. Retrieved from www.e.medicine.

Brender, J.D., Suarez, L., Langlois, P.H. (2008). Parental occupation, Hispanic ethnicity, and risk of selected congenital malformations in offspring. Ethn Dis, 18 (2), 218–224.

Brouwer, O.F., Burntinx, I.M., Willems, P.J. et al. (1990). Angelman's happy puppet syndrome. Tidjschr Kindergenesskd, 58 (3), 89–91.
Butler, M.G., Thompson, T. (2000). Prader-Willi syndrome: clinical findings. The Endocrinologist, 10 (4), 3S–16S.
Carey, J.C. (2003). Chromosomal disorders in Rudolph and Rudolph (Eds.), Rudolph's Pediatrics. New York: McGraw Hill, pp. 731–741.
Cassidy, S.B., Schwartz, S. (1998). Prader-Willi and Angelman syndromes: disorders of genomic imprinting. Medicine, 77, 140–151.
Cassidy, S.B., Schwartz, S. (2009). Prader-Willi syndrome. In: R.A. Pagon, et al. (Eds.), GeneReviews (Internet). Seattle, WA: University of Washington.
Cavanagh, J., Mathews, M. (2006). Maternal serum screening in Newfoundland and Labrador: do attitude and knowledge affect physicians' practice? Can Fam Physician, 52 (10), 1268–1269.
Cerrutti, M.P. (2006). Cri du chat syndrome. Orphanet J Rare Dis, 5, 1–33.
Chang, C.Y., Lin, S.P., Lin, H.Y. et al. (2007). Cri-du-chat syndrome. Acta Paediatr Taiwan, 48 (6), 328–331.
Chen, H. (2003). Wolf-Hirschhorn syndrome. Retrieved from www.e.medicine
Cicchetti, D. (1991). Fractures in the crystal: developmental psychopathology and the emergence of self. Devel Rev, 11 (3), 271–287.
Clarke, D.J., Boer, H. (1998). Problem behaviors associated with deletion Prader-Willi, Smith-Magenis, and cri du chat syndromes. Am J Ment Retard, 103 (3), 264–271.
Clayton-Smith, J., Laan, L. (2003). Angelman syndrome: a review of the clinical and genetic aspects. J Med Genet, 40 (2), 87–95.
Cornish, K.M., Cross, G., Green, A. et al. (1999). A neuropsychological-genetic profile of atypical cri du chat syndrome: implications for prognosis. J Med Genet, 36 (7), 567–570.
Curfs, L.M., Didden, R., Sikkema, S.P. et al. (1999). Management of sleeping problems in Wolf-Hirschhorn syndrome: a case study. Genet Couns, 10 (4), 345–350.
D'Antonio, L.L., Scherer, N.J., Miller, L.L. et al. (2001). Analysis of speech characteristics in children with velocardiofacial syndrome (VCFS) and children with phenotypic overlap without VCFS. Cleft Palate Craniofac J, 38 (5), 455–467.
Delatycki, M., Garder, R. (1997). Three case histories of trisomy 13 mosaicism and a review of the literature. Am J Med Genet, June, 403–407.
De Smedt, B., Reynvoet, B., Swillen, A. et al. (2009). Basic number processing and difficulties in single-digit arithmetic: evidence from velo-cardio-facial syndrome. Cortex, 45 (2), 177–188.
De Smedt, B., Swillen, A., Ghesquiere, P. et al. (2003). Pre-academic and early academic achievement in children with velocardiofacial syndrome (del22q11.2) of borderline or normal intelligence. Genet Couns, 14 (1), 15–29.
Descheemaeker, M.J., Vogels, A., Govers, V. et al. (2002). Prader-Willi syndrome: new insights in the behavioural and psychiatric spectrum. J Intellect Disabil Res, 46 (Pt 1), 41–50.
DeVore, G.R. (2003). Is genetic ultrasound cost-effective? Semin Perinatol, 27 (2), 173–182.
Drew, C.J. (1990). Down syndrome: best known but most misunderstood. PsycCritiques, 35 (8), 766–767.
Duarte, A.C., Menezes, A.I., Devens, E.S. et al. (2004). Patau syndrome with a long survival. A case report. Genet Mol Res, 3 (2), 288–292.
Dudley, O., McManus, B., Vogels, A. et al. (2008). Cross-cultural comparisons of obesity and growth in Prader-Willi syndrome. J Intell Disabil Res, 52 (5), 426–436.
Dykens, E.M., Clarke, D.J. (1997). Correlates of maladaptive behavior in individuals with 5p- (cri du chat) syndrome. Dev Med Child Neurol, 39 (11), 752–756.
Dykens, E., Schwenk, K., Maxwell, M. et al. (2007). The sentence completion and three wishes tasks: windows into the inner lives of people with intellectual disabilities. J Intell Disabil Res, 51 (8), 588–597.
Fang, J.S., Lee, K.F., Huang, C.T. et al. (2008). Cytogenetic and molecular characterization of a three-generation family with chromosome 5p terminal deletion. Clin Genet, 73 (6), 585–590.

Ferrier, L.J., Bashir, A.S., Meryash, D.L. et al. (1991). Conversational skills of individuals with fragile-X syndrome: a comparison with autism and Down syndrome. Dev Med Child Neurol, 33 (9), 776–788.

Fisch, G.S., Battaglia, A., Parrini, B. et al. (2008). Cognitive-behavioral features of children with Wolf-Hirschhorn syndrome. Am J Med Genet Semin Med Genet, 148C (4), 252–256.

Garcia-Ramirez, M., Csanyi, B., Martinez-Anton, J. et al. (2008). Genetic and clinical diagnosis of Angelman syndrome. An Pediatr (Barc), 69 (3), 232–238.

Ghosh, M., Shah, A.H., Dhir, K. et al. (2008). Behavior in children with Down syndrome. Indian J Pediatr, 75 (7), 685–689.

Giallo, R., Gavidia-Payne, S. (2006). Child, parent and family factors as predictors of adjustment of siblings of children with a disability. J Intellect Disabil Res, 50 (Pt 12), 937–948.

Gothelf, D., Feinstein, C., Thompson, T. et al. (2007). Risk factors for the emergence of psychotic disorders in adolescents with 22q11.2 deletion syndrome. Am J Psychiatry, 164 (4), 663–669.

Gothelf, D., Frish, A., Munitz, H. et al. (1997). Velocardiofacial manifestations and microdeletions in schizophrenic patients. J Am Child Adoles Psychiatry, 36 (11), 1020–1027.

Graham, A., Papalopulu, N., Lorimer, J. et al. (1988). Characterization of a murine homeo box gene, Hox 2-6, related to drosophila deformed gene. Genes Dev, 2 (11), 1424–1438

Hauser-Cram, P., Warfield, M.E., Shonkoff, J.P. et al. (2001). Children with disabilities: a longitudinal study of child development and parent well-being. Monogr Soc Res Child Dev, 66 (3), i–viii, 1–114.

Hay, B.N. (2007). Deletion 22Q11: spectrum of associated disorders. Semin Pediatr Neurol, 14 (3), 136–139.

Head, L.S., Abbeduto, L. (2007). Recognizing the role of parents in developmental outcomes: a systems approach to evaluating the child with developmental disabilities. Ment Retard Dev Disabil Res Rev, 13 (4), 293–301.

Heljic, S., Catibusic, F., Dozic, M. et al. (2004). Wolf-Hirschhorn syndrome. Med Arh, 58 (5), 318–320.

Hercher, L., Bruenner, G. (2008). Living with a child at risk for psychotic illness: the experience of parents coping with 22q11 deletion syndrome. Am J Med Genet A, 146A (18), 2355–2360.

Hirschorn, K., Cooper, H.L. (1961). Chromosomal aberrations in human disease: a review of the status of cytogenics in medicine. Nature, 31, 442–470.

Hirschhorn, K. (2008). A short history of the initial discovery of Wolf-Hirschhorn syndrome. Am J Med Genet C Semin Med Genet, 148C (4), 244–245.

Hodapp, R. (2008). Stress and coping by mothers of children with Prader-Willi, Williams and Down syndromes. Washington, DC: American Psychological Association.

Hodapp, R.M., Wijma, C.A., Masion, L.L. (1997). Families of children with 5p-(cri du chat) syndrome: familial stress and sibling reactions. Dev Med Child Neurol, 39 (11), 757–761.

Hoybye, C., Thoren, M., Bohm, B. (2005). Cognitive, emotional, physical, and social effects of growth hormone treatment in adults with Prader-Willi syndrome. J Intellect Disabil Res, 49 (Pt 4), 245–252.

Hu, Y.L. (2007). Serum screening of fetal chromosome abnormality during second pregnancy trimester: results of 26,803 pregnant women in Jiangsu Province. Zhonghua Yi Xue Za Zhi, 87 (35), 2476–2480.

Hunter, H. (1969). A controlled study of the psychopathology and physical measurement of Klinefelter's syndrome. Brit J Psychiatry, 115 (521), 443–448.

Jaruratanasirikul, S., Soponthammarak, S., Chanvitan, P. et al. (2004). Clinical abnormalities, intervention programs, an school attendance of Down syndrome children in southern Thailand. J Med Assoc Thai, 87 (10), 1199–1204.

Kessler, S., Moos, R. (1973). Behavioral aspects of chromosomal disorders. Ann Rev Med, 24, 89–102.

King, G.A., Zwaigenbaum, L., King, S. et al. (2006). A qualitative investigation of changes in the belief systems of families with autism or Down syndrome. Child Care Health Dev, May; 32 (3), 353–369.

Landry, S.H., Garner, P.W., Pirie, D. et al. (1994). Effects of social context and mother's requesting strategies on Down's syndrome children's social responsiveness. Develop Psychology, 30 (2), 293–302.

Mainardi, P.C. (2006). Cri du Chat syndrome. Orphanet J Rare Dis, 1, 33.

Marco, E.J., Skuse, D.H. (2006). Autism lessons from the X chromosome. Soc Cogn Affect Neurosci, 1 (3), 183–193.

Mazzocco, M., Ross, J.L. (2007). Neurogenetic developmental disorders: variations of manifestation in childhood. Cambridge: The MIT Press.

Miron, P., Cote, Y.P., Lambert, J. (2008). Effect of maternal smoking on prenatal screening for Down syndrome and trisomy 18 in the first trimester of pregnancy. Prenat Diagn, 28 (3), 180–185.

Moncia, A., Livet, M.O., Malzac, P. et al. (1994). Angelman syndrome. Arch Pediatr, 1 (12), 1118–1126.

Morava, E., Czako, M., Melegh, B. et al. (2000). Velo-cardio-facial phenotype and deletion of 22q11.2 in Hungarian children. Clin Genet, 58 (5), 403–405.

Morava, E., Lacassie, Y., King, A. et al. (2002). Scoliosis in velo-cardio-facial syndrome. J Pediatr Orthop, 22 (6), 780–783.

Moss, J., Oliver, C., Arron, K. et al. (2009). The prevalence and phenomenology of repetitive behavior in genetic syndromes. J Autism Dev Disord, 39 (4), 572–588.

Nadel, L. (1996). Learning, memory and neural function in Down's syndrome. In J.A. Rondal, J. Perera, L. Nadel, et al. (Eds.) Down's syndrome: psychological, psychobiological and socio-educational perspectives. Philadelphia: Whurr Publishers, 21–42.

Naguib, K.K., Al-Awadi, S.A., Moussa, M.A. et al. (1999). Trisomy 18 in Kuwait. Int J Epidemol, 28 (4), 711–716.

Nanjiani, A., Hossain, A., Mahgoub, M.D. (2007). Patau syndrome. J Neuropsychiatry Clin Neurosci, 19, 201–202.

National Down Syndrome Society. (2006). Questions and answers about Down syndrome. Retrieved from www.ndss.org

National Human Genome Research Institute. (2008). Retrieved from www.genome.gov

National Institute of Child Health and Human Development. (2006). Retrieved from www.nichd.nih/gov/publications

National Organization for Rare Disorders. (2003). Retrieved from http://www.rare diseases.org

Orsmond, G.I., Seltzer, M.M. (2007). Siblings of individuals with autism or Down syndrome. Effects on adult lives. J Intellect Disabil Res, 51 (Pt 9), 682–696.

Oskarsdottir, S., Belfrage, M., Sandstedt, E. et al. (2005). Disabilities and cognition in children and adolescents with 22q11 deletion syndrome. Dev Med Child Neurol, 47 (3), 177–184.

Paduch, D.A., Fine, R.G., Bolyakov, A. et al. (2008). New concepts in Klinefelter syndrome. Curr Opin Urol, 18 (6), 621–627.

Papolos, D.F., Faedda, G.L., Veit, S. et al. (1996). Bipolar spectrum disorders in patients diagnosed with velo-cardio-facial syndrome: does a hemizygous deletion of chromosome 22q11 result in bipolar affective disorder? Am J Psychiatry, 153 (12), 1541–1547.

Park, A., Mathews, M. (2009). Women's decisions about maternal serum screening testing: a qualitative study exploring what they learn and the role prenatal care providers play. Women Birth, 22 (2), 73–78.

Patau, K., Smith, D.W., Therman, E. et al. (1960). Multiple congenital anomaly caused by an extra autosome. Lancet, 1, 790.

Pelc, K., Cheron, G., Dan, B. (2008). Behavior and neupsychiatric manifestations in Angleman syndrome. Neuropsychiatr Dis Treat, 4 (3), 577–584.

Phelan, M.C. (2008). Deletion 22q13.3 syndrome. Orphanet J Rare Dis, 3, 14.

Polani, P.E. (1969). Abnormal sex chromosomes and mental disorder. Nature, 223 (5207), 680–686.

Prader-Willi Association. (2008). Prader-Willi syndrome. Retrieved from www.pwsausa.org

Price, J., Roberts, J., Vandergrift, N. et al. (2007). Language comprehension in boys with fragile X syndrome and boys with Down syndrome. J Intellect Disabil Res, 51 (Pt 4), 318–326.

Rahi, J.S., Manaras, I., Tuomainen, H. et al. (2004). Meeting the needs of parents around the time of diagnosis of disability among their children: evaluation of a novel program for information, support, and liaison by key workers. Pediatrics, 114 (4), e477–482.

Robb, S.A., Pohl, K.R., Baraitser, M. et al. (1989). The 'happy puppet' syndrome of Angelman: review of the clinical features. Arch Dis Child, 64 (1), 83–86.

Roser, P., Kawohl, W. (2008). Turner syndrome and schizophrenia: a further hint for the role of the X chromosome in the pathogenesis of schizophrenic disorder. World J Biol Psychiatry, 11, 1–4.

Ross, J.L., Roeitgen, D.P., Stefanatos, G. et al. (2008). Cognitive and motor development during childhood in boys with Klinefelter syndrome. Am J Med Genet A, 146A (6), 708–719.

Rubin, K.R. (2008). Turner syndrome: transition from pediatrics to adulthood. Endocr Pract, 14 (6), 775–781.

Sarimski, K. (2003). Early play behaviour in children with 5p- (Cri-du-Chat) syndrome. J Intellect Disabil Res, 47 (pt 2), 113–120.

Scherer, N.J., D'Antonio, L.L., Kalbfleisch, J.H. (1999). Early speech and language development in children with velocardiofacial syndrome. Am J Med Genet, 88 (6), 714–723.

Secretary of State (UK) for Health (2001). Valuing people – a new strategy for learning disability for the 21st century. The stationary office, Cm 5086. Retrieved March 1, 2010 from: http://www.archive.official-documents.co.uk/document/cm50/5086/5086.pdf

Shprintzen, R.J. (2008). Velo-cardio-facial syndrome: 30 years of study. Dev Disabil Res Rev, 14 (1), 3–10.

SOFT (Support Organization for Trisomy 18, 13 and Related Disorders). (2006). Retrieved from www.trisomy.org

Stuart, S.W., King, C.H., Pai, G.S. (2007). Autism spectrum disorder, Klinefelter syndrome, and chromosome 3p21.31 duplication. MedGenMed, 9 (4), 60.

Sugama, S., Namihira, T., Matsuoka, R. et al. (1999). Psychiatric inpatients and chromosome deletions within 22q11.2. J Neurol Neurosurg Psychiatry, 67 (6), 803–806.

Summers, J.A., Allison, D.B., Lynch, P.S. et al. (1995). Behaviour problems in Angelman syndrome. J Intellect Disabil Res, 39 (Pt 2), 97–106.

Tennakoon, J., Kandasamy, Y., Acock, G. et al. (2008). Edwards syndrome with double trisomy. Singapore Med J, 49 (7), e190–e191.

Tsai, C.H., Van Dyke, D.L., Feldman, G.L. (1999). Child with velocardiofacial syndrome and del (4) (q34.2): another critical region associated with a velocardiofacial syndrome-like phenotype. Am J Med Genet, 82 (4), 336–369.

Turchetti, D., Rezzaboni, E., Zomer, H. et al. (2006). Psychological consequences of prenatal diagnosis in a case of familial Angelman syndrome. Prenat Diagn, 26 (12), 1156–1159.

Walker, L.V., Miller, V.J., Dalton, V.K. (2008). The health-care experiences of families given the prenatal diagnosis of trisomy 18. J Perinatol, 28 (1), 12–19.

Walz, N.C., Baranek, G.T. (2006). Sensory processing patterns in persons with Angelman syndrome. Am J Occup Ther, 60 (4), 472–479.

Wang, Y.X., Li, R., Shao, J. et al. (2007). A study on the social adjustment and its affective factors in Down syndrome children. Zhonghua Yi Xue Za Zhi, 87 (20), 1402–1406.

Whitman, B.Y., Myers, S., Carrel, A. et al. (2002). The behavioral impact of growth hormone treatment for children and adolescents with Prader-Willi syndrome: a 2 year, controlled study. Pediatrics, 109 (2), E35.

Whittington, J., Holland, A., Webb, T. et al. (2004). Academic underachievement by people with Prader-Willi syndrome. J Intellect Disabil Res, 48 (Pt 2), 188–200.

Widdershoven, J.C., Stubenitsky, B.M., Breugem, C.C. et al. (2008). Outcome of velopharyngoplasty in patients with velocardiofacial syndrome. Arch Otolaryngol Head Neck Surg, 134 (11), 1159–1164.

Wisniewski, K.E., Kida, E., Brown, W.T. (1996). Consequences of genetic abnormalities in Down's syndrome on brain structure and function. In J.A. Rondal, J. Perera, L. Nadel, et al. (Eds.), Down's syndrome: psychological, psychobiological and socio-educational perspectives. Philadelphia: Whurr Publishers, 3–19.

Wright, I., Lewis, V., Collis, G.M. (2006). Imitation and representational development in young children with Down syndrome. Brit J Develop Psychology, 24 (2), 429–450.

Wustmann, T., Preuss, U.W. (2009). Turner syndrome and psychosis: a case report and brief review of the literature. Psychiatr Prax, July; 36 (5), 243–245.

Ysunza, A., Pamplona, M.C., Molina, F. et al. (2009). Surgical planning for restoring velopharyngeal function in velocardiofacial syndrome. Int J Pediatr Otorhinolaryngol, 73 (11), 1572–1575.

Zollino, M., Murdolo, M., Marangi, G. et al. (2008). On the nosology and pathogenesis of Wolf-Hirschhorn syndrome: genotype-phenotype correlation analysis of 80 patients and literature review. Am J Med Genet C Semin Med Genet, 148C (4), 257–269.

Chapter 3
Autism

Autistic spectrum disorders are lifelong severe brain-based heritable disabilities that have enormous impact on the affected individual, the individual's family, and the community. Autistic disorder, the formal name for classical autism, falls under the category of pervasive developmental disorders in the Diagnostic and Statistical Manual of Mental Disorders, Fourth Edition (American Psychiatric Association and American Psychiatric Association Task Force on DSM-IV, 2000). Disorders under this category also include Asperger syndrome, pervasive developmental disorder not otherwise specified, Rett syndrome, and childhood disintegrative disorder.

Autism is characterized by onset before age 3 of (1) stereotyped and repetitive patterns of behavior, interests, and activities, (2) significant impairment in reciprocal social interaction; and (3) significant deficits in verbal and nonverbal communication. Those with Asperger syndrome have communication difficulties that are more concentrated on nonverbal communication, although cognitive and verbal development is apparently normal before age 3. Individuals with pervasive developmental disorder not otherwise specified (PDD-NOS) have features of autistic disorder but do not meet the criteria for other autism subtypes. Individuals with Rett syndrome have gross and fine motor impairment, hand stereotypies, and growth failure (Percy and Lane, 2004). Childhood disintegrative disorder manifests between ages 2 and 10 (prior to that development is typical): the child's behavioral, cognitive, and verbal skills regress significantly.

When the term "autistic spectrum disorders" is used, it generally refers only to autistic disorder, Asperger syndrome, and PDD-NOS. While each of these disorders manifests differently, there is a central feature of social impairment. Although the word "spectrum" is used, this does not imply there is a shared etiology for these disorders.

Contributed by Emily Stumpf, M.S., University of California, San Francisco, CA, USA.

M.L. Goldstein, S. Morewitz, *Chronic Disorders in Children and Adolescents*,

DOI 10.1007/978-1-4419-9764-7_3,

Epidemiology of Autism: Is There an Autism Epidemic?

Headlines proclaim "Autism Increase Baffles Scientists" (Blakeslee, 2002) and "Autism Diagnoses Double in California" (Blakeslee, 2003). Over the past two decades, there has been a clear and dramatic increase in the number of children diagnosed with autism worldwide (Fombonne, 2009). The estimate of prevalence ranges from 0.7 to 72.6 per 10,000 (Fombonne, 2009). But does this reflect a true change in the risk of autism, or are there other reasons that might have caused this increase?

Higher rates of diagnosis may be due, at least in part, to expanded classification criteria. Classification criteria for autism were first outlined by Rutter (1978). With the advent of DSM-III in 1980, autism was formally described. In subsequent iterations of the DSM, classification criteria have been added. Despite the creation of new categories of Asperger syndrome, Rett syndrome, and child disintegrative disorder under DSM-IV in 1994, which would presumably reduce the number of children diagnosed with autism, the rates of diagnosis of autism have increased.

A second hypothesis to explain the increased rates of diagnosis is better detection and assessment. Perhaps the number of autism cases has gone up as rates of diagnosis of mental retardation have decreased: the so-called diagnostic substitution hypothesis. Studies have shown, though, that rates of autism have increased while rates of mental retardation have held constant (Croen et al., 2002).

A third hypothesis is that higher rates of diagnosis are caused by the inclusion of milder cases and earlier diagnosis. One large study conducted in California found that the inclusion of milder cases accounted for 56% of the increase and earlier diagnosis accounted for 12% of the increase (Hertz-Picciotto and Delwiche, 2009). This finding replicated earlier studies that showed that increased prevalence was attributable to diagnosis at an earlier age (Parner et al., 2008).

Finally, there could, of course, be a true increase in the prevalence of autism. The main identified risk factors are genetic, which should not change substantially over time. But this does not mean that other risk factors, such as environmental influences, are not contributing to the increase.

Genetics of Autism

Leo Kanner first described autism in 1943 (Kanner, 1943). Consistent with the psychoanalytic era, the early consensus was that psychogenic factors were the main causes of autism. For example, Bettleheim in *The Empty Fortress* popularized "refrigerator mothers" as the root cause (Bettelheim, 1967). As the field of psychiatry moved toward a more biochemical focus, autism increasingly became viewed as a disorder with biological underpinnings. Although geneticists were initially dismissive of this theory (Hanson and Gottesman, 1976), this began to change when the first study of autistic twins in 1977 showed a concordance rate of autism that was 36% in monozygotic pairs as opposed to 0% for dizygotic pairs (Folstein and Rutter, 1977). Subsequent early British and Scandinavian twin studies showed a concordance rate for monozygotic twins of 60% (Bailey et al., 1995) to 91% (Steffenburg et al., 1989), with 0% concordance for dizygotic twins. Familial studies, as summarized in *The Genetics of Autism*, show that autism in siblings recurs at 2–8%, a rate much higher than the prevalence of autism in the general population (Muhle et al., 2004). Familial studies and twin concordance rates thus point to a strong genetic component of autism.

With the exception of Rett syndrome, which is the result of mutations on the MECP2 gene (methyl-cPG-binding protein 2) on the X chromosome (Amir et al., 1999), there is no specific genetic cause for autism. Instead, many genes have been associated with the presence of autistic spectrum disorders. Currently, autism is generally considered to be a genetic disorder with a likely polygenic inheritance pattern (Folstein and Rosen-Sheidley, 2001) with multiple susceptibility loci (Grice and Buxbaum, 2006).

Chromosome 15 has repeatedly been linked to the development of autism. In particular, duplications in the 15q11–q13 region are frequent (Depienne et al., 2009). This region contains the Prader–Willi/Angelman syndrome critical region, which encodes for gamma-aminobutyric acid (GABA) receptor genes. GABA is an inhibitory neurotransmitter, and decreases in GABA receptors may explain both the comorbid seizures and the cognitive impairments characteristic of autism (Fatemi et al., 2009).

Chromosome 7 has also been implicated in the development of autism (Schellenberg et al., 2006). Several genes on this chromosome have been linked to language disorders and brain development. For instance, FOXP2 is associated with language disorder (Lai et al., 2001; MacDermot et al., 2005; Vernes et al., 2008), and RELN (Skaar et al., 2004), HOXA1 (Conciatori et al., 2004), and WNT2 (Wassink et al., 2001) are associated with both brain development and autism.

The presence of rare genetic disorders such as Fragile X (Hatton et al., 2006), Angelman syndrome (Steffenburg et al., 1996; Peters et al., 2004), and tuberous sclerosis (Baker et al., 1998) has been associated with autism, although these conditions constitute only about 1–2% of the cases (Abrahams and Geschwind, 2008). Rare nuclear and mitochondrial genetic defects may also contribute to autism (Smith et al., 2009).

The genetics of autism is not yet fully understood, and it is likely that environmental and epistatic interactions contribute to the complexity of autism's genetic basis. Despite the lack of consensus regarding the genetic etiology of the broad phenotype of autism, genetic research presents several consequences and potential benefits, as outlined by Rutter (2000). First, the focus on genetics has shifted our understanding of etiology from psychogenic to biological factors, although environmental influences and methods of child rearing are still being explored as possible causes. Genetic studies have also emphasized the importance of genetic counseling. A focus on genetics may produce further divisions of the broad phenotype of autism. Genetics may yield information on etiological processes, protective factors, and environmental risks, and genetic research on autism may provide information on genetically specific treatments and interventions.

Other Risk Factors Associated with Autism

Male sex appears to be a risk factor for autism. The male:female ratio is 4.2:1 (Fombonne, 2009). This sex ratio would suggest an X-linked disorder, but the data are inconclusive. A recent large linkage study found no evidence to support the X-linked hypothesis (Xiaohong et al., 2008), while other research has suggested such a linkage (Philippe et al., 1999). Similarly, research has shown that autism is not associated with the Y chromosome (Jamain et al., 2002). These findings do not rule out the possibility of susceptibility loci on the X and Y chromosomes.

In one large population-based study of autistic children in the USA, advanced maternal and paternal age were shown to be independent risk factors for the development of autism (Durkin et al., 2008). Population-based studies show no evidence for socioeconomic status as a significant risk factor (Larsson et al., 2005; Daniels et al., 2008). Although prevalence appears to vary by race and ethnicity, there is evidence that could be reflective of referral and diagnostic bias (Begeer et al., 2009).

Vaccines and Autism

Vaccines guard the health of the population. At the same time, there are adverse events, both acute and chronic, that are associated with their administration. There has been controversy as to whether the measles, mumps, and rubella (MMR) vaccine and the preservative thimerosal, often used in vaccines, have contributed to the development of autism. Others hypothesize that the administration of vaccines in quick succession during early childhood results in the development of autism if the immune system is overwhelmed.

The debate regarding the MMR vaccine and autism began in 1998 with a report by Andrew Wakefield, in *The Lancet*, that suggested autism was the result of gastrointestinal tract inflammation following MMR vaccination (Wakefield et al., 1998). This clinical case series had tremendous impact, and epidemiological studies of "autistic enterocolitis," the MMR vaccine, and autism soon followed. However, ecological studies (Dales et al., 2001; Farrington et al., 2001; Kaye et al., 2001; Madsen et al., 2002; Fombonne et al., 2006) provide convincing evidence that there is no link between the MMR vaccine and autism spectrum disorders (DeStefano and Thompson, 2004).

Another hypothesis is that the ethylmercury-based vaccine preservative thimerosal is responsible for autism. In 1997, the Food and Drug Modernization Act mandated that mercury compounds be quantified and identified in food and drugs (Buck, 2000). The FDA found young children may receive as much as 187.5 μg of mercury through vaccination (Gerber and Offit, 2009). In 1999, the American Academy of Pediatrics and the US Public Health service jointly called for the removal of mercury from children's vaccines, which was completed in the USA in 2001 (MMWR, 1999). However, that elimination has not altered the rates of diagnosis, casting further doubt on any link between autism and thimerosal (Committee, 2004).

As thimerosal and the MMR vaccine were being discredited as possible sources of autism, a third theory emerged: the administration of vaccines in quick succession in childhood led to a breakdown of the immune system and resulted in autism. This theory was popularized after the ruling in favor of Hannah Poling. Poling was developing normally before the administration of five vaccines at age 19 months. Shortly thereafter, she became lethargic, refused to walk, and was diagnosed with symptoms of autism and encephalopathy due to a mitochondrial enzyme disorder. Poling's family successfully sued the Department of Health and Human Services under the Vaccine Injury Compensation Program, based on evidence that the administration of multiple vaccines was implicated in aggravating her underlying mitochondrial disorder, which in turn produced autistic symptoms (Offit, 2008). A possible connection was thus established between vaccinations, breakdown of the immune system, and Poling's autistic symptoms. However, the idea that multiple vaccines can overwhelm the immune system is not otherwise supported; evidence suggests that autism is not an immune-mediated disease (Gerber and Offit, 2009).

Pathophysiology of Autism

Autopsy and neuroimaging studies have shown both macroscopic and microscopic abnormalities of the brains of persons with autistic spectrum disorders. Much attention has been devoted to macrocrania, or large head size, and its correlation to megalencephaly, or abnormally large brain size for age. Brain size has been studied using postmortem brain weights, head circumference, and magnetic resonance imaging. A meta-analysis by Redcay and Courchesne (2005) showed pathological brain growth occurred during early childhood. Autistic subjects were found to have reduced brain sizes at birth, followed by dramatically increased brain size from ages 2–4 (adult autistic brain sizes fell within normal ranges). The authors of this study point out that this period of pathological growth occurs before the typical onset age of autism, and thus the abnormal brain development as it relates to the etiology of autism may have already occurred (Redcay and Courchesne, 2005).

Microscopic anomalies in brain structures have also been noted in autistic brains. Studies have consistently noted decreased numbers of cerebellar Purkinje neurons and cortical dysgenesis, while increased cell packing in the limbic system and brain stem and olivary dysplasia have also been reported (DiCicco-Bloom et al., 2006). These findings may be indicative of atypical pruning or other brain development processes that could contribute to autism.

Serological research has shown that children with autism have elevated levels of certain kinds of chemicals in the brain and blood. Platelet hyperserotonemia has been a consistent finding since 1961 (Schain and Freedman, 1961). There are multiple genetic bases that could explain this elevation in relation to autism (Anderson et al., 2009; Huang and Santangelo, 2008), including epistatic interactions (Coutinho et al., 2007). Animal models suggest that during fetal brain development, high levels of serotonin may disrupt serotonergic functioning and lead to the behavioral and social dysfunction characteristic of autism (McNamara et al., 2008).

Beginning in 1979, Panksepp put forth the hypothesis that autism may be caused by an "opioid peptide excess," resulting in overactivity of the brain's endogenous opiate system. Researchers hypothesized that exogenous opioid peptides, such as those derived from casein or gluten, entered the circulatory system, accumulated, and resulted in permanent structural changes that produced autistic symptoms (Seim and Reichelt, 1995). Thus, Whiteley et al. (1999) supported gluten-free diets to reduce the opioid peptides that they believed contributed to autism. Many experts now follow gluten- and casein-free diets as an alternative treatment for autism (Millward et al., 2008). However, later studies have not shown hyperpeptiduria in autistic persons (Cass et al., 2008). Thus, the "opioid peptide excess" hypothesis and the potential for opioid peptides as a biomarker for autism are still controversial.

The hypothesis that autism is linked to autoimmune disorders was first put forth by Money et al. (1971). Since then, attention has been devoted to increased levels of cytokines and brain inflammation as a result of immune dysfunction. A subset of autistic individuals do have abnormal immune systems, but it is unclear how dysfunctional immunity contributes to the development and/or persistence of autistic symptoms (Wills et al., 2007).

Comorbidities of Autism

In addition to the triad of core deficits of autism, comorbid psychiatric and medical conditions are commonly associated with autism. One study found a psychiatric illness to be comorbid in 72% of children diagnosed with autism, with obsessive-compulsive disorder, attention-deficit hyperactivity disorder, separation anxiety, and specific phobias the most common (Leyfer et al., 2006). Mental retardation is present in approximately 26–30% of children with autistic spectrum disorders (Chakrabarti and Fombonne, 2001; 2005). Epilepsy is found in 20–25% of children with autistic spectrum disorders (Canitano, 2007). Sleep disorders, food intolerance, and gastrointestinal dysfunction have also been comorbidities noted in autism (Ming and Brimacombe, 2008). Behavioral abnormalities have been observed, including impaired attention, impaired fine and gross motor control, abnormal facial processing, sensory deficits (both hypo- and hyperresponsiveness to stimuli), and prosody (Hughes, 2008).

Imitation is also impaired in patients with ASDs (Williams et al., 2004). This deficit in imitation lends support to the hypothesis of the "theory of mind," or the ability to understand that others have beliefs, intentions, and emotional states different from one's own. In autistic individuals, deficient mirror neurons are understood to contribute to these imitation and communication deficits (Oberman and Ramachandran, 2007).

Physical Conditions Associated with Autism

In light of the "autistic enterocolitis" hypothesis, particular attention has been devoted to the gastrointestinal conditions and flora. An overabundance of bacteria such as *Clostridium histolyticum* (Parracho et al., 2005) has been found in autistic individuals' gastrointestinal tracts. Other chronic infections also have been associated with autism, including *Mycoplasma* spp., *Chlamydia pneumoniae*, herpes (Nicolson et al., 2007), and *Borrelia burgdorferi* (which causes Lyme disease) in the blood (Bransfield et al., 2008).

Beginning with Kanner's first description of the disorder, physical differences were noted to be a distinguishing feature in autism (Kanner, 1943). Attention has been devoted to identifying subtypes of autism based on physical dysmorphologies associated with autism beyond cranial size. For example, Miles and Hillman (2000) evaluated 94 autistic individuals with both an MRI and a physical morphology exam. They suggested genetic differences could differentiate between two subgroups: those with "idiopathic autism" who fell within the normal ranges of morphology and MRI-revealed brain structure and those who were phenotypically abnormal (Miles and Hillman, 2000). Similarly, Toriello discusses the importance of noting physical abnormalities for clinicians as a way of directing individuals to further testing options (Toriello, 2008). Assessing morphological differences may be especially important as dysmorphology has been shown to be predictive of poorer response to treatment and poorer prognosis (Stoelb et al., 2004).

Psychosocial Impact of Autism

The effect of having an autistic child can be felt throughout the family unit. As a result of their disability, children with autism are significantly more likely to suffer psychosocial consequences such as missing school or repeating a grade, and they are less likely to attend religious or community services (Lee et al., 2008). Trauma is frequent in children with autism; they have high rates of head, face, and neck injuries; poisoning; and self-inflicted injuries. In addition, children with autism are more likely to use emergency services as compared to controls (McDermott et al., 2008).

Parents are concerned with their autistic child's learning difficulties, social interactions, and achievement (Lee et al., 2008). Parents of children with autistic spectrum disorders have consistently reported parental stress (Davis and Carter, 2008): cognitive and language impairments appear to be particularly burdensome (Bebko et al., 1987). A child's behavior problems can lead to significant maternal stress and depression, while paternal stress can be predicted by their partner's depression (Hastings, 2002; Hastings et al., 2005). Marital relationship needs may be neglected due to the attention focused on the autistic child (Higgins et al., 2005). Additionally, parents have greater financial, employment, and time burdens as compared to families with children with other types of special health-care needs (Kogan et al., 2008).

During childhood and adolescence, siblings of children with autism have been found to interact less with their brothers and sisters than typically developing siblings: evidence suggests that it may be more difficult to interact and engage siblings as the level of disability increases (Stoneman, 2001). Although siblings report positive aspects of their relationship with an autistic sibling, nonetheless, siblings are concerned about being embarrassed or isolated and worry about destructive behavior and their sibling's future (Orsmond and Seltzer, 2007). Research on overall well-being of siblings of children with chronic disabilities has shown that siblings are at risk for negative psychological symptoms such as anxiety and depression (Sharpe and Rossiter, 2002). Siblings of autistic children may have adjustment difficulties that increase during adolescence, although study findings on this topic are inconsistent (Orsmond and Seltzer, 2007).

Screening

Because intervention has the potential to change the process of development and diagnosis for individuals with ASDs, there has been great effort devoted to early detection and screening of children. Two models of screening are widely employed. One is a population-based first-level screening that takes place as part of monitoring a child's developmental progress in the primary care setting. Another is second-level screening for children at high risk who are not progressing in a developmentally typical way (Oosterling et al., 2009).

Several first-level screening instruments exist, including the Modified Checklist for Autism in Toddlers (M-CHAT) (Robins et al., 2001) and the Early Screening of Autistic Traits Questionnaire (ESAT) (Swinkels et al., 2006). Second-level screening instruments for young children include the Pervasive Developmental Disorders Screening Test II – Developmental Clinical Screener (PDDST-II, DCS) (Siegel, 2004), the Autism Behavior Checklist (ABC) (Krug et al., 1980), and the Screening Tool for Autism in Two-Year-Olds (STAT) (Stone et al., 2004). Because deficient reciprocal social interaction is the shared feature in ASDs, screening and detection should focus on the recognition of impairments in this area.

Diagnosis

There are two commonly used instruments in the diagnosis of autism. One instrument is the Autism Diagnostic Interview – Revised (ADI-R) (Lord et al., 1994). This instrument is a structured interview with caregivers comprised of 93 items assessing the functional domains of communication, reciprocal social interaction, and patterns of behavior and interests. This tool is designed for those of 18 months of mental age or older. Use of this screening algorithm yields diagnoses consistent with both ICD-10 and DSM-IV classifications for subjects scoring at certain levels in the three domains.

The second instrument is the Autism Diagnostic Observation Schedule (ADOS) (Lord et al., 2000). This assessment is conducted by a trained clinician and can be used with both nonverbal and verbally competent children and adults. It focuses on the same three domains of communication, social interaction, and behavior, covered in four modules.

Course and Prognosis

Three distinct patterns of onset have been discussed in the pathogenesis of autism. First, in the "congenital" pattern of onset, behavioral abnormalities are present within the first year of life. In the second pattern, children may show normal early development, followed by a developmental plateau and failure to reach developmental milestones. The third pattern, "autistic regression," is characterized by abrupt or gradual loss of previously acquired abilities (Stefanatos, 2008).

To be able to cope with the various effects of autism, accurate information is needed about prognosis for autistic individuals. Research has shown that autism diagnoses are fairly stable over time, with diagnostic reclassification mainly resulting in movement from autism to PDD-NOS (Lord et al., 2006). Most individuals with autism remain autistic throughout their lifetimes.

Longitudinal studies reveal that for autistic adults, 30–50% have very poor outcomes, 15–25% have poor outcomes, 15–25% have fair outcomes, and only 10–15% have good outcomes (Broman and Fletcher, 1999). IQ and language development are the best predictors of outcome (Tsatsanis, 2003). Prognosis is known to be poor for children with an IQ less than 50, but even those with higher IQs may still be substantially impaired and rely heavily on family and other support systems (Howlin et al. 2004).

Opportunities for Intervention

Research has shown that core symptoms of autism are malleable and can improve with early and comprehensive treatments. In determining policies related to the interventions recommended for autistic children, several countries have established review groups (National Research Council, U.S., Committee on Educational Interventions for Children with Autism, 2001). Researchers have not conducted many longitudinal randomized controlled studies that compare comprehensive treatments (Rogers and Vismara, 2008). More research is needed to determine which pharmacotherapeutic and comprehensive intervention strategies are beneficial in targeting both core deficits and associated symptoms of autism.

Pharmacological Interventions

A sampling of pharmacological and comprehensive psychosocial interventions is outlined below.

Only risperidone has been FDA approved for the management of autism. An analysis of the use of risperidone for autistic children showed this medication resulted in a decrease in children's levels of irritability, repetitive behaviors, and social withdrawal, although weight gain was a side effect (Jesner et al., 2007). Other agents that are prescribed off-label may aid in treatment. Medication is typically targeted at symptoms of aggression, self-injury, anxiety, hyperactivity, and hyperarousal (Ozonoff et al., 2003). A review of Medicaid claims for autistic children found that the seven most common pharmacotherapies used were antidepressants, stimulants, tranquilizers/anti-psychotics, anticonvulsants, hypotensives, anxiolytic/sedative/hypnotics, and benzodiazepines. In this study, 83% of children were prescribed a drug from one of 125 medication classes, and 70% were prescribed some type of psychotropic medication during the course of 1 year (Oswald and Sonenklar, 2007).

Significantly, the effect of psychotropic medication has not been studied extensively on the developing brain in humans (with the exception of stimulants used for the treatment of attention-deficit hyperactivity disorder). Thus, short-term benefits of managing behavior with psychotropic medication must be weighed against the possibility and unknown risk of permanently altering the brain's neurochemistry.

Comprehensive Psychosocial Interventions

Discrete Trial Training

The approach of applying behavioral learning theory to interventions, or applied behavioral analysis (ABA), has been thoroughly researched and is widely employed in the treatment of autism. Applied behavioral analysis is based on B.F. Skinner's principles of operant conditioning (Skinner, 1938), which include shaping, discrimination training, and reinforcement. The use of ABA principles to treat autistic children has been adapted and formalized by Ivar Lovaas at the University of California, Los Angeles, Young Autism Project. The Lovaas method of discrete trial training (DTT) is not synonymous with ABA, but DTT is based on ABA principles.

The theory behind the Lovaas method is that autistic children can show broad improvements by addressing problematic behaviors individually within a specialized environment (Lovaas and Smith, 1989). The intervention is based on a series of antecedents and consequences presented in succession. DTT consists of four parts: the presentation of the instruction (SD – discriminative stimulus), the child's response (R), the consequence which is designed to reinforce the correct response (SR – reinforcing stimulus), and a pause between trials (ITI – intertrial interval) (Myles, 2007). The most recent meta-analysis of the efficacy of DTT showed that compared to no treatment, DTT-treated autistic subjects showed statistically significant improvements, particularly on motor and functional measures. Across studies, those treated with DTT improve in language, intelligence, and adaptive behaviors (Luiselli, 2008).

TEACCH

The *T*reatment and *E*ducation of *A*utistic and related *C*ommunication handicapped *CH*ildren (TEACCH) program, which was pioneered by Eric Schopler, is founded on the idea that rather than an emotional difficulty, autism is due to neurobiological abnormalities. TEACCH advocates community-based treatment, structured teaching, and parental involvement (Schopler, 1998).

In TEACCH, classrooms or homes are organized to differentiate learning areas and minimize distraction. Visual schedules show the sequence of daily events, work systems direct students to which activities will be completed independently, and task organization specifies subsections within each task. Activities are carried out in a predictable sequence within flexible routines. This system is designed to capitalize on the child's interests and learning strengths while reducing anxiety, fostering language skills, and compensating for difficulties in memory and attention (Mesibov et al., 2005).

Many studies have supported the efficacy of TEACCH, which can be implemented in the home, special and regular schools, and residential settings (Ozonoff and Cathcart, 1998; Probst and Leppert, 2008). A recent study, conducted over 3 years, showed autistic children improved with TEACCH, particularly in conjunction with inclusion programs (Panerai et al., 2009). TEACCH promotes improvement in some domains, such as developmental age, daily living skills, and socialization (Panerai et al., 2009). A meta-analysis showed that in comparison to standard care, there was no statistically significant difference between TEACCH and standard care for imitation skills and eye–hand coordination (Ospina et al., 2008).

The Learning Experiences, an Alternative Program for Preschoolers and Their Parents (LEAP)

The LEAP program, developed in 1982, uniquely places autistic children and typical children in the same learning environment. The program utilizes an integrated preschool, behavioral management skill training for parents and encourages national advocacy and outreach. LEAP is guided by the principles of inclusion, early and individualized intervention, parent–professional collaboration, and developmentally appropriate practice. LEAP includes components of Bandura's theory of social learning, where peers can learn through modeled behaviors (Bandura, 1969) and applied behavioral analysis. The program runs for 3 h a day, 5 days a week, year-round. The classroom combines 6 autistic children and 10 typically developing children. The curriculum balances child- and teacher-directed activities, and learning experiences are designed to foster cognitive, physical, language, social, and emotional skills.

The LEAP program has published longitudinal studies on the efficacy of their program. In an 18-year follow-up, the majority of participants significantly increased their social interaction, developmental functioning, appropriate behavior with caregivers, and decreased autistic behaviors (Strain and Hoyson, 2000). However, there are currently no controlled studies evaluating LEAP in comparison to other intervention programs.

"Floor Time"

Stanley I. Greenspan developed the "floor time" play-based therapy, which is at the center of his developmental, individual differences, relationship-based model intervention program (DIR). Greenspan theorized that providing positive learning and play interactions between a child and adult would foster the acquisition of abilities needed to increase functional and developmental capacities (Greenspan and Wieder, 1999). The intervention is intended to address the core deficits of autism by engaging children in problem solving and creative, emotional, and fun interactions (Greenspan et al., 2008). To date, there is no great body of rigorous scientific studies supporting the efficacy of this treatment (Simpson et al., 2005). But some research has shown that DIR can be effective (Greenspan and Wieder, 2005) and implemented at a modest cost (Solomon et al., 2007).

The Denver Model

The Denver model, developed by Sally Rogers and colleagues (Rogers et al., 1986), provides systematic instruction within a play-based developmental framework. The Denver model is eclectic in its basis on Jean Piaget's theory of cognitive development and Margaret Mahler's psychoanalytic theory of development of a self through interpersonal interactions. The Denver model focuses on play as a primary tool to develop emotional, social, cognitive, and communication skills. The INREAL intervention, which is designed to improve functional speech in natural settings, is also employed (Weiss, 1981). Successful implementation of the Denver model increases the functioning and understanding of symbolic communication.

Alternative Therapies

Alternative therapies abound in the treatment of autism. Acupuncture, massage, electroconvulsive therapy, music, and hyperbaric oxygen therapy have been shown to produce improvements in small studies of autistic children. Robots have also been used to elicit imitative behavior and expressiveness in autistic children (Hughes, 2008). Chelation, probiotic and vitamin supplements, antifungals, secretin, yoga, immune therapies, specialized diets, and auditory integration have also been used (Levy and Hyman, 2008). While some of the studies investigating these alternative therapies are rigorous, most are only specific case reports. Further investigation is needed on the usefulness of alternative treatments.

Whether pharmacologic, psychosocial, or alternative therapies are employed, cultural and socioeconomic considerations must be taken into account in autism interventions. Research has been conducted primarily in children from Anglo backgrounds and has failed to track autistic children with cultural considerations in mind (Dyches et al., 2004). Culture may be a modifier in the efficacy of autism intervention programs. Language barriers, conceptualizations of parental authority, views on autism etiology, stigma, and shame may contribute to different choices and utilizations of autism treatments. Socioeconomic status may also be a factor (Rogers and Vismara, 2008), particularly because of the high cost associated with affording treatments not covered through private insurance or government programs.

Given the complexity of the medical, psychological, and behavioral issues that autistic children present, it is crucial they establish a "medical home" where a primary care physician can address the multitude of needs and coordinate care. Research has shown that the presence of a "medical home" can improve coordination of care, while reducing the number of unmet needs for both parents and children (Kogan et al., 2008).

The Role of Parents

Parents have been essential in advancing research, promoting treatments, shifting understanding, and raising awareness of autism. Bernard Rimland, an experimental psychologist who had an autistic child of his own, directed attention away from a psychoanalytic to a biological understanding of autism's etiology (Rimland, 1964). Parents Jon Shestack and Portia Iverson founded the Cure Autism Now Foundation, which created a gene bank to assist researchers in investigating genetic bases of autism. The parent-run Autism Research Institute organizes highly publicized Defeat Autism Now! fundraisers and conferences to share information about medical treatments for autism. More recently, parents have been instrumental in lobbying for legislation, such as the Combating Autism Act (Silverman and Brosco, 2007).

Parents, observing the nuances of their children's behaviors and responses daily, often choose which modalities of treatment and education to employ for their children. Parents have popularized certain alternative treatments through networking with other autistic parents (Silverman and Brosco, 2007). Many parents supervise comprehensive home-based programs with the help of public or private autism treatment organizations. Parents can also be intimately involved in the implementation of treatment for their children. By teaching skills to parents, interventions can be structured in a way that increases parent empowerment and confidence and decreases stress, while improving autistic children's responsiveness, affect, and engagement (Brookman-Frazee, 2004).

Parents have contributed to the emerging culture of autism, which celebrates autistic individuals' unique personalities, perspectives, and contributions to society. As part of the autistic rights movement, parents have lobbied for increased services and sued government institutions, all the while advocating for increased self-determination for their children. Specialized terminology has grown from this culture; for example, the term "Autistic Cousins" is used to describe people without a primary diagnosis of autism and the phrase "differently brained" is preferred to "disordered" (Ward and Meyer, 1999).

Policy

Autism is now being diagnosed more frequently and at earlier ages. This calls for sweeping changes in both health care and educational policy. Understanding the laws related to children with autism is essential for their care and treatment. Recently, a number of laws have been passed that support treatment and research for autism. For example, the 2000 Children's Health Act established the National Center on Birth Defects and Developmental Disabilities at the CDC and NIH to promote research focusing on causes, detection, prevention, and interventions for autism. The Combating Autism Act of 2006 (Public Law No. 109–416) authorized nearly $1 billion over 5 years to fund research and provide education, screening, referrals, and intervention for people with ASDs, Rett syndrome, and childhood disintegrative disorder. Nonetheless, existing policies in health and education do not fully meet the needs of autistic children.

Health Care

Autistic children, with their frequent physical comorbidities, have extraordinary health-care needs that must be addressed. Currently, having a diagnosis of autism does not qualify patients for Medicaid or Medicare. If an autistic individual is otherwise covered under these programs, however, screening, diagnosis, and treatment are provided. Many states have developmental disability and autism-specific waivers that allow persons who would otherwise receive institutional services to receive services in their homes and communities.

Recently, a social movement developed to mandate the coverage of autism-related services for Medicaid, Medicare, and private health insurance recipients. Several states passed laws requiring private insurers to end these discriminatory practices by requiring the coverage of evidence-based treatment and screening techniques. Arguments against such bills are often based on a calculation that covering services will result in higher insurance premiums. Looking to Pennsylvania, a state where such laws have been enacted, premiums indeed increased by approximately 0.19–2.31% per year (Bouder et al., 2009). This minimal increase, however, must be weighed against the potential benefits of providing treatment services for such a disabling disorder.

Models of cost-effectiveness have demonstrated that with early intervention, cost savings ranges from $656,000–$1,082,000 per person over their lifetime (Jacobson et al., 1998). The expenditure of funds for prevention/treatment should be viewed as a fiscally responsible way of distributing the cost of care for affected citizens, particularly in shifting costs from special education to prevention and treatment. In the interests of a healthy community, the expense must also be weighed against the negative consequences that extend to individuals and families affected by autism.

Education

Public education is a vehicle for providing regular instruction in conjunction with treatment for psychosocial symptoms of autism. Over the past decade, the number of children diagnosed with autism who receive special education services in the USA has increased by 500% to approximately 120,000 (GAO, 2005). The cost of educating a child with autism is enormous. The average per pupil spending was $18,790 in the 1999–2000 school year, almost three times as great as the $6,556 per pupil expenditure for a student receiving regular educational services (GAO, 2005).

The Individuals with Disabilities Educational Act (IDEA) (Public Law No. 94–142) is the primary federal legislation under which individuals with autism and other disabilities receive educational services. The IDEA was first enacted in 1975 as the Education for All Handicapped Children Act, but was renamed in 1990 (Public Law No. 101–476).

This Act mandates the free and appropriate public education for students with disabilities in the least restrictive environment. Students served by IDEA are required to have individual education plans (IEPs) and are eligible for service such as counseling and speech and occupational, behavioral, and physical therapy. IDEA mandates that when possible, these services should be provided within the context of inclusion: providing special services in the regular classroom as opposed to separate classes or programs.

IDEA Part C funds early intervention services for children from birth to age 3. Services may be provided in the home or community setting. The American Recovery and Reinvestment Act of 2009 was signed into law by President Obama on February 17, 2009. One of its provisions is a $400 million expansion of Part C Early Intervention Program, in addition to $11.3 billion for the IDEA State Grant program. IDEA Part B is for children aged 3–21. Services are provided in preschool or school settings. The transition from services under Part C to services under Part B is often a point where lawsuits and parental dissatisfactions coalesce. Parents prefer the intensity of in-home services provided to younger children under Part C, whereas schools look to shift to group services under Part B (Gabriels and Hill, 2007).

Disabled individuals are also entitled to equal access to federally funded facilities and to participate equally in extracurricular activities, all pursuant to Section 504 of the Rehabilitation Act of 1973. This provision addresses the issue as one of civil rights. The mandated inclusion requires that the necessary accommodations be made.

> The No Child Left Behind Program (NCLB), which amended and reauthorized the Elementary and Secondary Education Act of 1965, also applies to the education of autistic students. The purpose of this program "is to ensure that all children have a fair, equal, and significant opportunity to obtain high-quality education and reach, at a minimum, proficiency on challenging State academic achievement standards and academic assessments" (cite 20 U.S.C. ∫ 6301). Under NCLB, by 2014, states must ensure that students are making adequate early progress and that they are proficient in reading, math, and science (cite 20 U.S.C. ∫ 6311). Parental involvement in education is encouraged under NCLB, and communication between parents and teachers is required (cite 20 U.S.C. ∫ 6318 (d)). Thus, parents may use NCLB to advocate for services and involvement in their child's education.

Autism is a neurologically based disability that profoundly affects children, adolescents, their families, and the community. Autism is characterized by a central impairment of communication. Over the past decades, autism rates have clearly increased worldwide, although the cause of this increase is unknown. There does appear to be a strong genetic basis for autism, and with the recognition that autism is a heritable biologically driven condition, research has focused on understanding the complex interaction of genetic and environmental influences that may be the cause of autism.

Significant physical and psychosocial complications are associated with autism. Autistic individuals show physical structural abnormalities and have comorbid psychiatric and medical conditions such as anxiety, phobias, ADHD, sensory deficits, and gastrointestinal problems. Autism results in dramatically reduced quality of life for affected individuals and their families, with increased parental stress, reduced sibling interaction, and limited normal social activities.

Early screening and diagnosis is critical for efficacious intervention. Pharmacological options and comprehensive programs such as discrete trial training, TEACCH, the Denver model, LEAP, and floor time have shown promise. Alternative therapies, such as specialized diets, may be used instead of or in conjunction with other interventions. Unfortunately, for most individuals, autism is a lifelong condition with a poor prognosis.

The rising rates of autism diagnoses call for dramatic changes in the existing educational and health-care policies for those with autism. Mandating that insurers cover autism-related services and fund comprehensive treatment and education for autistic children and adolescents is necessary. Most importantly, further research efforts to determine the cause, effective treatments, and prevention for autism will be crucial as society comes to terms with the enormous effects of these disabling disorders.

References

Abrahams, B.S., Geschwind, D.H. (2008). Advances in autism genetics: on the threshold of a new neurobiology. Nat Rev Genet, 9 (5), 341–355.

American Psychiatric Association. Task Force on DSM-IV. (2000). Diagnostic and statistical manual of mental disorders: DSM-IV-TR. Washington, DC: American Psychiatric Association.

Amir, R.E., Van den Veyver, I.B., et al. (1999). Rett syndrome is caused by mutations in X-linked MECP2, encoding methyl-CpG-binding protein 2. Nat Genet, 23 (2), 185–188.

Anderson, B., Schnetz-Boutaud, N., et al. (2009). Examination of association of genes in the serotonin system to autism. Neurogenetics, 10 (3), 209–216.
Bailey, A., Le Couteur, A., et al. (1995). Autism as a strongly genetic disorder: evidence from a British twin study. Psychol Med, 25 (1), 63–77.
Baker, P., Piven, J., et al. (1998). Autism and tuberous sclerosis complex: prevalence and clinical features. J Autism Dev Disord, 28, 279–285.
Bandura, A. (1969). Principles of behavior modification. New York, NY: Holt.
Bebko, J.M., Konstantareas, M.M., et al. (1987). Parent and professional evaluations of family stress associated with characteristics of autism. J Autism Dev Disord, 17 (4), 565–576.
Begeer, S., Bouk, S., et al. (2009). Underdiagnosis and referral bias of autism in ethnic minorities. J Autism Dev Disord, 39 (1), 142–148.
Bettelheim, B. (1967). The empty fortress: infantile autism and the birth of the self. New York, NY: The Free Press.
Blakeslee, S. (2002). Increase in autism baffles scientists. New York, NY: The New York Times.
Blakeslee, S. (2003). Autism diagnoses double in California. New York, NY: The New York Times.
Bouder, J., Spielman, S., et al. (2009). Brief report: quantifying the impact of autism coverage on private insurance premiums. J Autism Dev Disord, 39 (6), 953–957.
Bransfield, R.C., Wulfman, J.S., et al. (2008). The association between tick-borne infections, lyme borreliosis and autism spectrum disorders. Med Hypotheses, 70 (5), 967–974.
Broman, S.H., Fletcher, J. (1999). The changing nervous system: neurobehavioral consequences of early brain disorders. New York, NY: Oxford University Press.
Brookman-Frazee, L. (2004). Using parent/clinician partnerships in parent education programs for children with autism. J Posit Behav Interv, 6, 195–213.
Buck, M.L. (2000). The FDA Modernization Act of 1997: impact on pediatric medicine. Ped Pharmacotherapy, 6 (12), 1–4.
Canitano, R. (2007). Epilepsy in autism spectrum disorders. Eur Child Adolesc Psychiatry, 16 (1), 61–66.
Cass, H., Gringras, P., et al. (2008). Absence of urinary opioid peptides in children with autism. Arch Dis Child, 93 (9), 745–750.
Chakrabarti, S., Fombonne, E. (2001). Pervasive developmental disorders in preschool children. J Am Med Assoc, 285 (24), 3093–3099.
Chakrabarti, S., Fombonne, E. (2005). Pervasive developmental disorders in preschool children: confirmation of high prevalence. Am J Psychiatry, 162 (6), 1133–1141.
Committee, I.S.R. (2004). Immunization safety review: vaccines and autism. Washington, DC: National Academy Press.
Conciatori, M., Stodgell, C.J., et al. (2004). Association between the HOXA1 A218G polymorphism and increased head circumference in patients with autism. Biol Psychiatry, 55 (4), 413–419.
Coutinho, A., Sousa, I., et al. (2007). Evidence for epistasis between SLC6A4 and ITGB3 in autism etiology and in the determination of platelet serotonin levels. Hum Genet, 121 (2), 243–256.
Croen, L.A., Grether, J.K., et al. (2002). The changing prevalence of autism in California. J Autism Dev Disord, 32, 207.
Dales, L., Hammer, S.J., et al. (2001). Time trends in autism and in MMR immunization coverage in California. J Am Med Assoc, 285 (9), 1183–1185.
Daniels, J.L., Forssen, U., et al. (2008). Parental psychiatric disorders associated with autism spectrum disorders in the offspring. Pediatrics, 121 (5), e1357–1362.
Davis, N., Carter, A. (2008). Parenting stress in mothers and fathers of toddlers with autism spectrum disorders: associations with child characteristics. J Autism Dev Disord, 38 (7), 1278–1291.
Depienne, C., Moreno-De-Luca, D., et al. (2009). Screening for genomic rearrangements and methylation abnormalities of the 15q11-q13 Region in autism spectrum disorders. Biol Psychiatry, 66 (4), 349–359.

DeStefano, F., Thompson, W.W. (2004). MMR vaccine and autism: an update of the scientific evidence. Expert Rev Vaccines, 3 (1), 19–22.

DiCicco-Bloom, E., Lord, C., et al. (2006). The developmental neurobiology of autism spectrum disorder. J Neurosci, 26 (26), 6897–6906.

Dyches, T., Wilder, L., et al. (2004). Multicultural issues in autism. J Autism Dev Disord, 34 (2), 211–222.

Durkin M.S., Maenner M.J., Newschaffer C.J., et al. (2008, December 1). Advanced parental age and the risk of autism spectrum disorder. Am J Epidemiol, 168 (11), 1268–1276. Epub 2008 Oct 21.

Farrington, C.P., Miller, E., et al. (2001). MMR and autism: further evidence against a causal association. Vaccine, 19 (27), 3632–3635.

Fatemi, S., Folsom, T., et al. (2009). Expression of GABAB receptors is altered in brains of subjects with autism. Cerebellum, 8 (1), 64–69.

Folstein, S.E., Rosen-Sheidley, B. (2001). Genetics of autism: complex aetiology for a heterogeneous disorder. Nat Rev Genet, Nature Publishing Group (2), 943–955.

Folstein, S., Rutter, M. (1977). Infantile autism: a genetic study of 21 twin pairs. J Child Psychol Psychiatry, 18 (4), 297–321.

Fombonne, E. (2009). Epidemiology of pervasive developmental disorders. Pediatr Res, 65 (6), 591–598.

Fombonne, E., Zakarian, R., et al. (2006). Pervasive developmental disorders in Montreal, Quebec, Canada: prevalence and links with immunizations. Pediatrics, 118 (1), e139–e150.

Gabriels, R.L., Hill, D.E. (2007). Growing up with autism: working with school-age children and adolescents. New York, NY: Guilford Press.

GAO (2005). Report to the chairman and ranking minority member, subcommittee on human rights and wellness, committee on government reform, House of Representatives, Special education: children with autism. Washington, DC: United States Government Accountability Office.

Gerber, J.S., Offit, P.A. (2009). Vaccines: vaccines and autism: a tale of shifting hypotheses. Clin Infect Dis, 48 (4), 456–461.

Greenspan, S.I., Brazelton, T.B., et al. (2008). Guidelines for early identification, screening, and clinical management of children with autism spectrum disorders. Pediatrics, 121 (4), 828–830.

Greenspan, S.I., Wieder, S. (1999). A functional developmental approach to autism spectrum disorders. J Assoc Persons Severe Handicaps, 24 (3), 147–161.

Greenspan, S.I., Wieder, S. (2005). Can children with autism master the core deficits and become empathetic, creative, and reflective? A ten to fifteen year follow-up of a subgroup of children with Autism Spectrum Disorders (ASD) who received a comprehensive developmental, individual-difference, relationship-based (DIR) approach. J Dev Learn Disord, 9, 39–61.

Grice, D.E., Buxbaum, J.D. (2006). The genetics of autism spectrum disorders. Neuromolecular Med, 8 (4), 1159–1174.

Hanson, D.R., Gottesman, I. (1976). The genetics, if any, of infantile autism and childhood schizophrenia. J Autism Child Schizophr, 6 (3), 209–234.

Hastings, R.P. (2002). Parental stress and behaviour problems of children with developmental disability. J Intellect Dev Disabl, 27 (3), 149–160.

Hastings, R., Kovshoff, H., et al. (2005). Systems analysis of stress and positive perceptions in mothers and fathers of pre-school children with autism. J Autism Dev Disord, 35 (5), 635–644.

Hatton, D.D., Sideris, J., et al. (2006). Autistic behavior in children with fragile X syndrome: prevalence, stability, and the impact of FMRP. Am J Med Genet, Part A, 140A (17), 1804–1813.

Hertz-Picciotto, I., Delwiche, L. (2009). The rise in autism and the role of age at diagnosis. Epidemiology, 20 (1), 84–90.

Higgins, D.J., Bailey, S.R., et al. (2005). Factors associated with functioning style and coping strategies of families with a child with an autism spectrum disorder. Autism, 9 (2), 125–137.

Howlin, P., Goode, S., et al. (2004). Adult outcome for children with autism. J Child Psychol Psychiatry, 45 (2), 212–229.

Huang, C.H., Santangelo, S.L. (2008). Autism and serotonin transporter gene polymorphisms: a systematic review and meta-analysis. Am J Med Genet B Neuropsychiatr Genet, 147B (6), 903–913.

Hughes, J.R. (2008). A review of recent reports on autism: 1000 studies published in 2007. Epilepsy Behav, 13 (3), 425–437.

Jacobson, J.W., Mulick, J.A., et al. (1998). Cost-benefit estimates for early intensive behavioral intervention for young children with autism-general model and single state case. Behav Interv, 13 (4), 201–226.

Jamain, S., Quach, H., et al. (2002). Y chromosome haplogroups in autistic subjects. Mol Psychiatry, 7 (2), 217–219.

Jesner, O.S., Aref-Adib, M., Coren, E. (2007). Risperidone for autism spectrum disorder. Cochrane Database Syst Rev, Issue 1, Art. No.: CD005040. DOI: 10.1002/14651858.CD005040.pub2

Kanner, L. (1943). Autistic disturbances of affective contact. Nervous Child, 2, 217–250.

Kaye, J.A., Melero-Montes, M., et al. (2001). Mumps, measles, and rubella vaccine and the incidence of autism recorded by general practitioners: a time trend analysis. BMJ, 322 (7284), 460–463.

Kogan, M.D., Strickland, B.B., et al. (2008). A national profile of the health care experiences and family impact of autism spectrum disorder among children in the United States, 2005–2006. Pediatrics, 122 (6), e1149–1158.

Krug, D.A., Arick, J., et al. (1980). Behavior checklist for identifying severely handicapped individuals with high levels of autistic behavior. J Child Psychol Psychiatry, 21 (3), 221–229.

Lai, C.S., Fisher, S.E., et al. (2001). A forkhead-domain gene is mutated in a severe speech and language disorder. Nature, 413 (6855), 519–523.

Larsson, H.J., Eaton, W.W., et al. (2005). Risk factors for autism: perinatal factors, parental psychiatric history, and socioeconomic status. Am J Epidemiol, 161 (10), 916–925.

Lee, L., Harrington, C.R., et al. (2008). Children with autism: quality of life and parental concerns. J Autism Dev Disord, 38 (6), 1147–1160.

Levy, S.E., Hyman, S.L. (2008). Complementary and alternative medicine treatments for children with autism spectrum disorders. Child Adolesc Psychiatric Clinics North Am, 17 (4), 803–820.

Leyfer, O., Folstein, S., et al. (2006). Comorbid psychiatric disorders in children with autism: interview development and rates of disorders. J Autism Dev Disord, 36 (7), 849–861.

Lord, C., Risi, S., et al. (2000). The Autism diagnostic observation schedule – generic: a standard measure of social and communication deficits associated with the spectrum of autism. J Autism Dev Disord, 30 (3), 205–223.

Lord, C., Risi, S., et al. (2006). Autism from 2 to 9 years of age. Arch Gen Psychiatry, 63 (6), 694–701.

Lord, C., Rutter, M., et al. (1994). Autism diagnostic interview-revised: a revised version of a diagnostic interview for caregivers of individuals with possible pervasive developmental disorders. J Autism Dev Disord, 24 (5), 659–685.

Lovaas, O.I., Smith, T. (1989). A comprehensive behavioral theory of autistic children: paradigm for research and treatment. J Behav Ther Exp Psychiatry, 20 (1), 17–29.

Luiselli, J.K. (2008). Effective practices for children with autism: educational and behavioral support interventions that work. New York, NY: Oxford University Press.

MacDermot, K.D., Bonora, E., et al. (2005). Identification of FOXP2 truncation as a novel cause of developmental speech and language deficits. Am J Hum Genetics, 76 (6), 1074–1080.

Madsen, K.M., Hviid, A., et al. (2002). A population-based study of measles, mumps, and rubella vaccination and autism. N Engl J Med, 347 (19), 1477–1482.

MMWR (1999). Notice to readers: thimerosal in vaccines: a joint statement of the American Academy of Pediatrics and the Public Health Service. MMWR, 48 (26), 563–565.

McDermott, S., Zhou, L., et al. (2008). Injury treatment among children with autism or pervasive developmental disorder. J Autism Dev Disord, 38 (4), 626–633.

McNamara, I.M., Borella, A.W., et al. (2008). Further studies in the developmental hyperserotonemia model (DHS) of autism: social, behavioral, and peptide changes. Brain Res, 1189, 203–214.

Mesibov, G.B., Shea, V., et al. (2005). The TEACCH approach to autism spectrum disorders. New York, NY: Kluwer.

Miles, J.H., Hillman, R.E. (2000). Value of a clinical morphology examination in autism. Am J Med Genetics, 91 (4), 245–253.

Millward, C., Ferriter, M., Calver, S., et al. (2008, April 16). Gluten- and casein-free diets for autistic spectrum disorder. Cochrane Database Syst Rev, Issue 2, Art. No.: CD003498.

Ming, X., Brimacombe, M., et al. (2008). Autism spectrum disorders: concurrent clinical disorders. J Child Neurol, 23 (1), 6–13.

Money, J., Bobrow, N.A., et al. (1971). Autism and autoimmune disease: a family study. J Autism Dev Disord, 1 (2), 146–160.

Muhle, R., Trentacoste, S.V., et al. (2004). The genetics of autism. Pediatrics, 113 (5), e472–486.

Myles, B.S. (2007). Autism spectrum disorders: a handbook for parents and professionals. Westport, CT: Praeger.

National Research Council (U.S.). Committee on Educational Interventions for Children with Autism. (2001). Educating children with autism. Washington, DC: National Academy Press.

Nicolson, G.L., Gan, R., et al. (2007). Evidence for *Mycoplasma* ssp., *Chlamydia pneunomiae*, and human herpes virus-6 coinfections in the blood of patients with autistic spectrum disorders. J Neurosci Res, 85 (5), 1143–1148.

Oberman, L.M., Ramachandran, V.S. (2007). The simulating social mind: the role of the mirror neuron system and simulation in the social and communicative deficits of autism spectrum disorders. Psychol Bull, 133 (2), 310–327.

Offit, P.A. (2008). Vaccines and autism revisited –The Hannah Poling case. N Engl J Med, 358 (20), 2089–2091.

Oosterling, I.J., Swinkels, S.H., et al. (2009). Comparative analysis of three screening instruments for autism spectrum disorder in toddlers at high risk. J Autism Dev Disord, 39 (6), 897–909.

Orsmond, G.I., Seltzer, M.M. (2007). Siblings of individuals with autism or Down syndrome. Effects on adult lives. J Intellect Disabil Res, 51 (Pt 9), 682–696.

Ospina, M.B., Krebs Seida, J., et al. (2008). Behavioural and developmental interventions for autism spectrum disorder: a clinical systematic review. PLoS One, 3 (11), e3755.

Oswald, D.P., Sonenklar, N.A. (2007). Medication use among children with autism spectrum disorders. J Child Adolesc Psychopharm, 17 (3), 348–355.

Ozonoff, S., Cathcart, K. (1998). Effectiveness of a home program intervention for young children with autism. J Autism Dev Disord, 28 (1), 25–32.

Ozonoff, S., Rogers, S.J., et al. (2003). Autism spectrum disorders: a research review for practitioners. Washington, DC: American Psychiatric Pub.

Panerai, S., Zingale, M., et al. (2009). Special education versus inclusive education: the role of the TEACCH Program. J Autism Dev Disord, 39 (6), 874–882.

Parner, E.T., Schendel, D.E., et al. (2008). Autism prevalence trends over time in Denmark: changes in prevalence and age at diagnosis. Arch Pediatr Adolesc Med, 162 (12), 1150–1156.

Parracho, H.M., Bingham, M.O., et al. (2005). Differences between the gut microflora of children with autistic spectrum disorders and that of healthy children. J Med Microbiol, 54 (10), 987–991.

Percy, A.K., Lane, J.B. (2004). Rett syndrome: clinical and molecular update. Curr Opin Pediatrics, 16 (6), 670–677.

Peters, S., Beaudet, A., et al. (2004). Autism in Angelman syndrome: implications for autism research. Clin Genet, 66 (6), 530–536.

Philippe, A., Martinez, M., et al. (1999). Genome-wide scan for autism susceptibility genes. Paris Autism Research International Sibpair Study. Hum Mol Genet, 8 (5), 805–812.

Probst, P., Leppert, T. (2008). Brief report: outcomes of a teacher training program for autism spectrum disorders. J Autism Dev Disord, 38 (9), 1791–1796.

Redcay, E., Courchesne, E. (2005). When is the brain enlarged in autism? A meta- analysis of all brain size reports. Biol Psychiatry, 58 (1), 1–9.

Rimland, B. (1964). Infantile autism: the syndrome and its implications for a neural theory of behavior. New York, NY: Appleton-Century-Crofts.

Robins, D.L., Fein, D., et al. (2001). The modified checklist for autism in toddlers: an initial study investigating the early detection of autism and pervasive developmental disorders. J Autism Dev Disord, 31, 131.

Rogers, S.J., Herbison, J.M., et al. (1986). An approach for enhancing the symbolic, communicative, and interpersonal functioning of young children with autism or severe emotional handicaps. J Early Interv, 10 (2), 135–148.

Rogers, S.J., Vismara, L.A. (2008). Evidence-based comprehensive treatments for early autism. J Clin Child Adolesc Psychol, 37 (1), 8–38.

Rutter, M. (1978). Diagnosis and definitions of childhood autism. J Autism Child Schizophr, 8 (2), 139–161.

Rutter, M. (2000). Genetic studies of autism: from the 1970s into the millennium. J Abnorm Child Psychol, 28 (1), 3–14.

Schain, R.J., Freedman, D.X. (1961). Studies on 5-hydroxyindole metabolism in autistic and other mentally retarded children. J Pediatrics, 58 (3), 315–320.

Schellenberg, G.D., Dawson, G., et al. (2006). Evidence for multiple loci from a genome scan of autism kindreds. Mol Psychiatry, 11 (11), 1049–1060.

Schopler, E. (1998). Behavior and cognitive therapy today: essays in honor of Hans J. Eysenck: Selected proceedings of the XXVII Congress of the European Association for Behavioral and Cognitive Therapies, Venice 1997. Kidlington, Oxford, Pergamon: xv, 339.

Seim, A.R., Reichelt, K.L. (1995). An enzyme/brain-barrier theory of psychiatric pathogenesis: unifying observations on phenylketonuria, autism, schizophrenia and postpartum psychosis. Med Hypotheses, 45 (5), 498–502.

Sharpe, D., Rossiter, L. (2002). Siblings of children with a chronic illness: a meta- analysis. J Pediatr Psychol, 27 (8), 699–710.

Siegel, B. (2004). The pervasive developmental disorders screening test II (PDDST-II). San Antonio, TX: Harcourt Assessment.

Silverman, C., Brosco, J.P. (2007). Understanding autism: parents and pediatricians in historical perspective. Arch Pediatr Adolesc Med, 161 (4), 392–398.

Simpson, L., Owens, P.L., Zodet, M.W., et al. (2005). Health care for children and youth in the United States: annual report on patterns of coverage, utilization, quality, and expenditures. Ambul Pediatr, 5 (1), 6–44.

Skaar, D.A., Shao, Y., et al. (2004). Analysis of the RELN gene as a genetic risk factor for autism. Mol Psychiatry, 10 (6), 563–571.

Skinner, B.F. (1938). The behavior of organisms. New York, NY: Appleton-Century-Crofts.

Smith, M., Spence, M.A., et al. (2009). Nuclear and mitochondrial genome defects in autisms. Ann N Y Acad Sci, 1151 (The Year in Human and Medical Genetics 2009), 102–132.

Solomon, R., Necheles, J., et al. (2007). Pilot study of a parent training program for young children with autism: the PLAY Project Home Consultation program. Autism, 11 (3), 205–224.

Stefanatos, G. (2008). Regression in autistic spectrum disorders. Neuropsychol Rev, 18 (4), 305–319.

Steffenburg, S., Gillberg, C., et al. (1989). A twin study of autism in Denmark, Finland, Iceland, Norway and Sweden. J Child Psychol Psychiatry, 30 (3), 405–416.

Steffenburg, S., Gillberg, C.L., et al. (1996). Autism in Angelman syndrome: a population-based study. Pediatr Neurol, 14 (2), 131–136.

Stoelb, M., Yarnal, R., et al. (2004). Predicting responsiveness to treatment of children with autism: a retrospective study of the importance of physical dysmorphology. Focus on Autism Other Dev Disabl, 19 (2), 66–77.

Stone, W.L., Coonrod, E.E., et al. (2004). Psychometric properties of the STAT for early autism screening. J Autism Dev Disord, 34 (6), 691–701.

Stoneman, Z. (2001, May). Supporting positive sibling relationships during childhood. Mental Retardation Dev Disabil Res, 7 (2), 134–142.

Strain, P.S., Hoyson, M. (2000). The need for longitudinal, intensive social skill intervention: LEAP follow-up outcomes for children with autism. Topics Early Child Spec Educ, 20 (2), 116–122.

Swinkels, S.H.N., Dietz, C., van Daalen, E., et al. (2006). Screening for autistic spectrum in children aged 14 to 15 months. I: the development of the Early Screening of Autistic Traits Questionnaire (ESAT). J Autism Dev Disord, 36, 723–732.

Toriello, H.V. (2008). Role of the dysmorphologic evaluation in the child with developmental delay. Pediatr Clin of North Am, 55 (5), 1085–1098.

Tsatsanis, K.D. (2003). Outcome research in Asperger syndrome and autism. Child Adolesc Psychiatric Clin North Am, 12 (1), 47–63.

Vernes, S.C., Newbury, D.F., et al. (2008). A functional genetic link between distinct developmental language disorders. N Engl J Med, 359 (22), 2337–2345.

Wakefield, A.J., Murch, S.H., et al. (1998). Ileal-lymphoid-nodular hyperplasia, non-specific colitis, and pervasive developmental disorder in children. Lancet, 351 (9103), 637–641.

Ward, M.J., Meyer, R.N. (1999). Self-determination for people with developmental disabilities and autism: two self-advocates' perspectives. Focus Autism Other Dev Disabl, 14 (3), 133–139.

Wassink, T.H., Piven, J., et al. (2001). Evidence supporting WNT2 as an autism susceptibility gene. Am J Med Genetics, 105 (5), 406–413.

Weiss, R.S. (1981). INREAL intervention for language handicapped and bilingual children. J Early Interv, 4 (1), 40–51.

Whiteley, P., Rodgers, J., et al. (1999). A gluten-free diet as an intervention for autism and associated spectrum disorders: preliminary findings. Autism, 3 (1), 45–65.

Williams, J., Whiten, A., et al. (2004). A systematic review of action imitation in autistic spectrum disorder. J Autism Dev Disord, 34 (3), 285–299.

Wills, S., Cabanlit, M., et al. (2007). Autoantibodies in autism spectrum disorders (ASD). Ann N Y Acad Sci, 1107 (Autoimmunity, Part C The Mosaic of Autoimmunity), 79–91.

Xiaohong Gong, E.B., Blasi, F., Claudio Toma, C.B., et al. (2008). Analysis of X chromosome inactivation in autism spectrum disorders. Am J Med Genetics, Part B: Neuropsychiatr Genet, 147B (6), 830–835.

Chapter 4
Cerebral Palsy

Cerebral palsy (CP) is a group of physical disorders that affect an individual's ability to move and to maintain posture and balance. The disorder is a static encephalopathy (permanent or unchanging brain damage) caused by an insult to the brain during either the perinatal or the postnatal period. The condition appears during the first few years of life. Early signs usually appear before the age of 3. The condition affects the child's ability to coordinate body movements. As a result, affected babies are often slow in their ability to roll over, sit, crawl, walk, and/or smile. In the USA and around the world, the incidence of CP is 1.5–2 cases per 1,000 live births. CP is the most common cause of severe childhood disability.

Some babies are born with CP, while others get it after they are born. The damage can occur during fetal development, during the actual birth process, or during the first few months after birth. The majority of children with CP are born with it, although the condition may not be detected until months or even years later. The disorder is caused by an abnormality in or an injury to the cerebrum, the largest area of the brain and the area of the brain which controls sensation and voluntary motor function. Although CP impacts body movement, the underlying problem originates in the brain, rather than in the muscles.

Physicians and researchers have identified many possible causes of CP, including maternal infection during pregnancy (rubella or other viral infections), disturbance to brain circulation prior to birth (blood clot or artery spasm), severe jaundice (from infection, severe bruising, Rh incompatibility, or ABO incompatibility), or abnormal brain development prior to birth (genetic or metabolic disorders).

Some children have CP as a result of brain damage occurring in the first few months of life. Later development of the disorder may be caused by a head injury, from a fall or accident, child abuse, or a brain infection due to meningitis or viral encephalitis.

Thorgood and Alexander (2005) have cited additional prenatal, neonatal, and postnatal causes such as multiple births, maternal illness, abdominal trauma, congenital malformations, and toxic or teratogenic agents (Li et al., 2009). Neonatal causes include prematurity (less than 32 weeks gestation), low birth weight (less than 2,500 g), growth retardation, seizures, intracranial hemorrhage, bradycardia, hypoxia, and abnormal birthing presentations. Postnatal causes include coagulopathies (clotting disorders) and intracranial hemorrhage.

M.L. Goldstein, S. Morewitz, *Chronic Disorders in Children and Adolescents*,
DOI 10.1007/978-1-4419-9764-7_4, © Springer Science+Business Media, LLC 2011

Using data from Swedish hospitals from 1987 to 2001, Hemminki et al. (2007) analyzed almost 4,000 CP patients' records and compared them to a control group. They discovered that parents who had one child with CP had a 4.8-fold risk of having a second CP child. Twins have a 29-fold increased chance of developing the disorder.

CP has typically been classified in three main categories:

1. Approximately 75% of CP patients have spastic or pyramidal CP that causes muscles to stiffen, thus making movement difficult. Spastic CP has three subsets: spastic diplegia which can impact the lower part of the body, both legs, hips, and/or the pelvis; spastic hemiplegia, which affects only one side of the body; spastic quadriplegia, the most severe form of spastic CP, which can affect all four limbs as well as the trunk. Cognitive impairment is present in approximately 30% of individuals with spastic diplegia and in approximately 28% of those with hemiplegia.
2. A second type of CP is athetotic or dyskinesia cerebral palsy, which affects about one in five people with CP. The disorder is also referred to as extra pyramidal CP, and it affects the entire body and often causes uncontrolled, slow movements. Generally, the child is hypotonic (muscles appear "floppy") at birth with abnormal movement patterns emerging. Muscle tone is normal during sleep. Sensorineural hearing loss is common. Cognitive impairment is present in approximately 22% of the youngsters with this condition.
3. A third type of CP is known as ataxic CP. This condition is the least common of the major forms of CP and influences balance and coordination.

CP ranges from mild to severe. One child might be unable to walk and need extensive, long-term care, while another child might be only slightly awkward and require no special care. The condition does not appear to worsen with age. CP appears to be more common in males, but the reasons for this disparity are unclear (Johnston and Hagberg, 2007). Baby boys born preterm appear to be more vulnerable to both white matter injury and intraventricular hemorrhage. Furthermore, Johnston and Hagberg (2007) suggest that new data indicate that there are significant neurobiological differences between males and females in their response to brain injuries.

Symptoms and Risk Factors

The most commonly observed symptom is abnormal muscle tone. The child may present with lack of muscle coordination when performing voluntary movements (ataxia): stiff muscles and exaggerated reflexes (spasticity); asymmetrical walking gait, usually with one leg or foot dragging; and/or with difficulty with precise motions, such as writing or zipping or buttoning a coat. The child's muscle tone may vary from being too floppy to being too stiff. Furthermore, the child may exhibit excessive drooling or have difficulty in swallowing, sucking, or speaking.

If considerable spasticity occurs, CP may lead to joint deformities in addition to problems with movement and posture. These children are also at increased risk for osteoporosis. According to Gordon and Simkiss (2006), 60% of children who were not walking by age 5 were likely to develop subluxation of the hip, with the greatest risk in those with severe neurological involvement. If these CP children experience swallowing or feeding problems, they may have nutritional problems. GI symptoms, including reflux and constipation, as well as dysphagia (difficulty in swallowing), may cause failure to thrive. In addition, these children are at greater risk of experiencing pulmonary complications, including aspiration and oromotor dysfunction.

Some CP children have multiple handicaps which may include problems with vision, hearing, and speech; experiencing abnormal sensation and/or perception; having urinary incontinence; experiencing seizures; having pulmonary complications; and suffering from dental problems. Mental retardation is present in 30–50% of CP children (Mayo Clinic, 2006).

The health and social outcomes in children with CP vary depending on the severity of the condition, the type of treatments, and the children's environment (Liptak and Accardo, 2004). Because CP is highly variable, researchers have developed classification systems such as the Gross Motor Function Classification System, in an attempt to more accurately describe the childrens' conditions.

Quality of Life

Research on the physical effects of CP on children is plentiful, and it has long been thought that the many limitations imposed by those effects will have a negative effect on the children's quality of life (QOL). In the following text, we describe some of the more recent research into the psychological and/or cognitive effects caused by the condition. In a few cases, the findings are surprising, while in others they are not.

Based on a cross-sectional study of 1,174 CP children, in nine European regions, Fauconnier et al. (2009) discovered that CP children with high levels of pain and substantial impairment in walking, fine motor skills, communication, and intellectual functioning were unlikely to participate in most aspects of life activities. The researchers also found that type of CP and feeding and vision problems predicted lower rates of participation in daily activities. However, socioeconomic status (SES) and demographic characteristics were not related to specific domains of life activities.

Peeters et al. (2008a) examined children with CP who also had accompanying reading disabilities. They indicated that general intelligence and speech ability were important factors in developing phonological awareness and that children with CP with intellectual disabilities seem to have problems in acquiring phonological awareness.

Kozeis et al. (2007) investigated visual function and perception in 105 CP children and found that even in the absence of mental retardation, CP children had poor visual skills. They felt that since the deficient visual skills had a negative effect on those with normal cognitive abilities, this is a separate identifiable factor that will compound the adverse effects of mental retardation.

Based on a qualitative study of parents and CP children, Waters et al. (2005) identified 13 common themes of concern: physical health, pain, participation in social and physical activities, emotional well-being, self-esteem, relationships with the community, supportive physical environments, family health, communication, and accessing CP services.

Dickinson et al. (2007) evaluated 1,174 European CP children from 8 to 12 years of age and found that some children with CP had QOL similar to other children, with the exception of schooling. Dammann and O'Shea (2007), Reading (2007), and Sparkes and Hall (2007) all supported the findings. However, Dickinson et al. (2007) did find that CP children who had severely limited self-mobility had lower levels of physical well-being and intellectual functioning with impaired mood, emotions, and autonomy. Severely impaired self-mobility also predicted speech problems with lower quality relationships with parents. The authors noted that pain was common among CP children and contributed to lower QOL in different aspects of life activities.

Berrin et al. (2007) investigated the role of pain and fatigue, and school functioning in CP children and found that both fatigue and pain have a negative effect on school functioning.

Based on a sample of 818 CP children from Europe, Arnaud et al. (2008) showed that impairment in gross motor function and low IQ predicted lower parent-reported QOL for CP children. However, the investigators discovered that increased levels of impairment were not always related to lower QOL. Less severely disabled children also had reduced QOL in terms of their moods, emotions, self-perception, acceptance by others, and school factors.

In another study, Dunn et al. (2007) found that parents of CP children rated their child's abilities and attributes lower than the children did.

Nadeau and Tessier (2006) showed that CP children had fewer reciprocated friendships, exhibited fewer sociable/leadership behaviors, and felt more isolated and victimized in comparison to their classmates without a disability. The findings were particularly significant for females with CP, irrespective of their type of disability.

Based on a cross-sectional survey in Europe, Parkes et al. (2008) evaluated psychological symptoms in 818 CP children. The investigators discovered that approximately 25% of the children surveyed exhibited substantial psychological difficulties with peer relations. Risk factors associated with these difficulties among CP children were increased gross motor function; lower intellect; increased pain; having a sibling who is ill or disabled; and residing in a town. The authors conclude that a substantial percentage of children with CP have psychological or social difficulties severe enough to require referral to specialized services. They recommend that clinicians carefully assess and manage CP children to make sure that their psychosocial difficulties are minimized and that potentially modifiable risk factors like pain are treated.

Using data from the above study, Parkes et al. (2009) revealed that children with hemiplegia (paralysis of one side of the body) had more social and psychological difficulties compared to a normative sample. Those who had severe intellectual disability (IQ less than 50 compared to those with an IQ greater than 70) were more likely to have hyperactivity and problems with their peers. These difficulties were more likely to have a substantial social and psychological impact. Boys were more likely to suffer from conduct disorder and hyperactivity. Those with low self-esteem were more likely to have peer difficulties and low levels of pro-social skills. Communication deficits, substantial pain, and living with a single parent increased the risk of poor psychosocial adjustment.

Quadriplegia

Morrow et al. (2008) compared parents' perceptions of QOL in quadriplegic cerebral palsy with the perceptions of health professionals using focus groups. The investigators discovered that the parents' perceptions as well as those of the health professionals centered on the following five issues: interactions of parent–child; the provision of health services; the child's emotional status; the physical status of the child; and the process of socialization. However, parents differed from health professionals in the sub-themes that they emphasized and the values that they attached to these issues. Parents felt that it was more important that their child felt loved, while health professionals felt that weight gain for the child was important. Health professionals did not regard as many issues as important as did the parents. The authors also found that discrepancies in priorities for outcomes in treatment adversely influenced parent–provider interactions.

Adolescents

Livingston et al. (2007) postulated that adolescents with CP have different life issues than children or adults and that there has been limited research for this age range. In their review of eight cross-sectional surveys, nine validation studies and three qualitative reports, the authors discovered that the functional status measures are reliable indicators of physical function but do not consistently predict changes in psychosocial status.

Using semi-structured interviews with CP adolescents and their parents, Davis et al. (2009) discovered that participation in social, physical, and school activities, CP-associated topics (e.g., pain and communication), finances, and adolescent developmental issues, such as sexuality and independence, were some of the major QOL issues. The investigators found that many of the issues raised by the adolescents and their parents were similar to the QOL reports among younger children with CP.

Donkervoort et al. (2007) studied adolescents with CP and found that 20–30% encountered restrictions in daily activities (mobility, self-care, nutrition) and social participation (taking responsibility, community living, leisure activities, and employment). They concluded that a significant number of adolescents and young adults with CP without severe learning disabilities were restricted in their social participation. They also posited that these problems were mainly the result of restricted gross motor functioning and a low level of education.

In another study, Wiegerink et al. (2006) examined 14 studies on adolescents and young adults with CP and found that self-efficacy and sexual self-esteem as well as the interrelationships with the parents' way of raising their children and successful experiences in social situations were significant factors in the development of social and sexual relationships.

Treatment

Physical Therapy

The treatment for children with CP may include physical therapy, occupational therapy, speech therapy, medication, surgery, communication aids and assistive technology, vision and hearing aids, orthotic devices, and other equipment.

Physical therapy is a widely utilized treatment intervention for children with CP (Anttila et al., 2008; Patel, 2005). Treatment is aimed at promoting motor skills as well as developmental skills, and is designed to enhance functional independence. Approaches include exercise, mobility training, muscle training, and orthotics or braces, and other equipment. Daily range of motion exercises, stretching exercises, age appropriate play, and the use of adaptive toys and games are typically employed in a physical therapy regimen. Horseback riding therapy (hippotherapy), treadmill training, bicycling, adaptive downhill skiing, and aquatic intervention are more recent developments in physical therapy for CP children.

Based on a review of 23 randomized controlled trials and 104 observational investigations, Anttila et al. (2008) showed some data to support strength training, constraint-induced movement therapy, and hippotherapy in treating children with CP. However, their review of the literature did not find sufficient data to verify the effectiveness of comprehensive physiotherapy and occupational therapy. The authors recommend caution in drawing conclusions because of the poor quality of the studies.

The benefits of intense physical exercise programs such as strength training are becoming increasingly well regarded for use with CP patients, but there have been few studies on the positive effects of generalized activity programs conducted with CP patients (Damiano, 2006).

Weindling et al. (2007) assessed whether additional physical therapy of 1 h per week for 6 months helped motor functioning or the general development of young children with CP. Results indicated that there was no appreciable effect of additional physical therapy with the CP population and that there was also no significant effect on parental stress. However, Hoare et al. (2007) demonstrated that constraint-induced movement therapy was useful in children with hemiplegic CP.

Macgregor et al. (2007) utilized massage on the calf muscles of adolescents with CP and found that there was no increase in range of movement, but that the calf muscles were either shorter or longer after massage. In addition, the incidence of abnormal stretch reflexes decreased and the amplitude of alternating ankle rotation increased in the majority of participants.

Pin et al. (2006) found that sustained stretching of longer duration was preferable to improve range of movements and to reduce spasticity of muscles around targeted joints.

Engsberg et al. (2006) reported that ankle strength increases may lead to improved function, gait speed, and QOL in children with spastic diplegia.

Liao et al. (2007) investigated the effectiveness of a functional strengthening program for CP children. They concluded that loaded sit-to-stand (STS) resistance exercise improved basic motor abilities, functional muscle strength, and walking efficiency for children with mild spastic diplegia.

Unger et al. (2006) also evaluated the impact of an 8-week strength training program and found that there was an improved degree of crouch gait and improved perception of body image. However, walking velocity, cadence, and stride length, as well as perceived functional ability did not change.

In a preliminary study, Deluca et al. (2006) evaluated 18 children with hemiparesis CP and found that constraint-induced therapy produced significantly greater gains than conventional rehabilitation services.

Williams and Pountney (2007) investigated the effects of exercise on the motor function of youngsters with CP who were non-ambulating. This study showed that training on a static bicycle led to improvements in functional ability. The static bicycle provided a safe and effective means of exercise to a population with very limited opportunities for activity. Fowler et al. (2007) examined the benefits of limb strengthening through the use of a stationary cycling intervention and demonstrated the efficacy of such a protocol in leading to improved functional ability.

Cherng et al. (2007) assessed the effect of treadmill training with body weight support (TBWS) on gait and gross motor function in children with spastic CP. Results indicated that TBSW treatment improved some gait parameters and gross motor functions in children with spastic CP, but TBSW did not produce significant improvements in muscle tone or motor control.

A number of reports have demonstrated the efficacy of horseback riding therapy (hippotherapy) as an intervention with those with cerebral palsy. Snider et al. (2007) showed that hippotherapy was effective for treating muscle symmetry in the trunk and hip and in improving gross motor functioning when compared with regular therapy. Sterba (2007) concluded that horseback riding therapy improved gross motor function. The three-dimensional, reciprocal movement of the walking horse produced normalized pelvic movement in the rider, closely resembling pelvic movement during ambulation in those without a disability and improved joint stability, weight shift, postural and equilibrium responses, and co-contraction. Furthermore, Sterba added that hippotherapy enhanced dynamic postural stabilization, recovery from perturbations and anticipatory and feedback postural control.

In another report, Massaad et al. (2006) evaluated the influence of hippotherapy on the vertical displacement of the body's center of mass (COM). Their research demonstrated that horseback riding therapy reduced the vertical COM displacement and positively influenced the general gait pattern in children with CP.

Sterba (2006) investigated the effect of adaptive downhill skiing on gross motor functioning in children with spastic CP. The participant's gross motor function total scores increased and remained increased after 10 weeks of adaptive skiing.

Getz et al. (2007) studied the effects of aquatic intervention on perceived physical competence and social acceptance in CP children. Aquatic intervention appeared to have a positive effect on perceived social acceptance and social function, but not on perceived physical competence.

Speech Therapy

Many children with CP have problems with drooling and dysarthria (difficulty in articulating words caused by impairment of the speech muscles). Speech therapy may help with speech, as well as with issues related to feeding and swallowing. In addition, speech therapists can utilize augmentative communication devices or sign language as instructional devices to deliver services.

Clinicians describe children with CP as passive communicators (Pennington and McConachie, 2001). Affected children have problems acquiring communication skills and their conversation with familiar partners is restricted (Pennington et al., 2004a). The conversational partners of children with CP have a tendency to direct and control their interactions. Various factors, such as the degree of the child's motor disability, extent of speech intelligibility problems, and level of cognitive development, shape these restricted conversation patterns (Pennington and McConachie, 2001). In one pilot investigation, Pennington and McConachie (2001) discovered that poor speech intelligibility was the most important factor in producing restrictive communication and recommended therapy to improve the children's speech production. The authors recommended introducing communication aids and training programs for parents to supplement the children's formal speech training.

Based on a literature review, Pennington et al. (2004b) evaluated the effectiveness of speech and language therapy in improving the communication skills of children with CP. Strategies focus on the children directly or their familiar communication partners. With regard to the latter approach, researchers are evaluating the effectiveness of interaction training for conversational partners of children with CP (Pennington et al., 2004a). Researchers are studying such techniques as positioning the conversational partner and child for interaction, creating opportunities for communication, and responding to the child's communication signals. Based on their review of the literature, Pennington et al. (2004b) did not find that speech and language therapy produced positive effects for children with CP. However, positive trends were noted. The authors did not recommend changes in treatment practices, but they did call for more research to investigate the impact of therapy on communication outcomes in children with CP.

Depending on the severity of the disorder, the child may need eyeglasses or surgery to correct a condition, including cross-eyes or strabismus. Hearing aids may also be utilized to help correct any hearing problem

A variety of orthotics, braces, and splints may be utilized as well. These may be placed on the child's legs, arms, or trunk and may assist the child in ambulating, positioning joints, or stretching. A manual wheelchair with seating adaptations to keep the back straight or a power wheelchair (for children with severe spasticity or athetosis) is often needed. Walkers may also be prescribed to enhance mobility. Posterior walkers promote a more upright posture.

Devices and Gadgets

Assistive technology includes grab bars, magnifiers, rails, and Velcro grips for eating utensils and writing implements, as well as voice communication devices, computer software programs, customized wheelchairs and positioning equipment (for the correction of posture).

McDonald and Surtees (2007) evaluated whether adaptive seating pads, commonly used for children with CP, helped with pelvic and hip positioning. Results revealed that seating systems using a sacral pad and kneeblock may not improve overall posture, but may improve hip position in children with CP.

Bjornson et al. (2006) analyzed the utility of dynamic ankle–foot orthoses (DAFO) in children with CP. The authors related that there were significant improvements in crawling/kneeling, standing, walking, running, and jumping skills in children who utilized DAFO's. They also concluded that young children who were independent walkers benefited more than children using assistive devices.

In another report, van Roon and Steenbergen (2006) examined the effect of adapted spoons on food spilling and movement kinematics in adolescents with CP. The results demonstrated the benefits of the use of adapted spoons.

Surgical and Medical Interventions

The most common surgical strategies are for scoliosis and hip dislocation; for severe contractures or deformities on tendons, bones, and joints; for tendon lengthening or transfer; and for osteomy to realign a limb. Intraecal insertion of a baclofen pump has been proved to be useful to help decrease spasticity in the lower extremities and trunk. In this procedure, an intraspinal catheter is placed and connected to a reservoir under the skin of the abdomen. The mechanism then continuously pumps small amounts of antispastic medication (baclofen) into the fluid around the spinal chord. Another relatively common surgical procedure is dorsal rhizotomy, a procedure in which the surgeon cuts a portion of the spinal sensory roots that provide input to spastic leg muscles.

McNee et al. (2007) evaluated the impact of serial casting, specifically the effect of short-term stretch casting on gait in children with spastic CP. Results indicated that casting improved passive and dynamic ankle dorsiflexion, but the changes were small, were short-lived, and did not appear to affect function.

Van Munster et al. (2007) examined the literature on the effects of surgery of the spastic hand in children with CP on functional outcome and muscle coordination. Their review of literature revealed that surgery improved the position of the hand and might improve hand function.

Gannotti et al. (2007) examined the factors associated with longer term outcomes of multilevel surgery in ambulatory CP children. The findings showed that children who demonstrated faster postoperative gait velocity 4 or more years after surgery were younger at the time of the initial evaluation, had undergone fewer surgical procedures, used ankle–foot orthotics postoperatively, and had increased hip extension range of motion. Children who demonstrated greater knee flexion in stance four or more years after surgery had undergone more surgical procedures, greater postoperative popliteal angle, and less knee extension range of motion.

Kerr et al. (2006) investigated the efficacy of neuromuscular electrical stimulation (NMES) and threshold electrical stimulation (TES) in strengthening the leg muscles in children with CP. They concluded that further evidence is required to determine whether electrical stimulation may be helpful as an adjunctive therapy.

Muller-Bolla et al. (2006) assessed the efficacy and safely of hyperbaric oxygen therapy in children with CP. Their findings reveal that exposure to hyperbaric oxygen at medium level pressure was responsible for a significant increase in middle ear barotraumas compared to children who received very low pressure.

Most research on the use of medication with CP children has focused on the utility of intramuscular botulinum toxin. Satila et al. (2006) investigated the effects of botulinum toxin A (BTXA) on impairment and function of the upper limb during a 2-year follow-up period. All CP children benefited from BTXA treatment in terms of reduction in muscle tone and increase in active and passive range of motion. However, results also revealed that spasticity returned within 6 months.

Kawamura et al. (2007) compared the effects of high and low doses of BTXA in CP children and discovered that there were no differences between the high-dose and low-dose groups in upper extremity function.

Sanger et al. (2007) investigated the use of BTXA in children with CP and upper extremity dystonia. They found that BTXA was a safe and effective treatment for upper extremity dystonia in children with CP. Reaching speed improved in response to injection and dystonia scores on various scales improved.

Wallen et al. (2007) examined the use of BTXA in conjunction with occupational therapy. Results revealed that the combination of treatment modalities produced accelerated attainment of functional goals, but no change in active or passive range of motion.

Scheinberg et al. (2006) demonstrated that oral baclofen has an effect beyond placebo in improving goal-oriented tasks in children with CP. Children who were administered baclofen scored significantly higher on the Goal Attainment Scale compared to those children who received a placebo.

Symons et al. (2007) investigated the effects of methylphenidate on the classroom behavior of children with CP (methylphenidate is a psychostimulant drug approved for treatment of attention-deficit hyperactive disorder).

High doses of the medication were associated with exacerbated amounts of stereotyped and disruptive behavior, while low doses of the medication were associated with clinically significant reductions in stereotyped and disruptive behavior.

Ali et al. (2007) evaluated the use of growth hormone therapy (GHT) on children with CP and found that GHT was associated with significant improvement in spinal bone mineral density and linear growth. However, GHT did not improve QOL scores.

Other treatments for CP include craniosacral therapy, Feldenkrais therapy, and acupuncture. These and other complementary and alternative therapies have not been shown to be effective (Liptak, 2005).

Although there have been numerous physical treatment modalities delineated for children with CP, more research is needed on the psychological treatment of children with CP. Zabalia (2007) suggested that psychological intervention with children with CP requires a variety of approaches and that an integrative approach is the best.

Parents and Other Caregivers of Children with CP

The regular caregiving involved in being the parent of a young child can become much more complex and demanding when the child has sensory, communicative, and intellectual disabilities (Raina et al., 2005). Parents of children with severe CP must balance the demands of caring for their child's chronic problems with the usual roles of modern life.

Based on data from the Ontario Motor Growth Study, Raina et al. (2005) examined the health and well-being of caregivers (mainly mothers) of children with CP. The investigators found that the best predictors of caregivers' well-being were their charges' behavior, caregiving demands, and family function. Their results showed that as their children's negative behavior increased, the caregivers' psychological and physical health was reduced. In contrast, positive child behavior predicted the caregivers' higher levels of self-perception and increased ability to cope with stress. Fewer demands on caregivers were linked to their better physical and psychological health and more positive family functioning predicted increased physical and psychological health. The authors also discovered that the caregivers increase in self-perception and being able to manage stress predicted greater psychological healt, but did not directly affect the caregivers' physical health. In addition, the study showed that greater self-esteem and feeling of mastery over caregiving issues were linked to better psychological health. Income and social support had an indirect impact on the caregivers' psychological health, while self-perception, managing stress, income, and social support had an indirect impact on physical health.

Caregivers of children with CP can suffer lower income and disruption in their employment. In a Canadian investigation, Brehaut et al. (2004) discovered that caregivers of children with CP had lower income than the general population of caregivers, after controlling for educational differences between the two samples. Compared to the general population of caregivers, the caregivers of children with CP were less likely to work for pay, less likely to work full-time, and more likely to care for their family as their primary activity.

Based on a qualitative study of mothers and fathers caring for a CP child, Davis et al. (2009) demonstrated that caring for a CP child can have both positive and negative effects on their parents. In their investigation, parents stated that when they obtained CP services for their child, they often felt unsupported. The authors conclude that CP services can be improved for the child if parental concerns and QOL problems are incorporated into the planning of services.

Rentinck et al. (2007) examined the literature to assess parental adaptation to families with a CP child. They concluded that a parent's adaptation may change over time as a function of their child's development and changing stages of family life.

Skok et al. (2006) assessed the impact of stress and social support on mothers of children with CP. They found that social support had a slight to moderate impact on mediating the impact of stress on these mothers.

Education

A number of characteristics may predict school readiness of children with CP. Using a sample of children who survived respiratory distress syndrome after preterm birth, Patrianakos-Hoobler et al. (2010) discovered that impairment and developmental delay at the age of 2 years predicted lack of academic readiness at the age of 5 years and 6 months (92 and 50%, respectively). Among children who were normal at age of 2 years, only 15% were classified as not academically ready. Eleven percent of the 2-year-old children in the sample were classified as disabled and 23% were classified as delayed. When the children reached the age of 5 years and 6 months, 11% required intensive special education and 21% required some special education. Children who had a developmental delay at age 2 years had a greater likelihood of requiring special education if they were disadvantaged in terms of SES.

Intellectual and speech disabilities affect CP children's school readiness. Peeters et al. (2009a) evaluated predictors of verbal working memory (as measured by a forced-recognition task) in CP children in the first grade of special education. The authors demonstrated that intelligence, auditory perception, and speech ability were precursors to verbal working memory. Those CP children who exhibited impairments in intellectual and speech functioning were likely to have restricted verbal working memory.

Given CP children's special education needs, investigators are analyzing the effectiveness of schools in meeting their unique needs. Jenks et al. (2009) evaluated the quality of arithmetic education for CP children. The authors assessed individual education plans, the amount of arithmetic instruction time, arithmetical instructional grouping, and type of arithmetic teaching technique for CP children in special education schools, CP children in mainstream schools, and a control group of children in mainstream schools. The investigators discovered that most of the individual education plans had poorly defined arithmetic goals, and effective assessments were lacking in many of the individual education plans.

Compared to "regular" schools, special education schools devoted much less time to arithmetic instruction (Jenks et al., 2009). Many CP children in the mainstream schools were given individual instruction. The investigators suggest that the offering of individual instruction for these CP children may explain why their arithmetic performance was comparable to the students in the control group.

The authors also discovered that the arithmetic teaching technique for CP children in the special schools did not appear to be optimal, but more research is needed in this area (Jenks et al., 2009).

Epilepsy, which is related to CP and severe mental retardation, is prevalent among students in special schools (Somoza et al., 2009; Tidman et al., 2003), and schools may vary in how they manage this condition (Tidman et al., 2003). Tidman et al. (2003) compared the prevalence, type, and management of epilepsy in children attending mainstream schools and those placed in special education programs. They discovered that children's seizures were better controlled in the mainstream schools, but even so, 44% of these students had ineffectively controlled seizures. The authors recommend that education and health professionals should recognize the need for additional resources for children in this vulnerable group.

Putnam et al. (1996) compared peer acceptance of classmates in both competitive- and cooperative-learning settings. The investigators found that positive changes in peer ratings for both special education and regular education classmates were more likely to occur in cooperative-learning settings than in competitive-learning environments.

In a study of teacher literacy expectations for CP children and those without a disability, Peeters et al. (2009b) showed that teacher expectations for reading and writing success for CP children was lower than for non-disabled children. A number of teachers did not know what to expect about the development of reading and writing skills of CP children. Both student intelligence measures and developing literacy skills predicted teacher expectations about reading development, while student intelligence scores predicted teacher expectations about writing skills.

Peeters et al. (2008b) compared the home literacy environment of CP children with that of comparable peers without disabilities. The authors discovered that both groups had stimulating home literacy environments. However, CP children who had speech or fine motor disabilities had difficulty performing certain literacy tasks. These investigators suggested that teachers and speech and language therapists can offer parents techniques for improving the literacy activities for their children with speech and fine motor impairments.

Mainstreaming is a major educational policy that may help children with special educational needs meet their optimal educational goals. However, in a review of the literature on the effectiveness of mainstreaming/inclusive education, Lindsay (2007) found that studies do not provide conclusive evidence for the positive effects of mainstreaming. Research shows only marginal positive outcomes for children with special education needs. The author suggests that more research is needed to assess which factors impact the education of children with special educational needs.

Case Study

The following case describes a male adolescent with CP. Robert, now 16 years old, was born into an upper class family in a wealthy suburban area. He has two older sisters, who both attended Ivy League colleges. His mother developed a severe viral infection during pregnancy. Robert's pediatrician noted abnormal muscle tone relatively early and Robert was diagnosed with CP. As he grew, he exhibited severe problems with muscle coordination, including ataxia and spasticity, as well as variations in muscle tone. He also displayed difficulty in swallowing and sucking, as well as excessive drooling, particularly when younger.

Because of his parent's education and wealth, Robert received the best of care and education. He even had two aides to assist him at all times, including school. Robert showed no evidence of any significant cognitive impairment, but he was unable to use a writing implement in school, cut with a scissors, or take physical education classes. He attended physical therapy daily and later participated in swimming and hippotherapy. Robert also received speech therapy and occupational therapy several times per week, and underwent over 25 surgeries.

He attended private schools and was accompanied by an aide. His parents made sizable donations to schools to ensure that he was would be accepted and that appropriate accommodations would be made. He typically uses a scooter to get around, but can use a walker for limited movement.

Robert has a number of friends and appears to be well accepted by peers despite his physical limitations. He has strong family support, and gets along well with his older siblings. There is no evidence of enabling him; rather the family encourages independence.

He does not exhibit any evidence of any depression or other emotional disorder. His speech has improved significantly, with only minimal stammering at times. Robert's articulation is clear. His intelligence is average, and he expresses a desire to attend college.

References

Ali, O., Shim, M., Fowler, E., et al. (2007). Growth hormone therapy improves bone mineral density in children with cerebral palsy: a preliminary pilot study. J Clin Endocrinol Metab, 92 (3), 932–937.

Anttila, H., Suoranta, J., Malmivaara, A., et al. (2008). Effectiveness of physiotherapy and conductive education interventions in children with cerebral palsy: a focused review. Am J Phys Med Rehabil, 87 (6), 478–501.

Arnaud, C., White-Koning, M., Michelsen, S.I., et al. (2008). Parent-reported quality of life of children with cerebral palsy in Europe. Pediatrics, 121 (1), 54–64.

Berrin, S.J., Malcarne, V.L., Varni, J.W., et al. (2007). Pain, fatigue and school functioning in children with cerebral palsy. J Pediatr Psychol, 32 (3), 330–337.

Bjornson, K.F., Schamale, G.A., Adamczyk-Foster, A., et al. (2006). The effect of dynamic ankle foot orthoses on function in children with cerebral palsy. J Pediatr Orthop, 26 (6), 773–776.

Brehaut, J.C., Kohne, D.E., Raina, P., et al. (2004). The health of primary caregivers of children with cerebral palsy: how does it compare with that of other Canadian caregivers? Pediatrics, 114 (2), e182–191.

Cherng, R.J., Liu, C.F., Lau, T.W., et al. (2007). Effect of treadmill training with body weight support on gait and gross motor function in children with spastic cerebral palsy. Am J Phys Med Rehabil, 86 (7), 548–555.

Mayo Clinic (2006). Cerebral palsy. Retrieved February 20, 2010 from: http://www.mayoclinic.com/health/cerebral-palsy/DS00302.

Damiano, D.L. (2006). Activity, activity, activity: rethinking our physical therapy approach to cerebral palsy. Phys Ther, 86 (11), 1534–1540.

Dammann, O., O'Shea, T.M. (2007). Happiness reconsidered in children with cerebral palsy. Lancet, 369 (9580), 2137–2138.

Davis, E., Shelly, A., Waters, E., et al. (2009). The impact of caring for a child with cerebral palsy: quality of life for mothers and fathers. Child Care Health Dev, 36 (1), 63–73.

Deluca, S.C., Echols, K., Law, C.R., et al. (2006). Intensive pediatric constraint-induced therapy for children with cerebral palsy: randomized, controlled, crossover trial. J Child Neurol, 21 (11), 931–938.

Dickinson, H.O., Parkinson, K.N., Ravens-Sieberer, U., et al. (2007). Self-reported quality of life of 8–12 year-old children with cerebral palsy: a cross-sectional European study. Lancet, 369 (9580), 2137–2138.

Donkervoort, M., Roebroeck, M., Wiegerink, D., et al. (2007). Determinants of functioning of adolescents and young adults with cerebral palsy. Disabil Rehabil, 29 (6), 453–463.

Dunn, N., Shields, N., Taylor, N.F., et al. (2007). A systematic review of the self-concept of chil dren with cerebral palsy and perceptions of parents and teachers. Phy Occup Ther Pediatr, 27 (3), 55–71.

Engsberg, J.R., Ross, S.A., Collins, D.R. (2006). Increasing ankle strength to improve gait and function in children with cerebral palsy: a pilot study. Pediatr Phys Ther, 18 (4), 266–275.

Fauconnier, J., Dickinson, H.O., Beckung, E., et al. (2009). Participation in life situations of 8–12 year old children with cerebral palsy: cross sectional European study. BMJ, 338, b1458.

Fowler, E.G., Knutson, L.M., DeMuth, S.K., Sugi, M., Siebert, K., Simus, V., Azen, S.P., Winstein, C.J. (2007). Pediatric endurance and limb trengthening for children with cerebral palsy (PEDALS)—a randomized controlled trial protocol for a stationary cycling intervention. BMC Pediatr, 21, 7–14.

Gannotti, M.E., Gorton, G.E., Nahorniak, M.T., et al. (2007). Postoperative gait velocity and mean knee flexion in stance of ambulatory children with spastic diplegia four years or more after multilevel surgery. J Pediatr Orthop, 27 (4), 451–456.

Getz, M., Hutzler, Y., Vermeer, A. (2007). The effects of aquatic intervention on perceived physical competence and social acceptance in children with cerebral palsy. Eur J Special Needs Educ, 22 (2), 217–228.

Gordon, G.S., Simkiss, D.E. (2006). A systematic review of the evidence for hip surveillance in children with cerebral palsy. J Bone Joint Surg Br, 88 (11), 1492–1496.

Hemminki, K., Li, X., Sundquist, K., et al. (2007). High familial risks for cerebral palsy implicate partial heritable aetiology. Paediatr Perinat Epidemiol, 21 (3), 235–241.

Hoare, B.J., Wasiak, J., Imms, C., et al. (2007). Constraint-induced movement therapy in the treatment of the upper-limb in children with hemiplegic cerebral palsy. Cochrane Database Syst Rev, 18 (2), CD004149.

Jenks, K.M., de Moor, J., van Lieshout, E.C., et al. (2009). Quality of arithmetic education for children with cerebral palsy. Int J Rehabil Res, 33 (1), 19–25.

Johnston, M.V., Hagberg, H. (2007). Sex and the pathogenesis of cerebral palsy. Dev Med Child Neurol, 49 (1), 74–78.

Kawamura, A., Campbell, K., Lam-Damji, S., et al. (2007). A randomized controlled trial comparing botulinum toxin A dosage in the upper extremity of children with spasticity. Dev Med Child Neurol, 49 (5), 331–337.

Kerr, C., McDowell, B., Cosgrove, A., et al. (2006). Electrical stimulation in cerebral palsy: a randomized controlled trial. Dev Med Child Neurol, 48 (11), 870–876.

Kozeis, N., Anogeianaki, A., Antonia, M., et al. (2007). Visual function and visual perception in cerebral palsied children. Opthalmic Physiol Opt, 27 (1), 44–53.

Li, J., Vestergaard, M., Obel, C., et al. (2009). Prenatal stress and cerebral palsy: a nationwide cohort study in Denmark. Psychosom Med, 71, 615–618.

Liao, H.F., Liu, Y.C., Liu, W.Y., et al. (2007). Effectiveness of loaded sit-to-stand resistance exercise for children with mild spastic diplegia: a randomized clinical trial. Arch Phys Med Rehabil, 88 (1), 25–31.

Lindsay, G. (2007). Educational psychology and the effectiveness of inclusive education/mainstreaming. Br J Educ Psychol, 77 (Pt 1), 1–24.

Liptak, G.S. (2005). Complementary and alternative therapies for cerebral palsy. Ment Retard Dev Disabil Res Rev, 11 (2), 156–163.

Liptak, G.S., Accardo, P.J. (2004). Health and social outcomes of children with cerebral palsy. J Pediatr, 145 (2 Suppl), S36–41.

Livingston, M.H., Rosenbaum, P.L., Russell, D.J., et al. (2007). Quality of life among adolescents with cerebral palsy: what does the literature tell us? Dev Med Child Neurol, 49 (3), 225–231.

Macgregor, R., Campbell, R., Gladden, M.H., et al. (2007). Effects of massage on the mechanical behavior of muscles in adolescents with spastic diplegia: a pilot study. Dev Med Child Neurol, 49 (3), 187–191.

Massaad, F., van den Hecke, A., Renders, A., et al. (2006). Influence of equinus treatments on the vertical displacement of the body's center of mass in children with cerebral palsy. Dev Med Child Neurol, 48 (10), 813–818.

McDonald, R.L., Surtees, R. (2007). Longitudinal study evaluating a seating system using a sacral pad and kneeblock for children with cerebral palsy. Disabil Rehabil, 29 (13), 1041–1047.

McNee, A.E., Will, E., Lin, J.P., et al. (2007). The effect of serial casting on gait in children with cerebral palsy: preliminary results from a crossover trial. Gait Posture, 25 (3), 463–468.

Morrow, A.M., Quine, S., Loughlin, E.V., et al. (2008). Different priorities: a comparison of parents' and health professionals' perceptions of quality of life in quadriplegic cerebral palsy. Arch Dis Child, 93 (2), 119–125.

Muller-Bolla, M., Collet, J.P., Ducruet, T., et al. (2006). Side effects of hyperbaric oxygen therapy in children with cerebral palsy. Undersea Hyperb Med, 33 (4), 237–244.

Nadeau, L., Tessier, R. (2006). Social adjustment of children with cerebral palsy in mainstream classes. Dev Med Child Neurol, 48 (5), 331–336.

Parkes, J., White-Koning, M., Dickinson, H.O., et al. (2008). Psychological problems in children with cerebral palsy: a cross-sectional European study. J Child Psychol Psychiatry, 49 (4), 405–413.

Parkes, J., White-Koning, M., McCullough, N., et al. (2009). Psychological problems in children with hemiplegia: a European multicentre survey. Arch Dis Child, 94 (6), 429–433.

Patel, D.R. (2005). Therapeutic interventions in cerebral palsy. Indian J Pediatr, 72 (11), 979–983.

Patrianakos-Hoobler, Msal, M.E., Hua, D., Marks, J.D., Plesha-Troyke, S., Schreiber, M.D. (2010). Predicting school readiness from neurodevelopmental assessments at age two years after respiratory distress syndrome in infants born premature. Dev Med Child Neurol, 100 (4), 524–528.

Peeters, M., Verhoeven, L., de Moor, J. (2009a). Predictors of verbal working memory in children with cerebral palsy. Res Dev Disabil, 30 (6), 1502–1511.

Peeters, M., Verhoeven, L., de Moor, J. (2009b). Teacher literacy expectations for kindergarten children with cerebral palsy in special education. Int J Rehabil Res, 32 (3), 251–259.

Peeters, M., Verhoeven, L., van Balkom, H., de Moor, J. (2008a). Foundations of phonological awareness in pre-school children with cerebral palsy: the impact of intellectual disability. J Intellect Disabil Res, 52 (Pt 1), 68–78.

Peeters, M., Verhoeven, L., van Balkom, H., et al. (2008b). Home literacy environment: characteristics of children with cerebral palsy. Int J Lang Commun Disord, Dec. 19, 1–24.

Pennington, L., Goldbart, J., Marshall, J. (2004a). Interaction training for conversational partners of children with cerebral palsy: a systematic review. Int J Lang Commun Disord, 39 (2), 151–170.

Pennington, L., Goldbart, J., Marshall, J., et al. (2004b). Speech and language therapy to improve the communication skills of children with cerebral palsy. Cochrane Database Syst Rev, 2, CD003466.

Pennington, L., McConachie, H. (2001). Predicting patterns of interaction between children with cerebral palsy and their mothers. Dev Med Child Neurol, 43 (2), 83–90.

Pin, T., Dyke, P., Chan, M. (2006). The effectiveness of passive stretching in children with cerebral palsy: a cross-sectional European study. Dev Med Child Neurol, 48 (10), 855–862.

Putnam, J., Markovchick, K., Johnson, D.W., et al. (1996). Cooperative learning and peer acceptance of students with learning disabilities. J Soc Psychol, 136 (6), 741–752.

Raina, P., O'Donnell, M., Rosenbaum, P., et al. (2005). The health and well-being of caregivers of children with cerebral palsy. Pediatrics, 115 (6), e626–36.

Reading, R. (2007). Review of self-reported quality of life of 8-12 year-old children with cerebral palsy: a cross-sectional European study. Child Care Health Dev, 33 (6), 804–805.

Rentinck, I.C., Ketelaar, M., Jongmans, M.J., et al. (2007). Parents of children with cerebral palsy: a review of factors related to the process of adaptation. Child Care Health Dev, 33 (2), 161–169.

Sanger, T.D., Kukke, S.N., Sherman-Levine, S. (2007). Botulinum toxin type B improves the speed of reaching in children with cerebral palsy and arm dystonia: an open-label, dose-escalation pilot study. J Child Neurol, 22 (1), 116–122.

Satila, H., Kotamaki, A., Koivikko, M., et al. (2006). Upper limb function after botulinum toxin A treatment in cerebral palsy: two years follow-up of six cases. Pediatr Rehabil, 9 (3), 247–258.

Scheinberg, A., Hall, K., Lam, L.T., et al. (2006). Oral baclofen in children with cerebral palsy: a double-blind cross over pilot study. J Paediatr Child Health, 42 (11), 715–720.

Skok, A., Harvey, D., Reddihough, D. (2006). Perceived stress, perceived social support and wellbeing among mothers of children with cerebral palsy. J Intellect Dev Disabil, 31 (1), 53–57.

Snider, L., Korner-Bitensky, N., Kammann, C., et al. (2007). Horseback riding as therapy for children with cerebral palsy: is there evidence of its effectiveness? Phys Occup Ther Pediatr, 27 (2), 5–23.

Somoza, M.J., Forlenza, R.H., Brussino, M., et al. (2009). Epidemiological survey of epilepsy in the special school population in the city of Buenos Aires. A comparison with mainstream schools. Neuroepidem, 32 (2), 129–135.

Sparkes, J., Hall, D. (2007). Quality of life in children with cerebral palsy. Lancet, 370 (9588), 656.

Sterba, J.A. (2006). Adaptive downhill skiing in children with cerebral palsy: effect on gross motor function. Pediatr Phys Ther, 18 (4), 289–296.

Sterba, J.A. (2007). Does horseback riding therapy or therapist-assisted hippotherapy rehabilitate children with cerebral palsy? Dev Med Child Neurol, 49 (1), 68–73.

Symons, F.J., Tervo, R.C., Kim, O., et al. (2007). The effects of methylphenidate on the classroom behavior of elementary school-age children with cerebral palsy: a preliminary observational analysis. J Child Neurol, 22 (1), 89–94.

Thorgood, C., Alexander, M.A. (2005). Cerebral palsy. Retrieved from: www.emedicine.com

Tidman, L., Saravanan, K., Gibbs, J. (2003). Epilepsy in mainstream and special educational primary school settings. Seizure, 12 (1), 47–51.

Unger, M., Faure, M., Frieg, A. (2006). Strength training in adolescent learners with cerebral palsy. Clin Rehabil, 20 (6), 469–477.

Van Munster, J.C., Maathuis, K.G., Haga, N., et al. (2007). Does surgical management of the hand in children with spastic unilateral cerebral palsy affect functional outcome? Dev Med Child Neurol, 49 (5), 385–389.

Van Roon, D., Steenbergen, B. (2006). The use of ergonomic spoons by people with cerebral palsy: effects on food spilling and movement kinematics. Dev Med Child Neurol, 48 (11), 888–891.

Wallen, M., O'Flaherty, S.J., Waugh, M.C. (2007). Functional outcomes of intramuscular botulinum toxin type A and occupational therapy in the upper limbs of children with cerebral palsy: a randomized controlled trial. Arch Phys Med Rehabil, 88 (2), 1–10.

Waters, E., Maher, E., Salmon, L., et al. (2005). Development of a condition-specific measure of quality of life for children with cerebral palsy: empirical thematic data reported by parents and children. Child Care Health Dev, 31 (2), 127–135.

Weindling, A.M., Cunningham, C.C., Glenn, S.M., et al. (2007). Additional therapy for young children with spastic cerebral palsy: a randomized controlled study. Health Technol Assess, 11 (16), 1–71.

Wiegerink, D.J., Roebroeck, M.E., Donkervoort, M., et al. (2006). Social and sexual relationships of adolescents and young adults with cerebral palsy: a review. Clin Rehabil, 20 (12), 1023–1031.

Williams, H., Pountney, T. (2007). Effects of a static bicycling program on the functional ability of young people with cerebral palsy who are non-ambulant. Dev Med Child Neurol, 49 (7), 522–527.

Zabalia, M. (2007). Integrative therapeutic approach for the intervention with children with cerebral palsy. Neuropsychiatrie de l'Enfance et de l'Adolescence, 55 (1), 52–57.

Chapter 5
Attention-Deficit Hyperactivity Disorder

Attention-deficit/hyperactivity disorder (AD/HD or ADHD) is a disorder that affects neurobehavioral functioning and development (Banerjee et al., 2007; Zwi et al., 2000). In children, ADHD is the most prevalent diagnosed cognitive and behavior disorder among school children (Banerjee et al., 2007). ADHD consists of recurring problems with impulse control and inattention and can involve symptoms of hyperactivity (Biederman and Faraone, 2005; American Psychiatric Association, 2000).

Various epidemiological neuropsychological, neuroimaging, genetic, and treatment investigations reveal that ADHD is a legitimate medical condition (Banerjee et al., 2007). The disorder has been recognized as part of society for a long time. Crichton (1798, 2001) discussed the phenomenon of mental restless. In 1937, using stimulants to treat the condition was first discussed (Patrick et al., 2009).

Over time, the term for the disorder has changed. The condition has been described as learning/behavioral disabilities, hyperactivity, minimal brain damage, minimal brain dysfunction, or hyperkinetic reaction of childhood. The diagnosis, attention-deficit disorder (ADD) with or without hyperactivity, was introduced in the DSM-III. In the DSM-IV, the diagnosis was changed to ADHD.

Experts disagree about whether the symptoms and impairments of ADHD are expressed differently in various cultures (Caldararo, 2002, 2003). However, the condition is viewed in divergent ways depending on different factors. ADHD is viewed in certain ways depending on how experts relate to the topic. Specialists may use terms from the DSM-IV to describe the disorder. Some experts view the condition in regard to biological factors or character flaws (Danforth and Yogawin, 2001).

Some critics, including Fred Baughman and Peter Braggin, see ADHD as a fraud perpetrated by the psychiatric profession and pharmaceutical industry. They view the condition as a fraud perpetrated on families who try to make sense of their children's perplexing behaviors. Russell Barkley and Xavier Catellanos assert that the condition is a true psychiatric disorder. Castellanos, however, has pointed out that the phenomenon is poorly understood (Castellanos, 2000).

One of the problems associated with the disorder is that the recognition of ADHD as a problem has led to the development of ineffective school policies that may result in over diagnosing of the condition among some school children (Kidd, 2000).

M.L. Goldstein, S. Morewitz, *Chronic Disorders in Children and Adolescents*,
DOI 10.1007/978-1-4419-9764-7_5, © Springer Science+Business Media, LLC 2011

Regardless of treatment, children diagnosed with ADHD often have comorbid conditions and suffer substantial social, educational, and family problems and reduced health-related quality of life (HRQL) (Molina et al., 2009; Loe and Feldman, 2007; Breslau et al., 2009; Peters and Jackson, 2009; Klassen et al., 2004). Based on a cross-sectional survey of 165 children who were referred to an ADHD Clinic in British Columbia, Canada, Klassen et al. (2004) showed that children with ADHD had more parent-reported problems in behavioral and emotional functioning, emotional well-being, and self-esteem.

In Klassen et al. (2004)'s investigation, 131 children were diagnosed with ADHD. Of these, 68.7% had a comorbid psychiatric disorder. Twenty of these ADHD children had two comorbid conditions, five had three comorbid conditions, and one had four comorbid problems. Fifty-one ADHD children were diagnosed with a comorbid learning disorder (LD), 45 had either oppositional defiant disorder (ODD) or conduct disorder (CD), and 27 suffered from another type of comorbid problem. ADHD children with comorbid disorders tend to have lower psychosocial-related HRQL than those without comorbid conditions. ADHD children with two or more comorbid conditions had worse psychosocial health across a variety of psychosocial HRQL areas than ADHD children with none or one comorbid disorder.

Based on a sample of 105 Korean children, Byun et al. (2006) showed that 80 children had at least one comorbid problem such as ODD, anxiety disorders, and affective disorders.

ADHD children have an increased likelihood of having low grades, low standardized reading and mathematics scores, and increased grade retention (Loe and Feldman, 2007; Galera et al., 2009). Based on a sample of 1,264 individuals, aged 12–25 years of age, from the longitudinal GAZEL Youth study, Galera et al. (2009) revealed that childhood and adolescent hyperactivity-inattention symptoms increased the likelihood of grade retention, failure to graduate from secondary school, earning a lower level diploma, and worse academic achievement.

ADHD children are likely to have greater use of school services, higher rates of detention and expulsion, and low rates of graduation from high school and postsecondary schools (Loe and Feldman, 2007). The high rates of expulsion and school dropout explain why almost 50% of all students with ADHD never complete high school. Another report found that less than 5% of persons in the USA with the disorder graduate from college (Cimera 2002).

Both the problematic behaviors of the ADHD children and the educational practices of their teachers may affect the affected students' academic performance.

Using an ethnically diverse cohort of 693 children assessed at age 6 and 17, Breslau et al. (2009) discovered that teacher evaluations of student attention problems predicted subsequent achievement in mathematics and reading.

Child and family characteristics may influence the academic achievement and level of behavioral adjustment of children with the disorder. In a longitudinal investigation of 115 ADHD children and a 59 controls from elementary through secondary school, Latimer et al. (2003) discovered that positive emotional and behavioral status during middle school mediated their negative academic and behavioral functioning during high school. The researchers also demonstrated that family conditions during middle school influenced the behavior of both ADHD and non-ADHD children in high school. Moreover, the students' previous academic achievement predicted their subsequent performance levels.

Unfortunately, children with the disorder often have families that are characterized by varying degrees of impaired family and marital functioning, difficult parent–child interactions, and parents' beliefs about lower parenting self-efficacy (Johnston and Mash, 2001). Moreover, the presence of ADHD in children is related to increased parental stress and parental mental health problems (Peters and Jackson, 2009).

Based on in-depth interviews of 11 mothers of ADHD children, Peters and Jackson (2009) showed that these mothers experience substantial stress and role demands from parenting a child with this disorder. The mothers suffered from so much stress from these responsibilities that they felt marginalized, stigmatized, and criticized.

Parental coping styles may affect parent–child interactions, including how parents discipline their ADHD children (Modesto-Lowe et al., 2008; McKee et al., 2004; Harvey et al., 2003). In a literature review, Modesto-Lowe et al. (2008) demonstrated that ADHD symptoms in children produce high parental stress and dysfunctional parenting. Parents of children with the condition often have mental health problems that affect how they respond to their child's symptoms. McKee et al. (2004) discovered that mothers of ADHD children who relied on more dysfunctional coping styles were more likely to be associated with more self reported weak and over-reactive discipline, more observed coercive parenting, and more observed child misbehavior before parent training. Fathers of ADHD children who used more dysfunctional coping patterns were more likely to report using weak discipline before and after parent training.

Impaired parental coping styles and other family difficulties are especially prominent when the ADHD child has comorbid CD and ODD (Pfiffner et al., 2005; Kilic and Sener, 2005; Satake et al., 2004; Klassen et al., 2004). ADHD is highly comorbid with CD and ODD, and these comorbidities can negatively alter the response, course, and outcome of treatment (Chronis et al., 2004; Pfiffner et al., 2005).

Investigators have analyzed the nature of family characteristics and functioning in families with ADHD children who have comorbid CD and ODD. In a study of 92 Turkish children, aged 6–11, diagnosed with ADHD and ADHD with comorbid ODD/CD, Kilic and Sener (2005) reported that maternal depression and paternal alcoholic drinking difficulties were prevalent among parents of ADHD children with comorbid ODD and CD. Unhealthy functioning was evident in the families of ADHD children with comorbid ODD and CD. Children with ADHD and comorbid ODD and CD scored high on the Child Behavior List subscales except for the subscales dealing with social withdrawal and sexual difficulties.

Using a sample of 149 families, Pfiffner et al. (2005) showed that negative and ineffective discipline by mothers was linked to ADHD children with comorbid ODD and CD. Lack of maternal warmth and involvement, negative and ineffective discipline by fathers, and fathers with an antisocial personality disorder were related to comorbid CD, but not ODD in ADHD children.

ADHD is a life-long chronic problem (Van Cleave and Leslie, 2008; Van Ameringen et al., 2010). Between 30 and 50% of the children diagnosed with the condition continue to have related problems as adults (Balint et al., 2008; Elia et al., 1999). In the USA, an estimated eight million adults have ADHD.

Based on a sample of 129 patients who were referred to an anxiety disorders clinic, Van Ameringen et al. (2010) found that the rate of adult ADHD was 27.9%. Most of the sample was female and single. In their study, major depressive disorder, social phobia, generalized anxiety disorder, and impulse control disorders were the most prevalent comorbid conditions among the adult ADHD patients.

Adults with ADHD who are not treated frequently have lifestyles that are chaotic and seem disorganized. As they age, these individuals develop ways of coping with their disabilities (Gentile, 2004). Some of these individuals may cope by using non-prescription drugs and alcohol.

Researchers have assessed the possible link between ADHD in childhood and adolescence and suicidal behaviors (Sourander et al., 2009; Galera et al., 2008). Based on the results of the Finnish 1981 Birth Cohort Study, using a sample of 5,302 individuals who were born in 1981, Sourander et al. (2008) discovered that among males, living in a broken family, psychological, hyperkinetic, conduct, and emotional problems at age 8 years predicted completed or serious suicide attempts. Among females, no associations were found between study variables at 8 years of age and suicide behaviors.

Similar findings were obtained using a sample of 916 persons, aged 7–18 years, from the longitudinal GAZEL Youth study (Galera et al., 2008). This investigation revealed that among males, hyperactivity-inattention symptoms were associated with an increased risk of both lifetime suicide plans and attempts and 12-month prevalence rates of suicide plans and attempts among adolescents. In contrast, hyperactivity-inattention symptoms did not increase the risk of lifetime suicide plans and attempts among females or adolescent 12-month prevalence rates of suicide plans and attempts.

In terms of functioning in different work environments, adults with ADHD are more likely to function better in less structured work settings that have fewer workplace regulations. They do better in jobs that have substantial autonomy such as self-employment. Persons who have symptoms of hyperactivity have a greater chance of changing jobs frequently because of their recurring need for stimulation and new interests.

Controversies About ADHD

ADHD is a controversial condition and has been since the 1970s. The controversies have centered on issues of diagnosis and treatment and have involved parents, teachers, clinicians, policy makers, and the media (Mayes et al., 2008; Cohen and Cicchetti, 2006). Some individuals believe that the disorder does not exist. Niedermeyer and Naidu (1997) reported that persons with the condition do not have any brain dysfunction, and the cause of the disorder is still unknown. Others doubt whether ADHD continues into adulthood. Clinicians have difficulty diagnosing the condition in adults because of inadequate diagnostic criteria, developmental changes, comorbid disorders, and the fact that persons with high levels of intelligence or situational variables can hide symptoms of the disease.

Jadad et al. (1999) identified five aspects of the condition that help to make it a controversial disorder. First, there are no confirmatory tests or specific characteristics for the disorder. Second, the diagnostic criteria for the disorder have changed often. Third, there is no cure for the disease, necessitating long-term treatment. Fourth, treatment involves the use of stimulants which have potential for abuse. Finally, in various countries, the rates of diagnosing and treating ADHD vary.

In addition to causing drug addiction and withdrawal reactions, the adverse effects of stimulant medications can include psychosis and depression. However, their long-term impact and effects in pregnancy have not been researched extensively. Therefore, the long-term effects are mostly unknown (Ashton et al., 2006).

Other controversies focus on whether ADHD has genetic and physiological causes, while another question centers on whether the use of stimulants is an effective treatment. Most clinicians believe that condition is a real disorder. However, clinicians still disagree over how to best diagnose and treat ADHD (Sim et al., 2004; Schonwald and Lechner, 2006).

ADHD Symptoms

Impulsiveness, hyperactivity, and inattention are the most prevalent symptoms of ADHD (Paule et al., 2000). Problems of impulsiveness consist of such behaviors as engaging in activities without first thinking of the consequences, quickly moving from one activity to another, and interrupting the conversations of other persons. Indicators of hyperactive behavior include being distracted easily, fidgeting, squirminess, climbing on objects, and non-restful sleep. Inattention is characterized by being easily distracted, day-dreaming, not completing work, problems in listening, and clumsiness in motor activities.

According to the DSM-IV, three sub-types of ADHD symptoms exist: inattentive, hyperactive/impulsive, and combined. A majority of individuals experience some of these symptoms. However, their symptoms do not disrupt their social, family, educational, or occupational functioning.

In an investigation of 105 Korean children, Byun et al. (2006) discovered that 70 were diagnosed with the combined-type disorder, 22 with the predominantly inattentive subtype, and only one with the predominantly hyperactive-impulsive subtype.

Among children with ADHD, hyperactivity is a frequent problem. However, symptoms of hyperactivity tend to fade away in adults. With regard to the symptoms of inattention, more than 50% of children with ADHD continue to suffer from problems of inattention in adulthood.

Comorbid Disorders

Children with ADHD often suffer from co-existing disorders and substance abuse, making the diagnosis and treatment of the condition more challenging. According to Pliszka (2000), approximately 20–25% of children with ADHD have a diagnosable LD. Lamminmaky et al. (1995) found that when a child has inattention problems, she or he also is more likely to have LDs.

In boys, ADHD is not linked to an increased rate of substance abuse unless the boys also have a co-existing CD (Lynskey and Hall, 2001). Adults with ADHD may have an increased probability of substance abuse problems, but further research is needed in this area.

Persons with ADHD may suffer from anxiety, depression, and other comorbid conditions. As children with the condition get older, they may increasingly develop depression (Brunsvold and Oepen, 2008; Van Ameringen et al., 2010). As girls with the disorder get older, they have a higher rate of increase than boys. The prevalence of depression in children with ADHD differs depending on the sub-type of ADHD symptoms.

As discussed previously, ADHD children may exhibit ODD and CD, both of which consist of antisocial behaviors, including aggression, frequent temper tantrums, deceitfulness, and stealing (Klassen et al., 2004; Masi et al., 2008; Byun et al., 2006). Using a sample of 198 children and adolescents consecutively diagnosed as having CD, Masi et al. (2008) evaluated risk factors and responses to treatment. They reported that in children with pre-pubertal-onset CD, two types of aggressive behaviors, predatory (e.g., planned) and affective (e.g., impulsive), and ADHD comorbidity were more prevalent than in children who did not have pre-pubertal-onset of CD.

Children with ADHD may suffer from primary disorder of vigilance, which involves difficulties in staying awake, poor attention and concentration, yawning, fidgeting, and being hyperactive in order to stay alert.

Boys with the combined subtype of ADHD symptoms are more likely than girls with the same condition to have a mood disorder (Bauermeister et al., 2007). Bipolar disorder is another comorbid condition in children with ADHD. Up to 25% of these children suffer from bipolar disorder. Children with ADHD and bipolar disorder may exhibit more aggressive behaviors and other behavioral problems than children who only have ADHD without co-existing conditions.

ADHD children may also suffer from an anxiety disorder (Byun et al., 2006; Bauermeister et al., 2007). Girls who are diagnosed with the inattentive sub-type of ADHD symptoms are more likely than boys to have a higher rate of an anxiety disorder (Bauermeister et al., 2007). Obsessive-compulsive disorder (OCD) is a co-existing condition among children with ADHD. OCD may have some genetically similarity to ADHD and share many of the same attributes.

Using a sample of 257 consecutive pediatric patients who were diagnosed using a DSM-IV-based clinical protocol, Masi et al. (2010) discovered that patients with OCD with an onset before the age of 12 were more likely to have comorbid tic disorder and disruptive behavior disorders. Comorbid tic disorder was more prevalent in boys, started earlier, and was more related to comorbid ADHD and other disruptive behavior problems. Comorbid ADHD in these pediatric patients was related to an earlier onset of OCD and worse responses to therapy.

Epilepsy is a prevalent comorbid disorder among persons with ADHD (Tan and Appleton, 2005; Aldenkamp et al., 2006). In addition, patients with some types of epilepsy produce symptoms like ADHD, and these symptoms can lead clinicians to misdiagnose them as having ADHD.

In children, Tourette syndrome often occurs in combination with ADHD (Pollak et al., 2009). However, researchers are unsure of the etiology of this comorbidity (Pringsheim et al., 2009). Using a sample of 181 children with Tourette syndrome and ADHD and 172 controls, one report showed that children with Tourette syndrome and ADHD were more likely to be exposed to low birth weight, prematurity, breathing difficulties, and maternal smoking compared to children with Tourette syndrome only (Pringsheim et al., 2009). The authors conclude that since ADHD only and tic-related ADHD have common risk factors, both conditions may have a common underlying neurobiological origin.

How does the functioning of ADHD children compare with that of children who have other conditions? Using teacher ratings on the Strengths and Difficulties Questionnaire (SDQ), Iizuka et al. (2010) discovered that ADHD children had more evidence of hyperactivity, inattention, and conduct problems than children with high-functioning autism spectrum disorder (HFASD). However, according to the teacher ratings, HFASD children exhibited more peer problems than ADHD children. The parent ratings of the SDQ revealed that HFASD children had more emotional and peer problems. The teacher ratings of the SDQ indicated that both ADHD and HFASD children had more difficulties in engaging in pro-social behaviors than did the parent ratings.

Causes/Risk Factors

ADHD has no known cause (Bailly, 2005). Instead, a variety of genetic and environmental factors, e.g., diet, maternal, and social conditions, may influence the development of the disorder

Genetic Factors

ADHD is very heritable. Family investigations show that parents and siblings of ADHD children have a two to eight times increased risk for developing ADHD (Banerjee et al., 2007; NHS, 2008). Studies of twins and adoptions support the highly genetic nature of the condition, although environmental factors also contribute to the disorder. The average heritability of the disorder is 0.77, making it comparable to other neuropsychiatric problems such as schizophrenia and bipolar disorder.

A combination of different genes, especially those that influence dopamine transporters, may influence the development of the disorder. Dopamine transporter, dopamine receptor D4, dopamine beta-hydroxylase, monoamine oxidase A, catecholamine-methyl transferase, and serotonin transporter promoter (SLC6A4), 5-hydroxytryptamine 2A receptor (5-HT2A), 5-hydroxytryptamine 1B receptor (5-HT1B) are some of the candidate genes (Roman et al., 2004).

ADHD does not adhere to a traditional genetic disease model because of the variety of targets thought to cause the disorder. Therefore, the disorder is a consequence of a complex interaction among genetic and environmental variables. Even though genetic factors may play a role, no single gene has been identified as playing a part in the etiology of the disorder (Acosta et al., 2004).

Environmental Factors

According to twin studies, non-genetic factors may account for 9–20% of the symptoms of ADHD (Sherman et al., 1997). Fetal exposure to tobacco smoke and alcohol during pregnancy, environmental exposure to lead in very early life, social adversity (e.g., being young, single with low educational attainment), and maternal psychosocial stress may influence the development of ADHD (Rodriguez et al., 2009; Rodriguez and Bohlin, 2005; St. Sauver et al., 2004; Langley et al., 2005; Obel et al., 2009; Schmitz et al., 2006; Braun et al., 2006; Banerjee et al., 2007; Linnet et al., 2003; Ha et al., 2009).

Nicotine from cigarette smoke may cause hypoxia or lack of oxygen to the fetus in utero (BBC, 2005). Another possible explanation is that women with ADHD have a greater likelihood of smoking (Science Daily, November 24, 2008). Because of the strong genetic basis of ADHD, these women have a higher probability of having children who develop the disorder (Science Daily, April 11, 2007).

Using a case–control investigation, Schmitz et al. (2006) reported that the children of mothers who smoked 10 or more cigarettes per day during pregnancy were more likely to develop ADHD-1 than children who were not exposed to nicotine during pregnancy.

Maternal smoking and stress during pregnancy may increase the probability of ADHD symptoms in children (Rodriguez and Bohlin, 2005). Based on a sample of 290 nulliparous Scandinavian women and 208 teachers, Rodriguez and Bohlin (2005) showed that prenatal exposure to smoking and stress independently predicts ADHD symptoms in children.

In their review of five studies of maternal psychosocial stress and possible ADHD, Linnet et al. (2003) discovered that the association between psychosocial stress during pregnancy and later ADHD symptoms in children were inconsistent. However, the authors noted that maternal psychosocial stress may modestly contribute to the onset of ADHD symptoms in children.

Pregnancy-related complications, such as low birth weight, are linked to the symptoms of the disorder (Langley et al., 2007; Martel et al., 2007).

With regard to prenatal exposure to alcohol, researchers have found conflicting results about whether exposure to low levels of maternal alcohol use during pregnancy is associated with ADHD symptoms (Linnet et al., 2003; Rodriguez et al., 2009). Linnet et al. (2003), after reviewing nine investigations about the possible link between prenatal exposure to alcohol and the development of ADHD in children, discovered inconsistent results.

Based on 21,678 reports from the Strengths and Difficulties Questionnaire or the Rutter Scale using three pregnancy cohorts within the Nordic Network on ADHD, Rodriguez et al. (2009) discovered that exposure to low doses of alcohol during pregnancy was not associated with ADHD symptoms in children in the three cohorts after controlling for social adversity and smoking.

Low blood lead levels have been found to be linked to ADHD (Ha et al., 2009; Nigg et al., 2008). Based on a sample of 1,778 children from 10 elementary schools in South Korea, Ha et al. (2009) showed that blood lead concentrations, even at low levels, were related to ADHD symptoms. However, this investigation did not find an association between blood mercury levels and symptoms of ADHD.

Nigg et al. (2008), using a sample of 150 children, aged 8–17 years, showed that children with ADHD-combined type had higher blood lead levels than children without ADHD. Symptoms of hyperactivity–impulsivity were linked to blood lead levels. However, symptoms of inattention–disorganizations were not related to blood lead levels. Blood level was associated with lower IQ, and hyperactivity mediated the impact of blood lead concentrations on IQ. The researchers conclude that low concentrations of blood lead are a risk factor for ADHD. However, this association is mediated by less effective cognitive control.

One report showed that pre-pregnancy BMI is related to ADHD symptoms in children (Rodriguez et al., 2008). Based on a follow-up of prospective pregnancy cohorts (12,556 school children rated by teachers), Rodriguez et al. (2008) showed that children of mothers who were both overweight and acquired a large amount of weight during pregnancy were two times more likely to have symptoms of ADHD than children of normal-weight mothers.

Ray et al. (2009) discovered that compared to mothers of non-ADHD children, the mothers of ADHD children had a greater likelihood of being diagnosed with many medical and psychosocial problems in a 2-year period before their child was born. The mothers of ADHD children were diagnosed with such conditions as depression, anxiety, and musculoskeletal problems. In addition, the mothers of ADHD children were more likely than the mothers of non-ADHD children to have higher total health-care costs per person in the year before and the 2 years after their child's delivery.

Diet Factors

Various investigations have not found that sugar worsens the symptoms of children with ADHD or that it is a cause of the condition (Benton, 2008; Staudenmayer, 1999). Food additives are not linked to ADHD symptoms. However, according to

Kemp (2008), removing food additives from the diet of ADHD children might be useful.

Social and Behavioral Factors

Social adversity, which is reflected in lower socioeconomic status, is also associated with ADHD in children (Langley et al., 2007; St. Sauver et al., 2004). Researchers have examined the possible independent impact of maternal smoking and maternal socioeconomic status on ADHD symptoms in children. Based on a clinical sample of 356 children with ADHD, Langley et al. (2007) discovered that prenatal exposure to smoking and lower socioeconomic status predicted ADHD symptoms in children.

Using a case–control investigation of 305 children with ADHD and 5,326 controls, St. Sauver et al. (2004) discovered that male gender and low parental education were major risk factors for the development of ADHD. In their investigation, pregnancy and labor factors, low birth weight and twin births did not predict ADHD.

In their review of the literature, Linnet et al. (2003) found a modest association between psychosocial stress during pregnancy and ADHD in children. Rodriguez and Bohlin (2005) assessed the possible association between maternal smoking and stress during pregnancy and ADHD symptoms in children. They discovered that prenatal exposure to stress and smoking were independent predictors of ADHD, especially among boys.

In sexually abused children, ADHD and posttraumatic stress disorder (PTSD) are the most prevalent diagnosed conditions (Weinstein et al., 2000; Cuffe, 1994). These two conditions overlap in terms of symptoms and comorbid disorders. Weinstein et al. (2000) recommend changing assessment guidelines to better evaluate traumatic experiences in children who present with ADHD symptoms.

Based on a case–control sample of consecutive outpatient admissions to a child psychiatric program, Ford et al. (2000) discovered that children with ODD and ADHD, to a lesser degree, were more likely to have a history of physical or sexual abuse. Children were at greater risk for severe PTSD symptoms if they suffered both ADHD and physical or sexual abuse or if they suffered from ODD and trauma resulting from an illness or accident.

Children who are physically and sexually abused and experience parental disruption may be at increased risk for ADHD. Cohen et al. (2002), using a sample of 99 physically abused adolescents and 99 controls, discovered that both parental marital disruption and physical abuse increased 15 times the adolescents' lifetime risk of ADHD. However, the authors showed that parental marital status by itself did not increase the risk of psychosocial problems among adolescents.

Alternative Theories of ADHD

Various alternative theories about the etiology of ADHD have been proposed. Hartmann suggested that persons with this condition possess some of the traits of hunters from pre-agricultural societies (Hartmann, 2003). Others believe that

ADHD reflects neurodiversity or atypical neurological development. According to these critics, ADHD symptoms should be respected like other individual differences. Social critics stress the fact that children with ADHD symptoms may have difficulties in meeting the social expectations regarding their behaviors for a variety of social reasons, although biological factors may play a role as well.

Another perspective is that the condition is associated with creative activities. Smalley (2008) believes that genetic research will help us differentiate between the disorder and various normal or even creative processes.

Social construct theorists do not believe that the condition is mainly a biological condition (Stead et al., 2005). For example, Szasz asserts that the disorder is invented (Szasz, 2001; Chriss, 2007). These critics suggest that the disorder is better understood in terms of environmental causes or personality differences (National Institute of Clinical Excellence, 2009).

Another perspective is that the condition occurs because of an individual's abnormally low arousal state (incrediblehorizons.com; ADHD, sci.csuhayward.edu). According to this view, persons with the disorder cannot moderate their behaviors on their own. Instead, they seek to stimulate themselves or engage in excessive actions, e.g., fidget, walk around, and talk, to cope with their abnormally low state of arousal. This approach shows why stimulant medications are successful in calming children with ADHD. According to this perspective, ADHD results from problems with dopamine and are reflected in low-stimulation PET scan findings.

Diagnosis

The diagnosis of ADHD is a clinical one since there is no objective test for the condition (Joughin et al., 2003). Diagnosing ADHD should be based on history taking, standardized rating scales, and assessment of the patient's behaviors and reports from informants (Vierhile et al., 2009).

The DSM-IV criteria is used to make the clinical diagnosis in North America, while in Europe, the ICD-10 is used (Moffitt and Melchior, 2007). Most people have many ADHD symptoms occasionally. In persons with the condition, however, the symptoms are more frequent and they result in substantial disability in social, educational, occupational, and family functioning. To be classified as having ADHD, these symptom-related impairments must occur in different settings, e.g., school, family, and work settings.

According to the American Academy of Pediatrics (2001) Clinical Practice Guidelines for children with ADHD, an accurate diagnosis takes into account:

1. the DSM-IV-TR Manual.
2. findings about the child's symptoms in different settings.
3. comorbid conditions that may make the diagnosis more difficult or complicate the treatment plans.

A variety of medical, social, and psychological problems must be excluded before diagnosing ADHD. Hypothyroidism, anemia, lead poisoning, chronic disease, hearing or vision disability, and side effects from medications are some of the medical problems that must be considered (Smucker and Heydayat, 2001). Moreover, problems associated with substance abuse and child abuse must be excluded before diagnosing ADHD.

ADHD and sleep are linked in complex ways. The central nervous system mechanisms that regulate sleep overlap with those that regulate attention and arousal (Owens, 2005). Individuals with primary sleep disorders present various symptoms of inattention and difficulties in regulating behaviors. Children who are sleepy exhibit a range of behaviors from yawning and rubbing eyes to exhibiting inattentiveness, mood lability, and impulsive, hyperactive, and aggressive behaviors (Owens, 2005; Golan et al., 2004).

A number of conditions produce excessive daytime sleepiness (EDS). Chronic sleep deprivation leads to EDS. Sleep, which is fragmented or disrupted because of obstructive sleep apnea or periodic limb movement disorder, can cause EDS. In addition, narcolepsy or other primary clinical disorders of EDS can produce EDS. Moreover, circadian rhythm disorders including delayed sleep phase syndrome can lead to symptoms of EDS. These conditions can produce symptoms similar to ADHD symptoms (Owens, 2005; Walters et al., 2008).

Treatment

Clinicians often use a combination of behavior interventions, changing lifestyles, medication, and counseling. According to Jensen et al. (2005), combining behavior interventions with pharmacological treatment is the most effective strategy. The second most effective approach is medical management by itself, followed by behavior management by itself. Pharmacological treatment is the most cost-effective approach. The second most cost-effective strategy is behavior management and the third most cost-effective approach is combining behavior interventions with medications.

A number of reports have analyzed racial, gender, and socioeconomic disparities in ADHD services (Hillemeier et al., 2007; Foy and Earls, 2005; Pastor and Reubern, 2005). These reports suggest that girls, African-Americans, and low-income individuals have a particularly difficult time in accessing therapy.

Using population-based data from the 1997–2001 National Health Interview Survey, Pastor and Reubern (2005) discovered that Hispanic and African children were less likely than white children to have parent-identified reports of ADHD with a learning disability.

A longitudinal investigation of mainly low-income children revealed that parents of white children were more likely to endorse ADHD screening items from the Diagnostic Interview Schedule for Children than parents of African-American children (Hillemeier et al., 2007).

Ethnic and racial disparities in receiving ADHD services are due to a combination of access barriers and individual, cultural, organizational, and societal conditions (Eiraldi et al., 2006). School professionals' failure to identify and refer students for treatment, inadequate help-seeking patterns of parents, providers' difficulties in diagnosing the disorder, and societal acceptance of the disorder as a legitimate health problem lead to ethnic and racial disparities in ADHD services (Foy and Earls, 2005).

According to Bailey and Owens (2005), lack of information about symptoms, treatment, and the effects if the disorder is untreated, and negative feelings toward over-diagnosis and misdiagnosis are patient-related obstacles for African-Americans.

Other causes of health disparities in ADHD services can include a scarcity of culturally competent health-care providers and stereotypes and biases of providers (Bailey and Owens, 2005). Kendall and Hatton (2002) explore how racism is a source of health disparity in families with ADHD children.

The American Academy of Pediatrics (AAP) has guidelines for assessing and treating ADHD children that can be used to overcome these barriers to treatment (Foy and Earls, 2005). The AAP ADHD toolkit offers resources for implementing the AAP guidelines in clinical practice. These resources help providers improve their assessment and treatment of ADHD and comorbidities.

ADHD Medications

The most frequently prescribed medications for ADHD are stimulants. These drugs increase the extracellular concentrations of dopamine and norepinephrine, which result in an increase in neurotransmission. According to Solanto (1998), therapeutic effects result because of noradrenergic effects at the locus coeruleus and the prefrontal cortex and the dopaminergic effects at the nucleus accumbens.

The most common ones are methylphenidate (ritalin, metadate, concerta), dextroamphetamine (dexedrine), dextromethamphetamine (desoxyn), and mixed amphetamine salts (adderall) (Faraone, 2003). A non-stimulant approved for treating ADHD is atomoxetine (strattera). Some antidepressants such as tricyclic antidepressants, SNRIs, or MAOIs have been prescribed off-label for the condition (Stein, 2004; Christman et al., 2004; Hazell, 2005).

Studies comparing the effectiveness of medications have been inadequate. Moreover, more research is needed to evaluate the impact of medications on academic functioning and behavior (McDonagh et al., 2007). For example, researchers do not know about the long-term impact of ADHD medical treatment in pre-school children (NHS, 2008; Greenhill et al., 2008).

The use of stimulants for treating ADHD is controversial even though they are considered safe when taken under physician's supervision (American Academy of Pediatrics, 2001). However, the use of stimulants is controversial because they produce unwanted side effects, their long-term impact is unknown, and use of stimulants creates social and ethical concerns (Stern and Stern, 2002; King et al., 2006; Murphy and Barkley, 2005; Lerner and Wigal, 2008). Black box warnings to certain ADHD drugs have been added by the Food and Drug Administration (FDA), (FDA, 2007). The American Heart Association and the American Academy of Pediatrics recommend that children should be carefully evaluated for heart conditions before being treated with stimulant drugs (American Academy of Pediatrics/American Heart Association, 2008).

Researchers have not systematically studied physician perceptions about the use of medications for ADHD. A survey of 365 physicians by Stockl et al. (2003) revealed that more than 92% agreed or strongly agreed that symptoms of ADHD causes problems in pediatric patients and stimulant medications are effective in treating this disorder. In terms of the drugs' side effects, 32% of the physicians surveyed, expressed concern about decreased appetite or weight loss associated with the medications, 50% expressed concern about the side effect of disrupted sleep, and 22% reported concern about the side effect of increased anxiety. Nineteen percent of the physicians in the sample reported being concerned about diversion of ADHD drugs. Thirty-seven percent of those sampled indicated that prescribing controlled medications for children and adolescents is a burden for themselves, 37% prescribing these drugs was a burden for their staff, and 40% reported that it was a burden for the parents. About 38% of the physicians in the survey preferred treating ADHD children or adolescents with a non-stimulant. Fifty-eight percent preferred treating pediatric patients with a non-controlled that did not have abuse potential over a controlled drug with abuse potential.

Many parents are concerned about having their children treated with psychopharmacological drugs (dosReis and Myers, 2008). Parents have these concerns about using stimulant drugs in treating ADHD children, even though this treatment approach is based on scientific evidence. Parents' reluctance may be due to what they learn from friends and family members about the drugs' adverse effects. More research is needed to determine how parents decide on treatment decisions and the possible positive benefits of these drugs in treating their ADHD children.

Based on a sample of Canadian parents of 73 boys, aged 5–13 years of age, with ADHD, Johnston et al. (2005) evaluated possible association between parents' beliefs and attributions and their experiences with various treatments for their ADHD children. The authors showed that the parents reported mainly using behavioral management and stimulant drugs in treating their ADHD boys. About 50% of the parents indicated that they also use diet and vitamin treatments. The parents had knowledge about the condition and their beliefs were fairly accurate. The parents viewed their child's ADHD symptoms as internal in nature and as persistent and widespread. Their use of various therapies was associated with their beliefs about ADHD. Parents who thought that ADHD was internal in nature, persistent, and widespread were more likely to rely on less scientifically based therapies.

Behavior Treatment Approaches

A variety of behavioral interventions are employed to treat ADHD. These behavioral approaches include interpersonal psychotherapy (IPT), psychoeducational techniques, family therapy, school-based approaches, cognitive behavioral therapy

(CBT), behavior therapy, training in social skills, and parent management and education approaches (NHS, 2008).

Behavioral parent training (BPT) and behavioral classroom management have been found effective in treating ADHD children (Pelham and Fabiano, 2008; Chronis et al., 2004). According to Pliszka (2007), parent management training and education methods have resulted in positive short-term outcomes. Researchers in some studies have found that BPT is effective in reducing children's ADHD behaviors and maladaptive parental functioning (Chronis et al., 2004). Moreover, BPT has been found to be useful in treating parental stress and ADHD children's behavior in classrooms.

Various factors can limit the effectiveness of this type of intervention. Single parenthood, the mental health of parents, and comorbid conditions in the ADHD children can limit the success of BPT interventions (Chronis et al., 2004).

According to Chacko et al. (2009), households with single mothers are likely to experience poor outcomes during and after BPT. Chacko et al. (2009) demonstrated that traditional BPT, and an enhanced BPT program (the Strategies to Enhance Positive Planning-STEPP) immediately after treatment, enhanced parental and child outcomes. STEPP also produced more engagement to treatment. However, the researchers found that BPT does not lead to normal behaviors for a majority of the ADHD children and positive treatment outcomes were not permanent.

Few investigations have examined the effectiveness of BPT for fathers of ADHD children (Fabiano et al., 2009; Fabiano, 2007). Fabiano et al. (2009) analyzed father and child outcomes using a standard BPT program, an enhanced BPT program (COACHES) that included BPT and sports skills training for children and parent–child relations related to a soccer game. Fathers who attended the COACHES program were more likely to rate their children as more improved than those participating in the traditional BPT sessions. The parents who attended COACHES reported that their children were more engaged in treatment, e.g., the children had better attendance and completed more of their homework.

The effectiveness of BPT also may depend on whether the ADHD children have comorbid ODD and CD (Chronis et al., 2004). ADHD children with comorbid ODD and CD can reduce BPT treatment completion, participant compliance, and treatment outcomes.

The format and setting of BPT programs may also have an impact on treatment success. More research is needed to which formats and settings offer optimal treatment outcomes. Chronis et al. (2004) notes that program evaluation studies are limited by the high degree of comorbidity between ADHD and ODD/CD.

Investigators have also analyzed the impact of BPT on ADHD children as an adjunct to routine clinical care. One Dutch study compared the effectiveness of BPT (12 sessions using a group format) as adjunct to routine clinical care (RCC) (family support and medications when appropriate) (van den Hoofdakker et al., 2007). Ninety-four ADHD children, aged 4–12 years, who had been referred to a mental health service, were randomly assigned to 5 months of BPT and RCC concurrently ($N = 47$) or to 5 months of only RCC ($N = 47$). Children in both groups improved on all outcome measures, including child behavior problems, ADHD symptoms, internalizing problems, and parental stress. The BPT plus RCC condition was more effective than RCC by itself in reducing behavioral and internalizing problems. The findings were the same for ADHD children, whether or not they were treated with medications. Children assigned to just the RCC condition received more multiple medications. The investigator found that BPT as adjunctive therapy improves the effectiveness of RCC in terms of reducing behavioral and internalizing problems. However, BPT plus RCC does not improve ADHD symptoms or parental stress.

Research has shown that family therapy has not had an impact on children with ADHD symptoms (The Cochrane Collaboration, 2005). The effects of family therapy may be influenced by the divorce rate among parents whose children have ADHD. Wymbs et al. (2008) found that parents whose children have ADHD have a greater likelihood of getting a divorce, particularly when their children are under 8 years old.

Experimental Approaches

Some persons with ADHD take dietary supplements and follow special diets to help them reduce their symptoms. Johnson et al. (2009) found that the dietary supplement, Omega-3, may have a positive impact on children and adolescents with ADHD who have inattention symptoms and related disorders. Studies of dietary supplements and special diets are controversial because they have limited research methods and the follow-up investigations have produced inconsistent findings. No dietary supplement has been approved by the FDA for treatment of ADHD in the USA (FDA, 2007).

Hillman et al. (2009) report that EEG biofeedback, also called neurofeedback, is helpful in the treatment of problems related to inattention, impulse control, and hyperactivity. Although research is limited, no side effects of biofeedback have been identified.

Aerobic exercise has been studied as a treatment for ADHD. During preadolescence, aerobic exercise may enhance cognitive performance and neural processes associated with executive control (Hillman et al., 2009). However, more research is needed to study the role of aerobic exercise in this area of cognitive performance research. Another investigation by Lopez-Williams et al. (2005) demonstrated that among boys with ADHD, athletic activities may increase acceptance by peers when associated with less negative behaviors.

ADHD Children in School

ADHD is one of the most challenging problems for children, schools, families, and health-care providers (Dang et al., 2007). Professionals may mistake ADHD symptoms for other health problems. As a result, comprehensive evaluation is needed to provide an accurate diagnosis and treatment of children with this disorder and maximize their educational achievement.

A number of conditions such as teacher knowledge about ADHD; cooperation and communication among teachers, school psychologists, and nurses; and the quality of curricular methods and content can impact the diagnosis, management, and functioning of ADHD children attending school (Dang et al., 2007; Foy and Earls, 2005). In a study of knowledge, resources and cooperation among professionals involved in working with ADHD students, Schweifer (2009) discovered that the professionals felt that their knowledge about ADHD was acceptable. However, school psychologists and special education teachers reported that they were better able to rely on their resources and make use of opportunities for professional cooperation than school medics or regular teachers. The professionals surveyed indicated that the major difficulty in working with ADHD children in school settings is enhancing cooperation among professionals.

To help deal with difficulties in professional cooperation and communication, Dang et al. (2007) have developed a ADHD Identification and Management in Schools approach. This framework, which was designed by a pediatrician, school nurses, and school psychologists, seeks to improve professional communication, foster standard practices, and enhance the quality of care for ADHD children.

Foy and Earls (2005) describe a community protocol in Guilford County, North Carolina, that is designed to promote agreement among clinicians, teachers, and child advocates over the assessment and treatment of children with ADHD symptoms. This community protocol has the potential for increasing efficiencies in provider practices, enhance standards of practice, and improve the identification of ADHD in students. The community protocol is intended to increase knowledge of the disorder among school professionals and increase the rate of appropriate school-based referrals.

Other investigations have revealed knowledge deficits about the disorder among school teachers (Gonzalez et al., 2009). In a report on teachers' knowledge about ADHD in five schools in the metropolitan area of San Juan, Puerto Rico, Gonzalez et al. (2009) reported 72% having limited knowledge about the condition. However, 60% identified two out of three vignettes about children with symptoms of the disorder. Various characteristics such as teacher age, gender, college alma mater, years of teaching experience did not predict the teachers' knowledge level about ADHD.

Researchers have analyzed the attitude and knowledge of ADHD and learning disabilities among high school teachers. Ghanizadeh et al. (2006) studied 196 Iranian elementary school teachers' knowledge and attitudes toward ADHD. The authors found that the elementary school teachers had low knowledge about the condition. For example, 53.1% thought that the disorder was due to spoiling of the children by parents. The teachers surveyed indicated that they received their information about ADHD primarily from television, radio, friends, relatives, periodicals, newspapers, and magazine.

Teacher attitude and knowledge about ADHD may influence how they evaluate the behavior, IQ, and personality of students with this diagnosis. Batzle et al. (2010) gave hypothetical descriptions of a male or female child with or without an ADHD label or an ADHD with treatment label to K through 12 teachers and asked them to rate the child in terms of behavior, IQ, and personality. The teachers evaluated the child with both an ADHD label and an ADHD stimulant treatment label more negatively than the child without any label. The teachers also rated a child with the ADHD label somewhat more negatively than one who had an ADHD with stimulant treatment label.

Case Study

The following case study describes a boy with ADHD. Nick is an 8-year-old, second-grade Caucasian youngster, who lives with his father and maternal grandmother. His biological mother died in an automobile accident when he was only 6 months old. His father is a construction worker. The family lives in a working class suburb.

Developmental milestones were all within normal limits. When Nick began preschool, at age 2, he was seen as aggressive with other children. In particular, he would get angry easily if he did not get his way, take toys away from classmates, and throw things. He also had a tendency to hug others and touch other children, despite the teachers reminding him to keep his hands to himself.

Nick also had difficulty following rules. He would run in the hallway, refuse to come in from playing outside, and had difficulty waiting his turn. In addition, he would often interrupt the teacher and peers and talk during rest time.

As he entered kindergarten, his teacher noted problems with attention. He would rush through his work, had difficulty in following directions, displayed problems with concentration, and was easily distracted. Problems with impulsivity and aggression continued. Then during first grade, his teacher noted that he attended better if placed physically closer to her and if he made eye contact with her. Concerns about organization emerged and assignments were routinely not completed, not turned in, lost or sloppily done. Nick also had significant issues in staying in his seat, blurting out answers, and talking during quiet times in class. At his parent teacher conference in the fall of first grade, his teacher suggested the possibility of ADHD to Nick's father. He subsequently contacted the pediatrician. Nick's doctor then referred Nick to a child psychologist for an evaluation.

As part of the evaluation, Nick was observed in several settings in school, including structured and unstructured settings. Nick's father, grandmother, and teacher all completed the BASC and Hawthorne ADDES, and both Nick and his father were interviewed. Nick was diagnosed with ADHD and the pediatrician subsequently utilized Aderall for medication. However, Nick had significant side effects, including loss of appetite and sleep disturbance. He was subsequently placed on Focalin, with similar results. At that juncture, the pediatrician referred Nick's family to a pediatric neurologist, who placed Nick on Strattera, with somewhat positive results. Nick also began individual counseling, and Nick's father and grandmother also had some parenting therapy to support Nick's counseling and provide education to the family.

Nick's aggressive behavior has dissipated, but there is still evidence of some impulsive behavior. In particular, he has difficulty waiting his turn and periodically blurts out answers. Disorganization and work completion remain significant problems. He continues with individual counseling and medication.

References

Acosta, M.T., Arcos-Burgos, M., Muenke, M. (2004). Attention deficit/hyperactivity disorder (ADHD): complex phenotype, simple genotype? Genet Med, 6 (1), 1–15.

Aldenkamp, A.P., Arzimanoglou, A., Reijs, R., et al. (2006). Optimizing therapy of seizures in children and adolescents with ADHD. Neurology, 67 (12 Suppl 4), S49–S51.

American Academy of Pediatrics (2001). Clinical practice guideline: treatment of the school-aged child with attention-deficit/hyperactivity disorder. Pediatrics, 108 (4), 1033–1044.

American Academy of Pediatrics/American Heart Association (2008). American Academy of Pediatrics/American Heart Association clarification of statement on cardiovascular evaluation and monitoring of children and adolescents with heart disease receiving medications for ADHD: May 16, 2008. J Dev Behav Pediatr, 29 (4), 335.

American Psychiatric Association. Task Force on DSM-IV (2000). Diagnostic and statistical manual of mental disorders: DSM-IV-TR. Washington, DC: American Psychiatric Association.

Ashton, H., Gallagher, P., Moore, B. (2006). The adult psychiatrist's dilemma: psychostimulant use in attention deficit/hyperactivity disorder. J Psychopharmacol (Oxford), 20 (5), 602–610.

Bailey, R.K., Owens, D.L. (2005). Overcoming challenges in the diagnosis and treatment of attention-deficit/hyperactivity disorder in African Americans. J Natl Med Assoc, 97 (10 Suppl), 5S–10S.

Bailly, L. (2005). Stimulant medication for the treatment of attention-deficit hyperactivity disorder: evidence-b(i)ased practice? Psychiatric Bull (The Royal College of Psychiatrists), 29 (8), 284–287.

Balint, S., Czobor, P., Meszaros, A., et al. (2008). Neuropsychological impairments in adult attention deficit hyperactivity disorder: a literature review. Psychiatr Hung, 23 (5), 324–335.

Banerjee, T.D., Middleton, F., Faraone, S.V. (2007). Environmental risk factors for attention-deficit hyperactivity disorder. Acta Paediatr, 96 (9), 1269–1274.

Batzle, C.S., Weyandt, L.L., Janusis, G.M., et al. (2010, September). Potential impact of ADHD with stimulant medication label on teacher expectations. J Atten Disord, 14 (2), 157–166. Epub 2009 Sep 22.

Bauermeister, J., Shrout, P., Chavez, L., et al. (2007). ADHD and gender: are risks and sequela of ADHD the same for boys and girls? J Child Psychol Psychiatry, 48 (8), 831–839.

BBC (2005, July 31). Bad behaviour linked to smoking. Retrieved from: http://news.bbc.co.uk/1/hi/health/472719.stm

Benton, D. (2008). Sucrose and behavioral problems. Crit Rev Food Sci Nutr, 48 (5), 385–401.

Biederman, J., Faraone, S. (2005). Attention deficit hyperactivity disorder (abstract). Lancet, 366 (9481), 237–248.

Braun, J.M., Kahn, R.S., Froehlich, T., et al. (2006). Exposures to environmental toxicants and attention deficit hyperactivity disorder in U.S. children. Environ Health Perspect, 114 (12), 1904–1909.

Breslau, J., Miller, E., Breslau, N., et al. (2009). The impact of early behavior disturbances on academic achievement in high school. Pediatrics, 123 (6), 1472–1476.

Brunsvold, G.L., Oepen, G., et al. (2008). Comorbid depression in ADHD: children and adolescents. Psychiatric Times, 25 (10). Retrieved from: http://www.psychiatrictimes.com/adhd/article/10168/1286863.

Byun, H., Yang, J., Lee, M., et al. (2006). Psychiatric comorbidity in Korean children and adolescents with attention-deficit hyperactivity disorder: psychopathology according to subtype. Yonsei Med J, 47 (1), 113–121.

Caldararo, N. (2002–2003). Comment on Brewis et al. Am Anthropol, 104 (1), 282–283.

Castellanos, X. (2000). Interviews: Xavier Castellanos, M.D. PBS. 2000–10–10.
Chacko, A., Wymbs, B.T., Wymbs, F.A., et al. (2009). Enhancing traditional behavioural parent training for single mothers of children with ADHD. J Clin Child Adolesc Psychol, 38 (2), 206–218.
Chriss, J.J. (2007). Social control: an introduction. Cambridge, UK: Polity.
Christman, A.K., Fermo, J.D., Markowitz, J.S., et al. (2004). Atomoxetine, a novel treatment for attention-deficit-hyperactivity disorder. Pharmacotherapy, 24 (8), 1020–1036.
Chronis, A.M., Chacko, A., Fabiano, G.A., et al. (2004). Enhancements to the behavioral parent training paradigm for families of children with ADHD: review and future directions. Clin Child Fam Psychol Rev, 7 (1), 1–27.
Cimera, R. (2002). Making ADHD a gift: teaching superman how to fly. Lanham, MD: Scarecrow Press, Inc.
Cohen, A.J., Adler, N., Kaplan, S.J., et al. (2002). Interactional effects of marital status and physical abuse on adolescent psychopathology. Child Abuse Negl, 26 (3), 277–288.
Cohen, D.J., Cicchetti, D. (2006). Developmental psychopathology. Chichester: Wiley.
Crichton, A. (1798, 2001). Dr Alexander Crichton and 'mental restlessness. Child Adolesc Ment Health, 6 (2), 66–73.
Cuffe, S.P. (1994). Comorbidity of attention deficit hyperactivity disorder and post traumatic stress disorder. J Child Fam Stud, 3 (3), 327–336.
Danforth, S., Yogawin, J. (2001). Hyper talk: sampling the social construction of ADHD in everyday language. Anthro Educ Q, 32 (2), 167–190.
Dang, M.T., Warrington, D., Tung, T., et al. (2007). A school-based approach to early identification and management of students with ADHD. J Sch Nurs, 23 (1), 2–12.
dosReis, S., Myers, M.A. (2008). Parental attitudes and involvement in psychopharmacological treatment for ADHD: a conceptual model. Int Rev Psychiatry, 20 (2), 135–141.
Eiraldi, R.B., Mazzuca, L.B., Clarke, A.T., et al. (2006). Service utilization among ethnic minority children with ADHD: a model of help-seeking behavior. Adm Policy Ment Health, 33 (5), 607–622.
Elia, J., Ambrosini, P.J., Rapoport, J.L. (1999). Treatment of attention-deficit-hyperactivity disorder. N Engl J Med, 340 (10), 780–788.
Fabiano, G.A. (2007). Father participation in behavioral parent training for ADHD: review and recommendations for increasing inclusion and engagement. J Fam Psychol, 21 (4), 683–693.
Fabiano, G.A., Chacko, A., Pelham, W.E., Jr., et al. (2009). A comparison of behavioral parent training programs for fathers of children with attention-deficit/hyperactivity disorder. Behav Ther, 40 (2), 190–204.
Faraone, S.P. (2003). Retrieved from Medscape Today. http://www.medscape.com/viewarticle/461543.
FDA (2007, February 21). FDA news. Retrieved from: http://www.fda.gov/bbs/topics/NEWS/2007/NEW01568.html
Ford, J.D., Racusin, R., Ellis, C.G., et al. (2000). Child maltreatment, other trauma exposure, and posttraumatic symptomatology among children with oppositional defiant and attention deficit hyperactivity disorders. Child Maltreat, 5 (3), 205–217.
Foy, J.M., Earls, M.F. (2005). A process for developing community consensus regarding the diagnosis and management of attention-deficit/hyperactivity disorder. Pediatrics, 115 (1), e97–e104.
Galera, C., Bouvard, M.P., Encrenaz, G., et al. (2008). Hyperactivity-inattention symptoms in childhood and suicidal behaviors in adolescence: the Youth Gazel Cohort. Acta Psychiatr Scand, 118 (6), 480–489.
Galera, C., Melchior, M., Chastang, J.F., et al. (2009). Childhood and adolescent hyperactivity-inattention symptoms and academic achievement 8 years later: the GAZEL Youth Study. Psychol Med, 39 (11), 1895–1906.
Gentile, J. (2004). Adult ADHD: diagnosis, differential diagnosis and medication management. Psychiatry, 3 (8), 24–30.

Ghanizadeh, A., Bahredar, M.J., Moeini, S.R. (2006). Knowledge and attitudes towards attention deficit hyperactivity disorder among elementary school teachers. Patient Educ Couns, 63 (1–2), 84–88.

Golan, N., Shahar, E., Ravid, S., et al. (2004). Sleep disorders and daytime sleepiness in children with attention-deficit/hyperactivity disorder. Sleep, 27 (2), 261–266.

Gonzalez Tejera, G., Gonzalez, M., Ramirez, B., et al. (2009). Attention deficit hyperactivity disorder in five schools of the San Juan metropolitan area: assessment of teacher's knowledge. Bol Assoc Med P R, 101 (1), 31–35.

Greenhill, L.L., Posner, K., Vaughan, B.S., et al. (2008). Attention deficit hyperactivity disorder in preschool children. Child Adolesc Psychiatr Clin N Am, 17 (2), 347–366.

Ha, M., Kwon, H.J., Lim, M.H., et al. (2009). Low blood levels of lead and mercury and symptoms of attention deficit hyperactivity in children: a report of the children's health and environment research (CHEER). Neurotoxicology, 30 (1), 31–36.

Hartmann, T. (2003). The Edison gene: ADHD and the gift of the hunter child. Rochester, VT: Park Street Press.

Harvey, E., Danforth, J.S., McKee, T.E., et al. (2003). Parenting of children with attention-deficit/hyperactivity disorder (ADHD): the role of parental ADHD symptomatology. J Atten Disord, 7 (1), 31–42.

Hazell, P. (2005). Do adrenergically active drugs have a role in the first-line treatment of attention-deficit/hyperactivity disorder? Expert Opin Pharmacother, 6 (12), 1989–1998.

Hillemeier, M.M., Foster, E.M., Heinrichs, B., et al. (2007). Racial differences in parental reports of attention-deficit/hyperactivity disorder behaviors. J Dev Behav Pediatr, 28 (5), 353–361.

Hillman, C., Buck, S.M., Themanson, J.R., et al. (2009). Aerobic fitness and cognitive development: event-related brain potential and task performance indices of executive control in preadolescent children. Dev Psychol, 45 (1), 114–125.

Iizuka, C., Yamashita, Y., Nagamitsu, S., et al. (2010, September). Comparison of the strengths and difficulties questionnaire (SDQ) scores between children with high-functioning autism spectrum disorder (HFASD) and attention-deficit/hyperactivity disorder (AD/HD). Brain Dev, 32 (8), 609–612. Epub 2009 Oct 13.

incrediblehorizons.com (no date). Attention deficit hyperactivity disorder is neurologically based disorder. Retrieved from: http://www.incrediblehorizons.com/Understanding%20Add.htm

Jadad, A.R., Booker, L., Gauld, M., et al. (1999). The treatment of attention-deficit hyperactivity disorder: an annotated bibliography and critical appraisal of published systematic reviews and metaanalyses. Can J Psychiatry. Revue Canad de Psychiatrie, 44 (10), 1025–1035.

Jensen, P.S., et al. (2005). Cost-effectiveness of ADHD treatments: findings from the multimodal treatment study of children with ADHD. Am J Psychiatry, 162, 1628–1636.

Johnson, M., Ostlund, S., Fransson, G., et al. (2009). Omega-3/omega-6 fatty acids for attention deficit hyperactivity disorder: a randomized placebo-controlled trial in children and adolescents. J Atten Disord, 12 (5), 394–401.

Johnston, C., Mash, E.J. (2001). Families of children with attention-deficit/hyperactivity disorder: review and recommendations for future research. Clin Child Fam Psychol Rev, 4 (3), 183–207.

Johnston, C., Seipp, C., Hommersen, P., et al. (2005). Treatment choices and experiences in attention deficit and hyperactivity disorder: relations to parents' beliefs and attributions. Child Care Health Dev, 31 (6), 669–677.

Joughin, C., Ramchandani, P., Zwi, M. (2003). Attention-deficit/hyperactivity. Am Fam Physician, 67 (9), 1969–1670.

Kemp, A. (2008). Food additives and hyperactivity. BMJ, 336 (7654), 1144.

Kendall, J., Hatton, D. (2002). Racism as a source of health disparity in families with children with attention deficit hyperactivity disorder. ANS Adv Nurs Sci, 25 (2), 22–39.

Kidd, P.M. (2000). Attention deficit/hyperactivity disorder (ADHD) in children: rationale for its integrative management. Altern Med Rev, 5 (5), 402–428.

Kilic, B.G., Sener, S. (2005). Family functioning and psychosocial characteristics in children with attention deficit hyperactivity disorder with comorbid oppositional defiant disorder or conduct disorder. Turk Psikiyatri Derg, 16 (1), 21–28.

King, G.A., Zwaigenbaum, L., King, S., et al. (2006). A qualitative investigation of changes in the belief systems of families of children with autism or Down syndrome. Child Care Health Dev, 32 (3), 353–369.

Klassen, A.F., Miller, A., Fine, S. (2004). Health-related quality of life in children and adolescents who have a diagnosis of attention-deficit/hyperactivity disorder. Pediatrics, 114 (5), e541–547.

Lamminmaky, T., et al. (1995). Attention deficit hyperactivity disorder subtypes: are there differences in academic problems? Dev Neuropsychol, 11, 297–310.

Langley, K., Holmans, P.A., van den Bree, M.B., et al. (2007). Effects of low birth weight, maternal smoking in pregnancy and social class on the phenotypic manifestation of attention deficit hyperactivity disorder and associated antisocial behavior: investigation in a clinical sample. BMC Psychiatry, 7, 26.

Langley, K., Rice, F., van den Bree, M.B., et al. (2005). Maternal smoking during pregnancy as an environmental risk factor for attention deficit hyperactivity disorder behavior. A review. Minerva Pediatr, 57 (6), 359–371.

Latimer, W.W., August, G.J., Newcomb, M.D., et al. (2003). Child and familial pathways to academic achievement and behavioral adjustment: a prospective six-year study of children with and without ADHD. J Atten Disord, 7 (2), 101–116.

Lerner, M., Wigal, T. (2008). Long-term safety of stimulant medications used to treat children with ADHD. Pediatr Ann, 37 (1), 37–45.

Linnet, K.M., Dalsgaard, S., Obel, C., et al. (2003). Maternal lifestyle factors in pregnancy risk of attention deficit hyperactivity disorder and associated behaviors: review of the current evidence. Am J Psychiatry, 160 (6), 1028–1040.

Loe, I.M., Feldman, H.M. (2007). Academic and educational outcomes of children with ADHD. Ambul Pediatr, 7 (1 Suppl), 82–90.

Lopez-Williams, A., Chacko, A., Wymbs, B.T., et al. (2005). Athletic performance and social behavior as predictors of peer acceptance in children diagnosed with attention-deficit/hyperactivity disorder. J Emot Behav Disorders, 13 (3), 173–180.

Lynskey, M.T., Hall, W. (2001). Attention deficit hyperactivity disorder and substance use disorders: is there a causal link? Addiction, 96 (6), 815–822.

Martel, M.M., Lucia, V.C., Nigg, J.T., et al. (2007). Sex differences in the pathway from low birth weight to inattention/hyperactivity. J Abnorm Child Psychol, 35 (1), 87–96.

Masi, G., Milone, A., Manfredi, A., et al. (2008, March–April). Conduct disorder in referred children and adolescents: clinical and therapeutic issues. Compr Psychiatry, 49 (2), 146–153. Epub 2007 Oct 24.

Masi, G., Millepiedi, S., Perugi, G., et al. (2010). A naturalistic exploratory study of the impact of demographic, phenotypic and comorbid features in pediatric obsessive-compulsive disorder. Psychopathology, 43 (2), 69–78.

Mayes, R., Bagwell, C., Erkulwater, J., et al. (2008). ADHD and the rise in stimulant use among children. Harv Rev Psychiatry, 16 (3), 151–166.

McDonagh, M.S., Peterson, K., Dana, T., et al. (2007). Drug class review on pharmacologic treatment for ADHD (Final Report, December 2007). Portland, OR: Oregon Health & Science University.

McKee, T.E., Harvey, E., Danforth, J.S., et al. (2004). The relation between parental coping styles and parent-child interactions before and after treatment for children with ADHD and oppositional behavior. J Clin Child Adolesc Psychol, 33 (1), 158–168.

Modesto-Lowe, V., Danforth, J.S., Brooks, D. (2008). ADHD: does parenting style matter? Clin Pediatr, 47 (9), 865–872.

Moffitt, T.E., Melchior, M. (2007). Why does the worldwide prevalence of childhood attention deficit hyperactivity disorder matter? Am J Psychiatry, 164 (6), 856–858.

Molina, B.S., Hinshaw, S.P., Swanson, J.M., et al. (2009, May). The MTA at 8 years: prospective follow-up of children treated for combined-type ADHD in a multisite study. J Am Acad Child Adolesc Psychiatry, 48 (5), 484–500.

Murphy, K.R., Barkley, R.A. (2005). Attention-deficit hyperactivity disorder, A clinical workbook (3rd ed.). New York, NY: Guildford Press.

National Institute of Clinical Excellence (2009). Attention deficit hyperactivity disorder: the nice guideline on diagnosis and management of ADHD in children, young people and adults. NHS, p. 121. Retrieved from: http://www.nice.org.uk/nicemedia/pdf/ADHDFullGuideline.pdf.

NHS (2008, September 24). Attention deficit hyperactivity disorder (ADHD): full guidelines (PDF). Retrieved from: http://www.nice.org.uk/nicemedia/pdf/CG72FullGuideline.pdf

Niedermeyer, E., Naidu, S.B. (1997). Attention-deficit hyperactivity disorder (ADHD) and frontal-motor cortex disconnection. Clin Electroencephalogr, 28 (3), 130–136.

Nigg, J.T., Knottnerus, G.M., Martel, M.M., et al. (2008). Low blood lead levels associated with clinically diagnosed attention-deficit/hyperactivity disorder and mediated by weak cognitive control. Biol Psychiatry, 63 (3), 325–331.

Obel, C., Linnet, K.M., Henriksen, T.B., et al. (2009). Smoking during pregnancy and hyperactivity-inattention in the offspring – comparing results from three Nordic cohorts. Int J Epidemiol, 38 (3), 698–705.

Owens, J.A. (2005). The ADHD and sleep conundrum: a review. J Dev Behav Pediatrcs, 26 (4), 312–322.

Pastor, P.N., Reubern, C.A. (2005). Racial and ethnic differences in ADHD and LD in young school-age children: parental reports in the National Health Interview Survey. Public Health Rep, 120 (4), 383–392.

Patrick, K.S., Straughn, A.B., Perkins, J.S., et al. (2009). Evolution of stimulants to treat ADHD: transdermal methylphenidate. Hum Psychopharmacol, 24 (1), 1–17.

Paule, M.G., Rowland, A.S., Ferguson, S.A., et al. (2000). Attention deficit/hyperactivity disorder: characteristics, interventions and models. Neurotoxicol Teratol, 22 (5), 631–651.

Pelham, W.E., Jr., Fabiano, G.A. (2008). Evidence-based psychosocial treatments for attention-deficit/hyperactivity disorder. J Clin Child Adolesc Psychol, 37 (1), 184–214.

Peters, K., Jackson, D. (2009). Mothers' experiences of parenting a child with attention deficit hyperactivity disorder. J Adv Nurs, 65 (1), 62–71.

Pfiffner, L.J., McBurnett, K., Rathouz, P.J., et al. (2005). Family correlates of oppositional and conduct disorders in children with attention deficit/hyperactivity disorder. J Abnorm Child Psychol, 33 (5), 51–563.

Pliszka, S. (2000). Patterns of psychiatric comorbidity with attention-deficit/hyperactivity disorder. Child Adolesc Psychiatr Clin N Am, 9 (3), 525–540.

Pliszka, S. (2007). Practice parameter for the assessment and treatment of children and adolescents with attention-deficit/hyperactivity disorder. J Am Acad Child Adolesc Psychiatry, 46 (7), 894–921.

Pollak, Y., Benarroch, F., Kanengisser, L., et al. (2009). Tourette syndrome-associated psychopathology: roles of comorbid attention-deficit hyperactivity disorder and obsessive-compulsive disorder. J Dev Behav Pediatr, 30 (5), 413–419.

Pringsheim, T., Sandor, P., Lang, A., et al. (2009). Prenatal and perinatal morbidity in children with Tourette syndrome and attention-deficit hyperactivity disorder. J Dev Behav Pediatr, 30 (2), 115–121.

Ray, G.T., Croen, L.A., Habel, L.A. (2009). Mothers of children diagnose with attention-deficit/hyperactivity disorder: health conditions and medical care utilization in periods before and after birth of the child. Med Care, 47 (1), 105–114.

Rodriguez, A., Bohlin, G. (2005). Are maternal smoking and stress during pregnancy related to ADHD symptoms in children? J Child Psychol Psychiatry, 46 (3), 246–254.

Rodriguez, A., Miettunen, J., Henriksen, T.B., et al. (2008). Maternal adiposity prior to pregnancy is associated with ADHD symptoms in offspring: evidence from three prospective pregnancy cohorts. Int J Obes (Lond), 32 (3), 550–557.

Rodriguez, A., Olsen, J., Kotimaa, A.J., et al. (2009). Is prenatal alcohol exposure related to inattention and hyperactivity symptoms in children? Disentangling the effects of social adversity. J Child Psychol Psychiatry, 50 (9), 1073–1083.

Roman, T., Rohde, L.A., Hutz, M.H. (2004). Polymorphisms of the dopamine transporter gene: influence on response to methylphenidate in attention deficit-hyperactivity disorder. Am J Pharmacogenomics, 4 (2), 83–92.

Satake, H., Yamashita, H., Yoshida, K. (2004, Spring). The family psychosocial characteristics of children with attention-deficit hyperactivity disorder with or without oppositional or conduct problems in Japan. Child Psychiatry Hum Dev, 34 (3), 219–235.

Schmitz, M., Denardin, D., Laufer Silva, T., et al. (2006). Smoking during pregnancy and attention-deficit/hyperactivity disorder, predominantly inattentive type: a case-control study. J Am Acad Child Adolesc Psychiatry, 45 (11), 1338–1345.

Schonwald, A., Lechner, E. (2006). Attention deficit/hyperactivity disorder: complexities and controversies. Curr Opin Pediatr, 18 (2), 189–195.

Schweifer, C. (2009). Attention deficit and hyperactivity in school children – knowledge, resources and cooperation among professions concerned. Wien Med Wochenschr, 159 (7–8), 183–187.

sci.csuhayward.edu (no date). *ADHD*. Retrieved from: http://www.sci.csuhayward.edu/~dsandberg/CHLDPATHLESCTS/ChldPathLect05ADHD.htm

Science Daily (2007, April 11). Prenatal smoking increases ADHD risk in some children. Retrieved from: http://www.sciencedaily.com/releases/2007/04/070410190421.htm

Science Daily (2008, November 24). Ability to quit smoking may depend on ADHD symptoms, researchers find. Retrieved from: http://www.sciencedaily.com/releases/2008/11/081121125602.htm

Sherman, D.K., Iacono, W.G., McGue, M.K. (1997). Attention-deficit hyperactivity disorder dimensions: a twin study of inattention and impulsivity-hyperactivity. J Am Acad Child Adolesc Psychiatry, 36 (6), 745–753.

Sim, M.G., Hulse, G., Khong, E. (2004). When the child with ADHD grows up. Aust Fam Physician, 33 (8), 615–618.

Smalley, S. (2008). Reframing ADHD in the genomic era. Psychiatric Times, 25 (7). Retrieved from http://www.psychiatrictimes.com/adhd/article/10168/1163208.

Smucker, W.D., Heydayat, M. (2001). Evaluation and treatment of ADHD. Am Fam Physician, 64 (5), 817–829.

Solanto, M.V. (1998, July). Neuropsychopharmacological mechanisms of stimulant drug action in attention-deficit hyperactivity disorder: A review and integration. Behav Brain Res, 94 (1), 127–152.

Sourander, A., Niemelä, S., Santalahti, P., et al. (2008, March). Changes in psychiatric problems and service use among 8-year-old children: a 16-year population-based time-trend study. J Am Acad Child Adolesc Psychiatry, 47 (3), 317–327.

Sourander, A., Klomek, A.B., Niemela, S., et al. (2009). Childhood predictors of completed and severe suicide attempts: findings from the Finnish 1981 Birth Cohort Study. Arch Gen Psychiatry, 66 (4), 398–406.

Staudenmayer, H. (1999). Environmental illness: myth and reality. Boca Raton, FL: CRC Press.

Stead, J., Gwynedd, L., Cohen, D. (2005). Critical new perspectives on ADHD. New York, NY: Routledge.

Stein, M.A. (2004). Innovations in attention-deficit/hyperactivity disorder pharmacotherapy: long-acting stimulant and nonstimulant treatments. Am J Manag Care, 10 (4 Suppl), S89–S98.

Stern, H.P., Stern, T.P. (2002). When children with attention-deficit/hyperactivity disorder become adults. South Med J, 95 (9), 985–991.

Stockl, K.M., Hughes, T.E., Jarrar, M.A., et al. (2003). Physician perceptions of the use of medications for attention deficit hyperactivity disorder. J Manag Care Pharm, 9 (5), 416–423.

St. Sauver, J.L., Barbaresi, W.J., Katusic, S.K., et al. (2004). Early life risk factors for attention-deficit/hyperactivity disorder: a population-based cohort study. Mayo Clin Proc, 79 (9), 1124–1131.

Szasz, T.S. (2001). Pharmacracy: medicine and politics in America. New York, NY: Praeger.

Tan, M., Appleton, R. (2005). Attention deficit and hyperactivity disorder, methylphenidate, and epilepsy. Arch Dis Child, 90 (1), 57–59.

The Cochrane Collaboration (2005, April 20). Family therapy for attention-deficit disorder or attention-deficit/hyperactivity disorder in children and adolescents. Retrieved from: http://www.cohrane.org/reviews/en/ab005042.html

Van Ameringen, M., Mancini, C., Simpson, W., et al. (2010, April 8). Adult attention deficit hyperactivity disorder in an anxiety disorders population. CNS Neurosci Ther, [Epub ahead of print]

Van Cleave, J., Leslie, L.K. (2008). Approaching ADHD as a chronic condition: implications for long-term adherence. J Psychosoc Nurs Ment Health Serv, 46 (8), 28–37.

van den Hoofdakker, B.J., van der Veen-Mulders, L., Sytema, S., et al. (2007). Effectiveness of behavioral parent training for children with ADHD in routine clinical practice: a randomized controlled study. J Am Acad Child Adolesc Psychiatry, 46 (10), 1263–1271..

Vierhile, A., Robb, A., Ryan-Krause, P. (2009). Attention-deficit/hyperactivity disorder in children and adolescents: closing diagnostic, communication, and treatment gaps. J Pediatr Health Care, 23 (1 Suppl), S5–S23.

Walters, A.S., Silvestri, R., Zucconi, M., et al. (2008). Review of the possible relationship and hypothetical links between attention deficit hyperactivity disorder (ADHD) and the simple sleep related movement disorders, parasomnias, hypersomnias, and circadian rhythm disorders (review abstract). J Clin Sleep Med, 4 (6), 591–600.

Weinstein, D., Staffelbach, D., Biaggio, M. (2000). Attention-deficit hyperactivity disorder and posttraumatic stress disorder: differential diagnosis in childhood sexual abuse. Clin Psychol Rev, 20 (3), 359–378.

Wymbs, B.T., Pelham, W.E., Jr., Molina, B.S.G., et al. (2008). Rate and predictors of divorce among parents of youths with ADHD. J Consult Clin Psychol, 76 (5), 735.

Zwi, M., Ramchandani, P., Joughin, S. (2000). Evidence and belief in ADHD. BMJ, 321 (7267), 975–976.

Chapter 6
Sensory Integration Dysfunction

Sensory integration dysfunction (SID) (also known as regulatory sensory processing disorder, sensory processing dysfunction, or sensory processing dysfunction) is a neurological disorder that involves impairment in processing data from the different senses (vision, auditory, touch, olfaction, and taste), the vestibular system (movement), and proprioception (body awareness).

Sensory integration problems are prevalent in children and adults (Kane, 2004). Pediatric neurologists, pediatricians, child psychologists, and other clinicians are increasingly diagnosing SID. It is not a diagnosis in the DSM-IV. However, regulatory sensory processing disorder is a diagnosis in the Diagnostic Manual for Infancy (by Stanley Greenspan) and the Zero to Three's Diagnostic Classification.

Individuals who have SID are able to receive sensory information. However, they perceive this sensory information in a dysfunctional way. In persons with SID, the brain may process the sensory information in an irregular way, possibly causing disorientation and anxiety.

SID can be associated with other neurological disorders, such as attention-deficit hyperactive disorder (ADHD), autism, developmental dyspraxia, dyslexia, speech delays, and Tourette syndrome. Those with SID can meet the criteria for Asperger syndrome as classified by the DSM-IV (Rogers and Ozonoff, 2005). A variety of therapies are available for SID. However, there is no known cure.

Children with multiple disabilities frequently have sensory motor integration problems (Kane, 2004). These children may have problems with motor planning and positional awareness. They frequently have problems with balance and feel anxious and uncomfortable in crowded situations.

Three Types of SID

SID has been classified into three diagnostic groups (Case-Smith, 2005; Miller et al., 2007):

Type 1: sensory modulation disorder
Type 2: sensory-based motor disorder
Type 3: sensory discrimination

M.L. Goldstein, S. Morewitz, *Chronic Disorders in Children and Adolescents*,
DOI 10.1007/978-1-4419-9764-7_6, © Springer Science+Business Media, LLC 2011

Children and some adults with a Type 1 disorder: Sensory modulation disorder may over- or underrespond to sensory stimuli or engage in behaviors to stimulate their senses (Case-Smith, 2005; Miller et al., 2007).

Children with sensory modulation disorders, because of their impaired central nervous system, have difficulty in determining the intensity frequency, duration, complexity, and novelty of various sensory stimuli. As a consequence, they are not able to grade their behavior responses to incoming sensations and underrespond or overrespond to incoming stimuli.

Children and some adults can experience different types of sensory modulation difficulties. One component of sensory modulation disorder consists of sensory registration problems, which refers to difficulties with which a child's central nervous system attends to sensory stimuli. Sensory registration problems involve a child's failure to notice sensory stimuli that most individuals usually notice.

Another aspect of sensory modulation disorders is sensory defensiveness, in which children and some adults overrespond to sensory stimuli.

Gravitational defensiveness is another component of sensory modulation difficulties. Gravitational defensiveness occurs when a child or adult tends to respond negatively and with fear to different movements. Gravitational defensiveness is especially likely to occur when a child's head position is changed or the child moves backward or forward through space.

Children with Type 1 disorder: Sensory modulation disorder may become fearful or anxious and develop negative and/or stubborn-type behaviors. Children with this disorder also may exhibit self-absorbed behaviors, making them difficult to engage socially. They also may pursue behaviors that are creative or sensation seeking.

Children with a Type 2 disorder: Sensory-based motor disorder exhibits motor behavior that is disorganized (Case-Smith, 2005). This disorganization occurs because the person cannot process sensory data correctly.

Those who have impairment in discriminating different sensory information, difficulties in controlling posture, and dyspraxia are classified as having Type 3 disorder: sensory discrimination disorder (Case-Smith, 2005). As a result, children with these disabilities tend to be inattentive and disorganized and perform poorly in school.

Hyposensitivity and Hypersensitivity

Children and adults may be mildly affected by SID, while others suffer significant disruption in their social, school, work, and family functioning. Children and adults can vary widely in the extent to which they are hyposensitive or hypersensitive. They also vary in the degree to which they have impairments in processing various sensory stimuli. These persons may have disability in only one sensory modality, a few modalities, or all of their sensory modalities.

Children and adults may be hypersensitive (Kane, 2004). Hypersensitivity, also known as sensory defensiveness, can involve feeling pain from clothes that rub against one's skin, not liking to be touched, difficulties tolerating normal lighting, and experiencing problems when someone looks them directly in the eye.

Other children and adults may be hyposensitive in which they have a very high tolerance for sensory stimuli. Hyposensitive children may seem restless and go after sensory stimulation.

Other Disorders

Some children with SID may be misdiagnosed as having autism since children with autistic disorders frequently have unusual responses to sensory stimuli. Compared to children with other developmental conditions, there is some evidence that autistic children may be more likely to underrespond to sensory stimuli, e.g., walk into objects, than overrespond to sensory stimuli, e.g., experience discomfort from loud sounds or seek sensory stimulation, such as making rhythmic movements (Ben-Sasson et al., 2008). Unusual responses to sensory stimuli may be more prevalent in autistic children than in autistic adults. For example, Williams et al. (2006) reported that tactile perception was dysfunctional in autistic children, while it was not in autistic adults.

Certain children with sensory-associated problems also may be misdiagnosed as having ADHD. In other instances, children with SID can have ADHD and other conditions, such as speech-related problems, e.g., apraxia, emotional difficulties, and aggressive tendencies. Likewise, a child may be misdiagnosed as having SID when she or he actually has attention difficulties.

Children with SID symptoms may have fetal alcohol syndrome (FAS). These children can experience a number of sensory integration difficulties.

Processing sensory stimuli is a foundational process and dysfunction in this processing of sensory stimuli can produce a wide range of symptoms, including speech delay, aggression, and hyperactivity. A child may seem to be hyperactive when she or he actually has SID. This child's vestibular system may be underresponding and may require extra stimuli for her or his motion sensor so that the child can be comfortable.

Another possibility is that a child has a disorder that fits the diagnostic criteria for both ADHD and SID. Siegel (2007) found that the disease hypokalemic sensory overstimulation meets the criteria for both disorders.

Assessment of a child with possible symptoms of SID may benefit from an interdisciplinary assessment to rule out other disorders, such as autism, ADHD, apraxia and other speech-related conditions, aggressiveness, anxiety, and behavioral disorders. For example, a child with possible SID symptoms might be seen by an occupational therapist, audiologist, speech pathologist, pediatric neurologist, and pediatric psychologist.

If the child cannot repeat what a teacher says in class, the child may be bored or distracted. The child can be evaluated by a pediatric neurologist or pediatric psychologist for SID. An occupational therapist may then evaluate the child to ascertain why the child is having trouble focusing and attending. An audiologist and a speech pathologist also can assess the child for difficulties in auditory processing or language processing.

During an auditory evaluation, the child may be asked to listen to signals from headphones and determine where the signals are originating. The auditory evaluation may be inconclusive if the child is distracted or bored or unsure about the test's oral instructions. In evaluating the child's performance on the test, the tester should consider both sensory issues and language variables.

In addition, other clinicians may be needed to diagnose other possible disorders, such as food intolerances, FAS, and genetic problems such as the Fragile X syndrome. In other instances, children may appear to have SID symptoms when they are simply bored because they are intellectually challenged during school or other settings.

Sensory Integration Treatment

Children and adults typically can become annoyed and distracted by noisy sounds or the discomfort of certain types of sweaters. Interventions are only warranted when the child is so affected by these stressful sensory stimuli that she or he withdraws from social interactions, engages in hyperactive and impulsive behaviors, and becomes aggressive, which may result from a "flight or fight" response to uncomfortable sensory stimuli. A child also can develop hyposensitivity to sensory stimuli. For example, a child may be insensitive to pain, e.g., may not blink after being burned.

A number of sensory integration therapies have been developed. There is a paucity of studies that show the effectiveness of these treatment modalities (Baranek, 2002; Schaaf and Miller, 2005; Hodgetts and Hodgetts, 2007). Treatments such as the use of prism lenses, physical exercise, and training in auditory integration have been investigated but methodological problems limit their validity. Sensorimotor handling has not been supported by research (Baranek, 2002).

Occupational therapy is the main type of treatment for SID. Occupational therapy consists of putting a child in a room that is set up to stimulate and challenge the child's five senses, sense of movement, and proprioception. The child is offered a degree of sensory stimulation that she or he can handle and is also encouraged by the therapist to move within the room. The emphasis is on improving the child's ability to tolerate and integrate sensory stimuli.

There are four principles that underlie occupational therapy for SID patients. First, according to the "just right challenge" principle, the child participates in play and must be able to handle the tasks that are presented to him or her during these play activities. Second, in the adaptive response principle, the child formulates new and effective techniques to the tasks that are offered. The third principle, "active engagement," assumes that if the play activities are fun, then the child will want to engage in these activities. Finally, according to the "child directed" principle, the wishes of the child are followed in developing play activities or tasks for the treatment.

The occupational therapist can treat children with hyposensitivity by presenting the children with strong sensory stimuli, e.g., use of vibrations or rubbing items. The therapist should design play activities that promote stimulation of the senses, e.g., finger painting or playing with play dough.

For children with hypersensitivity, the occupational therapist can offer the children peaceful activities such as listening to quiet music or gentle rocking in a room that has soothing lighting. The therapist can use rewards and treats to get children to engage in activities that they usually would refrain from doing.

In addition to improving the child's ability to tolerate and integrate sensory stimuli, occupational therapists and other clinicians focus on changing the environment to improve the way the child functions in different settings (Biel and Peske, 2005; Kane, 2004). Parents and teachers can change the child's environment in many ways to help them cope with sensory integration problems (Kane, 2004). Children can be given soft, tag-free clothing so that they do not feel pain from their clothes rubbing their skin. Kane (2004) recommends that for children who have sensitivity to touch, teachers should never touch the child from behind and when they do touch the child, they should use firm pressure on the back or shoulder instead of using a gentle touch. Teachers should line up children with sufficient space between themselves to minimize touching. Kane (2004) also recommends the use of chair pillow or cushion for children with sensitivity to touch.

For children who have problems with positional awareness, it is recommended that teachers use markers or masking tape to delineate the child's personal space (Kane, 2004). Teachers should place these children's desks along the side of the room away from student traffic, and they should ensure that the children be allowed an ample view of where other students are walking. The teacher should also permit children to select where they sit during story time.

Some children at school need more sensory stimuli to help them maintain their focus. Kane (2004) recommends that teachers permit these children to sit on an air cushion pillow that is filled slightly with air. This type of cushion enables children to experience movement without them leaving their desks. For children who need more sensory stimuli, teachers should allow them to climb or run during breaks and exercise periods. The teachers should also give these students opportunities to perform repetitive movements, e.g., washing their desk or erasing the blackboard. Kane (2004) also recommends that teachers should never discipline these children by taking away their recess or physical education periods.

Some children at school may also need additional sensory stimulation of their hands and mouths (Kane, 2004). These children should be permitted to keep a water bottle at their desks. They should be allowed to chew on a straw, coffee stick, or other suitable item. In addition, these children should be encouraged to have a small squeeze ball in their pocket.

At home, non-fluorescent lighting can be used to minimize the child's inability to tolerate room lighting. Children also can be given ear plugs to cope with emergency drills during school time.

Some occupational therapists also develop treatment approaches for adults with sensory integration difficulties.

References

Baranek, G.T. (2002). Efficacy of sensory and motor interventions for children with autism. J Autism Dev Disord, 32 (5), 397–422. doi:10.1023/A:1020541906063. PMID 12463517.

Ben-Sasson, A., Hen, L., Fluss, R., et al. (2008). A meta-analysis of sensory modulation symptoms in individuals with autism spectrum disorders. J Autism Dev Disord, 39 (1), 1–11. doi:10.1007/s10803-008-0593-3. PMID 18512135.

Biel, L., Peske, N.K. (2005). Raising a sensory smart child: the definitive handbook for helping your child with sensory integration issues. London, England: Penguin Books, Ltd.

Case-Smith, J. (2005). Occupational therapy for children, 5th edn. St. Louis, MO: Elsevier Mosby.

Hodgetts, S., Hodgetts, W. (2007, December). Somatosensory stimulation interventions for children with autism: literature review and clinical considerations. Can J Occup Ther, 74 (5), 393–400.

Kane, A. (2004). Teaching children with sensory motor integration deficits. ADD ADHD Advances, October 11 2004, http://addadhdadvances.com/sensory-integration-disorder-tips.html

Miller, L.J., Anzalone, M.E., Lane, S.J., et al. (2007, March–April). Concept evolution in sensory integration: a proposed nosology for diagnosis. Amer J Occup Therapy, 61 (2), 135–140.

Rogers, S.J., Ozonoff, S. (2005, December). Annotation: what do we know about sensory dysfunction in autism? a critical review of the empirical evidence. J Child Psychol Psychiatry, 46 (12), 1255–1268.

Schaaf, R.C., Miller, L.J. (2005). Occupational therapy using a sensory integrative approach for children with developmental disabilities. Ment Retard Dev Disabil Res Rev, 11 (2), 143–148.

Siegel, D.M. (2007). Chronic arthritis in adolescence. Adolesc Med State Rev, 18 (1), 47–61.

Williams, D.L., Goldstein, G., Minshew, N.J. (2006). Neuropsychologic functioning in children with autism: further evidence for disordered complex information-processing. Child Neuropsychol, 12 (4–5), 279–298. doi:10.1080/09297040600681190. PMC 1803025. PMID 16911973.

Chapter 7
Conduct Disorder and Oppositional Defiant Disorder

Conduct disorder (CD) is a behavioral disorder that occurs during childhood and adolescence where children repeatedly act aggressively and express anger inappropriately. The disorder can start in either childhood or adolescence (Conner, 1998–2000).

Children with CD display many different forms of antisocial and destructive behaviors. They violate the rights of others and do not follow accepted social and behavioral norms. They may commit violence against people and animals, destroy property, lie, steal, skip school, and run away from home. At a young age, many of these children start to use and abuse alcohol and drugs and experiment with sex. They commonly exhibit irritability, temper tantrums, and have low self-esteem.

Oppositional defiant disorder (ODD) (The International Classification of Diseases 10th Revision (ICD-10)) is a less serious form of CD (Turgay, 2009). Children and adolescents with ODD exhibit a recurring pattern of hostility, defying authority, and engaging in negative actions (Office of Child and Family Policy, 2008). Examples of ODD include persistent arguments with adults and persons in authority, violating rules, and being non-compliant, vindictive, or spiteful. As in the case of CD, youngsters with ODD frequently lose their tempers and display their anger and/or resentment in other ways. However, when compared to CD, ODD youngsters reflect a lesser opposition to social norms.

Increasingly, researchers have discovered that ODD has considerable overlap with CD (Turgay, 2009; Maughan et al., 2004). ODD may be a precursor to CD and antisocial personality (ASP). About 60% of persons with ODD will acquire CD (Turgay, 2009). Some younger boys with ODD will develop CD as they grow older, but others will not. Among boys with ODD, Biederman et al. (2008a) found that having ODD increases the probability of later development of CD and ASP for boys. Current data are inadequate to determine the trends for girls.

Demographic Characteristics

In the USA, 2–6% or 1–4 million children and adolescents have CD (Kazdin, 1994). The prevalence is the same during pre-adolescence and adolescence.

M.L. Goldstein, S. Morewitz, *Chronic Disorders in Children and Adolescents*,
DOI 10.1007/978-1-4419-9764-7_7,

The disorder exists in about 6–16% of boys and in 2–9% of girls younger than 18 years of age (Siminoff et al., 1997; Carlson et al., 1997).

Using a representative sample of 10,438 children, ages 5–15 years, from the 1999 British Child Mental Health Survey, Maughan et al. (2004) found that CD was more prevalent among boys than girls. As children get older, they are more likely to develop CD (Maughan et al., 2004). Girls are more likely than boys to acquire CD at age 12 or older. Approximately 40% of CP children will develop ASP as adults. Maughan et al. (2004) discovered that as 5- to 15-year-old CD children with status violations and other non-aggressive conduct-related difficulties grew older, their problems increased in prevalence with age. However, their aggressive behaviors decreased in prevalence with age.

ODD age patterns vary depending on its overlap with how CD is classified and diagnosed (Maughan et al., 2004). When guidelines from the DSM-IV are used, the rates of ODD became lower with age.

Causes of CD

The following researchers and articles have described a variety of factors that seem to increase the risk of CD development in children and adolescents (Encyclopedia of Children's Health, no date). Cognitive problems leading to school failures increase the probability that a child will develop CD. Children with a normal IQ may have trouble with verbal and abstract reasoning and thus lag behind their classmates academically. Their academic difficulties in turn can result in low self-esteem, social rejection, and increasing frustration, all of which can lead to the onset of CD.

Moffitt (1993) found that having a learning disorder (LD) is associated with developing CD. Her research demonstrates that learning impairments and minimal brain dysfunction (MBD) are highly related to the initiation of aggressive behavior, deviant behavior, and hyperactivity. A number of studies have found a link between attention-deficit/hyperactivity disorder (ADHD) and CD.

Byun et al. (2006) discovered that 53 or 50.5% of 105 patients in Korea diagnosed with ADHD had ODD.

In a study of 131 children in British Columbia, Canada, with ADHD, Klassen et al. (2004) found that 45 or 34.4% were diagnosed with CD or ODD.

Kilic and Sener (2005) evaluated family functioning and psychosocial attributes of 92 children, aged 6–11 years, diagnosed with ADHD and ADHD with co-existing ODD/CD. Based on the parents' completion of the Child Behavior Checklist, the authors reported that children with ADHD and comorbid ODD/CD scored high in dysfunctional behavior. However, these children had low scores related to social withdrawal and sexual problems. The researchers discovered a high degree of maternal depression and paternal alcohol difficulties among the children with ADHD and co-existing ODD/CD. In addition, the families of children with ADHD and ODD/CD demonstrated a high degree of dysfunctional family functioning based on the Roles and Behavior Control subscales of the Family Assessment Device.

Cunningham and Boyle (2002) evaluated mothers and their 4-year-old children at risk for ADHD, both ADHD and ODD, and a comparison group of mothers with symptom-free children. They found that mothers of children at risk for ODD had more family problems, perceived themselves as less capable as parents, and had fewer strategies for resolving their children's behavior difficulties than the control group. Moreover, mothers of children at risk for ODD were not as assertive in managing their children, showed higher levels of individual depression, and indicated that their children were more likely to internalize their problems than the mothers of children in the control group.

Relative to the control group, the children at risk for ADHD were more likely to have behavioral difficulties in school such as classroom management and social interaction problems.

When dealing with discipline problems, mothers in all groups used twice as many negative or controlling approaches as preventive or positive management approaches. Interestingly, the mothers of daughters at risk for the different disorders rewarded their daughters more often for each example of positive conduct than did the boys' mothers.

Youth diagnosed with CDs often have co-existing mental disorders, including anxiety and depressive disorders and substance abuse problems (Boylan et al., 2007; Turgay, 2005). Boylan et al. (2007) suggest that young children with ODD have an increased likelihood of developing internalizing conditions, such as anxiety and depression. In addition, mania is present in 40% of children and adolescents with CD (Biederman et al., 1999; Wrowley and Riggs, 1995; Young et al., 1995).

Conner (1998–2000) suggests that some of the following interactions can lead to CD:

1. Inadequate parent–child relationships and inappropriate or inconsistent parenting.
2. Negative reinforcement, such as harsh and/or inconsistent discipline toward the child and/or other family members.
3. Parents or significant others who model aggressive and coercive behaviors increase the risk that the child will imitate these antisocial behaviors.
4. Family environments characterized by emotional, physical, or sexual abuse.
5. Parental alcoholism and a family history of antisocial personality.
6. Adverse characteristics of the school environment.
7. Negative influences from peers and friends.

Based on a sample of 1,162 female and male twin pairs, aged 12–19 years, and 429 siblings, Ehringer et al. (2006) found that both genetic and non-shared environmental influences may contribute to the development of common adolescent disorders, including CD, ODD, and ADHD.

However, other researchers have emphasized the impact of environmental influences on these behavioral problems. For example, a meta-analysis of twin and adoption studies by Burt (2009) demonstrated that environmental influences, which produced similarities between siblings, accounted for 10–30% of the variability within CD, ODD, anxiety, depression, and other internalizing and externalizing conditions. In contrast, ADHD seemed to be caused largely by genetic factors.

Diagnosis

If a CD is suspected, the child should be evaluated promptly by her or his health practitioner and possibly a mental health professional (Encyclopedia of Children's Health, no date). Admission to an inpatient mental health facility may be necessary if a child diagnosed with CD has thoughts of self-injury or suicide or is a danger to other people.

A diagnosis of CD is made if the person repeatedly engages in aggressive and antisocial behaviors that disrupt social, family, and educational functioning as well as job-related performance. Individuals with CD may bully and threaten other people; start fights; be cruel to animals and people; coerce individuals into having sex; deliberately destroy other people's property; be frequently truant; have run away from home overnight at least twice or once for a long time period (Encyclopedia of Children's Health, no date). Three of these types of behaviors must have occurred over the prior 12 months, and one of the three behaviors must have taken place in the previous 6 months.

A diagnosis of ODD is made if the child or adolescent commits negative, defiant, and hostile behaviors more frequently than normal for the individual's age and developmental stage and that these actions substantially impair the individual's functioning (Office of Child and Family Policy, 2008).

A person is not diagnosed with both CD and ODD. Those who fulfill the criteria for both disorders are diagnosed with CD (Office of Child and Family Policy, 2008).

Clinicians need to consider the age of onset when diagnosing CD or ODD. Individuals with ODD have a younger age of onset than persons with CD (Office of Child and Family Policy, 2008).

Youth with CD often have a history of ODD, but not all children with ODD will develop CD (Loeber et al., 1991). Children with ODD who develop CD initially exhibit problems, such as being a bully, fighting, being dishonest, and destruction of property. These individuals later engage in CD-related behaviors including truancy, school vandalism, breaking and entering, aggravated assault, rape, and homicide.

Persons with child-onset CD must have one criterion of the condition before the age of 10 (Office of Child and Family Policy, 2008). Persons with adolescent-onset CD do not meet any criteria for the condition before 10 years of age.

Some researchers believe that youth with child-onset CD initially acquire their disruptive behaviors in their family environment (Office of Child and Family Policy, 2008). They then expand their deviant behaviors as they interact with antisocial peer groups, e.g., gangs, and isolate themselves from conventional peer groups. It is important to distinguish between child- and adult-onset CD, since studies show that persons with adolescent-onset CD are less likely to continue their antisocial behaviors as adults than those with child-onset CD (Grizenko, 1997; Robins, 1981). Another investigation found that children in preschool and elementary school who display antisocial conduct have a higher probability of engaging in antisocial behaviors in adulthood than preschool and elementary school children who do not exhibit antisocial behaviors (Kazdin, 1987).

Assessment

The following measurements are used to assess CD and ODD: (1) reports and evaluations; (2) direct observation; (3) institutional records; and (4) self-report instruments (Turgay, 2005; Patterson et al., 1992). The assessment should cover all behavioral and psychiatric problems since CD by itself is rare (Turgay, 2005).

Reports and evaluations from parents, teachers, counselors, and others familiar with the child or adolescent can help to determine if she or he has CD or ODD. However, these reports can offer conflicting results. For example, certain adults may perceive the child's actions as antisocial, while other adults may view her or his behaviors as normal (Reid et al., 1987; Lorber, 1981; Hart et al., 1994).

Direct observation of children's actions in different contexts, such as the family, community, and school, and in different time periods can provide data on the youth's overt actions, such as getting into arguments, bullying, and fighting (Office of Child and Family Policy, 2008).

School records, police records, and other institutional records can offer information about problems that the child is experiencing in different settings (Office of Child and Family Policy, 2008).

The above data sources may miss covert activities, such as drug use, vandalism, and sexual activities (Office of Child and Family Policy, 2008). To help correct this problem, self-report checklists, scales, and questionnaires can be employed. CD-related behaviors can be assessed with the Child Behavior Checklist, which can yield detailed information about the youth's normal social functioning, academic performance, delinquent behaviors, aggressive conduct, and attention problems. Clinicians can compare the child's performance on the checklist with the scores of children in the general population. In addition, parents, teachers, and children can use different forms of the checklist. Scales of the Minnesota Multiphasic Personality Inventory Adolescent version (MMPI-A) also provide information on CD-related behaviors.

Treatment

Early treatment for behavior problems is essential to restore social, family, school, and occupational functioning and avoid a wide range of problems during adulthood (Office of Child and Family Policy, 2008). Children with conduct-related behaviors are more likely to have substance abuse, psychiatric disorders, marital difficulties, impaired occupational functioning, and poor health as adults than those without early behavior problems (Goldstein et al., 2006; Lahey et al., 1995; Biederman et al., 1999; Young et al., 1995).

Using a national, representative sample, Goldstein et al. (2006) found that compared to persons with adolescent-onset CD, individuals with childhood-onset CD were more likely to show aggression against people and animals and vandalize property before the age of 15. Those with childhood-onset CD were more likely to exhibit violent behaviors throughout their lifetime than those with adolescent-onset CD. Persons with childhood-onset CD were more likely to have a variety of disorders, including lifetime social phobias, generalized anxiety disorder, substance dependence, and personality disorders, such as paranoid personality disorder.

Donovan et al. (2000) showed that adolescent girls with conduct-related problems had a greater likelihood of becoming young, single mothers and to have children with behavioral difficulties at an early age.

Because of the overlap of ODD with CD and the high prevalence of co-existing disorders, especially ADHD, treatment of CDs requires different types of psychosocial interventions and psychopharmacology (Kutcher et al., 2004; Maughan et al., 2004; Office of Child and Family Policy, 2008). Psychosocial methods include parent and child training, dyadic skill training, cognitive behavior therapy (CBT), family therapy, multi-system therapy (MST), group therapy, day treatment, and wilderness training. Medication also may be employed under certain conditions, especially to control symptoms related to the behavioral problem or co-existing medical problems. (Please note that all of the interventions mentioned above are discussed in detail further on in this section.)

Behavioral parent training is an effective treatment for parents of children with ODD and CD (Chronis et al., 2004). Parent and child training seek to modify inadequate parenting, which has been found to be a risk factor for CD and ODD (Office of Child and Family Policy, 2008; Conner, 1998–2000).

Parent training for families of children with ADHD and conduct-related problems includes training sessions that discuss the characteristics and causes of ADHD and its association with defiant and aggressive behaviors as well as techniques to enhance parenting skills (Danforth et al., 2006).

The Triple P Positive Parenting program, a multi-level parent training program, is designed to prevent and treat severe behavioral, emotional, and developmental difficulties in children aged 0–16 years (de Graaf et al., 2008; Sanders, 1999). The program attempts to improve parents' knowledge, skills, and confidence. The Triple P Positive program takes into account the fact that children experience different levels of behavioral dysfunction and parents may have varying needs in terms of the intervention's type and intensity. The program is based on social learning principles, child and family behavior therapy, developmental research, and social information-processing models.

The Triple P Positive program offers five levels of intervention (de Graaf et al., 2008; Sanders, 1999). Level 1 offers psychoeducational information on parenting skills to parents who are interested in the intervention. In Level 2, one to two sessions are offered to parents of children with mild conduct problems. Level 3, a four-session program, provides an intervention for children with mild to moderate behavioral problems. This intervention also offers parents active skills training.

In Level 4, parents of children with more severe conduct problems or who are at risk for developing these difficulties receive eight to ten intensive training sessions. These parent training sessions focus on child management skills and can be presented to individual parents or to groups of parents. Level 5, an enhanced behavioral family intervention, is designed to assist families who have parenting problems that are complicated by other stressors, such as domestic violence and parental depression.

Hahlweg et al. (2010) assessed the effectiveness of the Triple P Positive program using a sample of 280 families randomly assigned to either the Triple P Positive program or control group. At a 2-year follow-up, both the mothers and fathers in the Triple P Positive program had fewer dysfunctional parental behaviors, and mothers in the intervention reported more positive parenting behaviors. Mothers in the experimental group also indicated that their children exhibited fewer internalizing and externalizing behaviors. However, single-parent mothers in the Triple P Positive program did not experience changes in parenting behaviors or child behavior difficulties. The lack of changes in single-parent mothers and their children may be due to the high positive effects in the single-parent mothers in the control group.

Based on a meta-analysis of 15 studies, de Graaf et al. (2008) evaluated the effectiveness of the Triple P Positive Level 4 intervention. The authors found that the Triple P Positive Level 4 programs limited the children's conduct problems. These reductions in the children's behavior problems were maintained over time and additional improvements occurred in follow-up over the long term.

Sanders et al. (2000) evaluated the effectiveness of the delivery modes of the Triple P Positive Level 4 intervention using a sample of 305 preschoolers at high risk for acquiring behavior problems. Children in Level 5 (enhanced behavioral family intervention), Level 4 (standard behavioral family intervention), and Level 3 (self directed behavioral family interventions) and those on the waitlist improved in their disruptive behaviors. However, the children in the enhanced behavioral family intervention (Level 5) and standard behavioral family intervention (Level 4) improved more in parent-observed child behavior problems than children on the waitlist.

Parent–child interaction therapy (PCIT), a family-centered treatment approach, is designed to treat major behavior problems, such as CD and ODD, and ADHD in children aged 2½ to 12 years and dysfunctional parenting behaviors (Child Welfare Information Gateway, 2007). The program is designed for abused and at-risk children and their biological or foster parents. PCIT involves having therapists coach parents while they relate to their children. Therapists help parents adopt strategies that reinforce their children's positive behaviors. Therapists may sit behind a one-way mirror and coach the parent using "ear bug" audio equipment.

PCIT seeks to reduce negative parent–child interactions that may cause behavior difficulties in young children (Child Welfare Information Gateway, 2007). The approach is designed to help parents learn to model and reinforce positive parenting techniques for responding to negative emotions. Children, in turn, will develop positive behaviors because of these healthier parent–child interactions.

The therapy is delivered in 14–20 sessions that last about 1 h. Additional therapy may be added as needed. The intervention consists of two phases: (1) relationship enhancement and (2) discipline and compliance. Phase 1 seeks to enhance the parent–child relationship by helping parents follow the acronym "PRIDE" (praise, reflection, imitation, description, and enthusiasm). In Phase 2, parents are taught to discipline their child in a structured and consistent manner. For example, parents learn how to give clear and direct commands to their child and offer consistent consequences for their child's compliance or non-compliance. Parents learn these skills in play situations where they must give commands and discipline or reward their child appropriately.

Investigations have shown that PCIT can reduce children's conduct problems at home and in school settings (Thomas and Zimmer-Gembeck, 2007; Gallagher, 2003; Child Welfare Gateway Information, 2007). In a review and meta-analysis of 24 investigations of PCIT and Triple P Positive parenting programs, Thomas and Zimmer-Gembeck (2007) discovered that participation in PCIT programs resulted in significantly fewer parent-reported child conduct and parent difficulties. However, the abbreviated PCIT program was associated with only moderate effect sizes. All types of the Triple P Positive parenting programs, except the Media Triple P Positive parenting program, had moderate to large effect sizes based on parent-reported child activities and parenting behaviors. The Media Triple P Positive parenting had only small effect sizes.

Based on a review of 17 studies that included 628 preschool-aged children, Gallagher (2003) showed that PCIT programs produced significant improvements in child functioning. The investigations revealed that children who participated in the PCIT programs had less frequent and less intense conduct problems based on teacher and parent reports. Participation in PCIT interventions also was associated with more behavioral compliance in the clinics, less inattention problems and hyperactivity, less crying or whining, and less disruptive behavior.

In an investigation of families of children with ADHD and conduct-associated problems, Danforth et al. (2006) evaluated the outcome of group parent training which used the parameters of the Behavior Management Flow Chart. The use of skills learned in the group parent training not only reduced the children's symptoms of ADHD and CDs, but succeeded in having a favorable impact on parenting behavior and lowering the stress among parents.

Social skills training for youth is another type of intervention for children with CD and ODD (Maughan et al., 2004; Conner, 1998–2000). This strategy emphasizes social skills training and experiences that help the youngsters deal effectively with conflict. For example, children are taught how to start conversations, react to the needs of others, and set limits on their behavior.

The Incredible Years (IY) training program is a program for parents, teachers, and children (The Incredible Years, 2009, http://www.incredibleyears.com). The IY parent training program attempts to enhance parents' competencies, including their ability to provide positive discipline for their child and facilitate parents' involvement in their child's educational experiences. The goals of the curriculum are to foster their children's success in educational, social, and emotional functioning and limit the development of conduct-related problems.

The IY training for babies and toddlers, aged 0–3, is designed to support parents and their babies (The Incredible Years, 2009, http://www.incredibleyears.com). Consisting of a six-part curriculum, the IY Parents and Babies program seeks to help parents learn how to observe and identify their babies' behavioral cues and learning processes so that the parents can be more responsive in terms of the physical, tactile, and visual stimulation and verbal communication.

The IY teacher training curricula help teachers to improve their classroom management techniques, foster appropriate children's behaviors, improve the children's reading skills and other school readiness skills, and limit children's aggressive and non-compliant behavior in the classroom (The Incredible Years, 2009, http://www.incredibleyears.com). The IY teacher intervention program also helps teachers to work effectively with parents to enhance their school involvement and foster consistency in behavioral management and skill improvement from the school to the home.

The IY Dina Dinosaur classroom-based curriculum is designed to enhance peer interactions and limit aggressive behaviors for students aged 4–8 years (The Incredible Years, 2009, http://www.incredibleyears.com). Based on 120 lesson plans, the curriculum teachers can present the curricula two to three times a week using 15–20 min circle time discussions, which is followed by small group exercises. The program also consists of children's home detective club activities manuals, which are designed to foster parents' participation in educating their children about school rules, social skills, and problem-solving techniques.

Based on a total of 153 teachers and 1,768 socioeconomically disadvantaged students, Webster-Stratton et al. (2008) evaluated the IY teacher classroom management and the Dinosaur programs. They discovered that teachers who participated in the intervention relied on more positive classroom management techniques than the control teachers. Intervention teachers were more likely to have students who were more socially competent, more likely to control their emotions, and less likely to have behavioral problems.

Jones et al. (2007, 2008) analyzed the efficacy of the IY basic parent training program using a sample of families with preschool children who were at risk for acquiring CDs and ADHD. The findings indicated that participation in the IY basic parent training was related to a decrease in ADHD and conduct problems, such as inattention and impulsive behaviors.

Using a sample of students from five basic schools in Kingston, Jamaica, Baker-Henningham et al. (2009) assessed the impact of the IY teacher training program supplemented by 14 lessons on social and emotional skills presented in the classroom. The investigators discovered that the intervention reduced behavior problems, hyperactivity, and peer difficulties. In addition, the intervention produced more positive teacher–parent contacts than the control group.

Since symptoms of ODD are prevalent in clinical samples of children with tic disorders, Scahill et al. (2006) evaluated the impact of a structured parent training on the children's disruptive behaviors. Using data from the parent-rated

Disruptive Behavior Rating Scale, the researchers discovered that disruptive behavior decreased significantly. Parents also showed improvement in managing their children's negative behavior based on the Improvement scale of the Clinical Global Impression instrument.

A study of children with early-onset behavioral problems revealed that combining both child training and parent training produced better outcomes than either intervention by itself (Webster-Stratton and Hammond, 1997). According to Maughan et al. (2004), parent training is most beneficial for controlling oppositional conduct. Kazdin and Wassell (2000) showed that skills training for young people that consisted of cognitive problem-solving, along with parent management training, yielded positive results. The investigators found that parents who were willing to take part in the training were more likely to have children who maintained long-range positive effects of the intervention.

Dyadic skill training consists of 12–18 1-h sessions per week for children of preschool age and their parents (Speltz, 1990). This method assumes that the children's behavior problems are due to the fact that they had faulty caregiving.

Researchers have not found that CBT consistently controls children's conduct problems (Koegl et al., 2008; Munoz-Solomando et al., 2008; van de Wiel et al., 2002). In their meta-analysis of randomized controlled studies, Munoz-Solomando et al. (2008) discovered that CBT has not been shown to be effective in the treatment of conduct-related behaviors. However, they suggest that clinical guidelines and systematic literature reviews can enhance the mental health of children and adolescents.

Turner et al. (2005) assessed the usefulness of CBT in assisting foster carers in the management of foster children's difficult behavior. Based on a review of five eligible trials ($N = 443$), they showed that CBT-based training did not significantly improve the foster children's conduct problems and relationship difficulties. However, the CBT-based programs were associated with some improvement in the foster carers' behavioral management skills, attitudes, and psychological functioning. Nevertheless, the authors conclude that the effectiveness of CBT for foster carers has not been demonstrated.

Maughan et al. (2004) found that CBT, along with social skills training, was useful in treating aggressive and impulsive behaviors. CBT tries to solve disruptive behaviors and impaired emotional expressions using a systematic, goal-oriented approach. CBT consists of a variety of approaches, including cognitive therapy, rational emotive behavior therapy, and multimodal therapy. These techniques vary in the extent to which they rely on a combination of behavioral and cognitive research findings. Some CBT techniques are based on manuals and provide the patients with brief, direct, and time-limited therapies. CBT approaches may consist of having the patients keep a diary of major events and related feelings and have the patients test their cognitions, assumptions, and beliefs. CBT techniques may also use relaxation, mindfulness, and distraction methods.

Another method that has produced some favorable results for children with antisocial behavior is family therapy (Kazdin, 1985; Jacob, 1987). This approach seeks to modify problematic family systems and improve roles and communication within families. Adolescents who have not evidenced the most severe conduct behaviors such as being truant and running away may benefit the most from family therapy. Alexander and Parsons (1982) showed that for youth who committed low-level conduct problems, family therapy produced lower rates of repeat offenses for a 6–18 month period after therapy. In follow-up investigations, siblings in family therapy also had lower rates of contact with police.

MST has produced favorable results for treating mid-to-late age adolescent youth who engage in antisocial behaviors and externalize their problems (Schoenwald and Henggeler, 1999). The goal of this approach is to alter systems such as family, school, peers, and community that foster antisocial behaviors. MST offers parents and caregivers the resources, including skill development, and referrals to help them resolve their children's difficulties. Clinicians can make changes in the child's school environment. Also, therapists can assist the caregiver by finding suitable transportation, childcare, and other services. Clinicians provide action and treatment plans for the family and assign goals for the family and themselves. The therapists provide on-going treatment and assessment.

Some research has shown that MST has been useful with children who face institutionalization because of their persistent antisocial behaviors. According to Henggeler et al. (1999), MST costs less than a psychiatric hospitalization and seems to lead to improvements in school attendance and family dynamic and a reduction in the negative behaviors exhibited by the youth. MST has also been found to be more effective in reducing repeat offenses than eclectic individual therapy that involved psychodynamic, client-focused, or behavior-based approaches (Office of Child and Family Policy, 2008).

Group therapy is another form of treatment for children with externalizing and antisocial behaviors (Office of Child and Family Policy, 2008). Group therapy is designed for school-age children and can include community center groups. It tries to change the youth's behaviors in different group situations. The community-center form of group therapy assumes that conduct-related problems occur in large part because of involvement with deviant subcultures (Feldman, 1992; Office of Child and Family Policy, 2008). The community-center approach, therefore, uses a supervised setting to reduce the youth's relationship with antisocial friends and acquaintances and foster relationship with conventional peers. This type of group therapy can follow either the social learning model or the traditional model (Office of Child and Family Policy, 2008). In the social learning model, antisocial behaviors are controlled through the principles of behavior modification, such as reinforcement and modeling of appropriate behaviors. In contrast, the traditional model relies on rules and consequences. Groups of 10–15 children meet for 3 h weekly during the school year for both the social learning and traditional approaches.

Dishion and Andrews (1995) found that youth with CDs are more likely to benefit from group therapy if they are placed with conventional youth than if they are exposed to other children who exhibit antisocial behaviors.

Community-based residential programs have been used in the treatment of children with CD and ODD (Conner, 1998–2000). In these community-based residential programs, children and parents participate in a home or residential treatment setting. Facilitators serve as teaching parents. To achieve behavior change, youth with CDs participate in a point system, family conferences and other forms of self-government, and training in social skills. These young people are tutored in academic subjects and their progress is carefully monitored. Home-based reinforcement strategies are used to encourage that progress.

School-based interventions can be employed to treat youth with ODD and CD (Conner, 1998–2000). These strategies rely on classroom contingency management. However, Conner (1998–2000) notes that these school-based approaches can be difficult to initiate for certain youth since Public Law 94-142 excludes children who only suffer from behavioral problems.

For CD youth who do poorly in outpatient settings, day treatment has shown to be helpful (Kolko et al., 1999; Grizenko, 1997). Based on a study of a day treatment program that consisted of drug therapy, different types of individual and group therapy, and family therapy, Grizenko (1997) discovered that the positive outcomes lasted over 5 years. In an investigation of the effectiveness of a partial hospitalization program, Kolko et al. (1999) discovered that combining the medication, methylphenidate, with behavior treatment reduced ODD-related behaviors and increased conventional behavior.

Wilderness school interventions can help youth with CD and ODD (Conner, 1998–2000). These programs remove the child from environmental influences that promote or maintain antisocial and externalizing behaviors. Wilderness school programs seek to develop and maintain new conventional attitudes, behaviors, and skills. Counselors and therapists seek to achieve these goals by creating a structured and rigorous environment for the youth. Effective programs use themes such as honesty, awareness, skills, and responsibility.

Cowles et al. (1995), Steiner (1997), and Kazdin (1985) have found no evidence for the use of psychodynamic or insight-oriented individual and group psychotherapy in treating CD or ODD.

According to Conner (1998–2000), family-based treatments are more beneficial than individual-based interventions that involve the child only and not the parents and family. For pre-adolescent youth, training parents to use behavioral approaches can be effective. Peer group-based interventions and individual approaches are effective for adolescents with CDs. Family-based strategies are less effective with older children because the negative family interactions probably have lasted for much of the adolescents' life, and they are beginning to rebel against family pressure. If other strategies have been ineffective and the antisocial behavior continues or escalates, wilderness training can be helpful.

Drug therapy by itself has not been shown to be effective in the treatment of CD and ODD (Office of Child and Family Policy, 2008). Conner (1998–2000) notes that medication is ineffective when treating CDs since the conditions deal with behaviors. However, psychopharmacological interventions may be useful in treating co-existing mental disorders, such as ADHD, and some symptoms of conduct-related behaviors (Turgay, 2009). Controlling ADHD symptoms could make it easier to treat conduct-related behaviors.

Among preschool children with signs of ADHD, Daley et al. (2009) suggest that parent training should be initiated as the first line of treatment. Medications should not be used unless this parent training is ineffective.

A few investigations have discovered that psychostimulants or atomoxetine has produced positive outcomes in treating ODD related to ADHD (Turgay, 2009).

A pilot study of the medication, bupropion, revealed that it was helpful in treating ADHD symptoms among youth with CD and substance abuse disorders (Riggs et al., 1998). In addition, for patients with ODD and comorbid conditions, mood regulators, alpha (2) agonists, and antidepressants may be useful as secondary therapies (Turgay, 2009).

Another pilot investigation of methylphenidate, clonidine, and the combination of these drugs used to treat young people with ADHD and co-existing CD and ODD showed that these medications reduced symptoms related to each condition over a period of 3 months (Connor et al., 2000).

Treating comorbid substance abuse disorders, anxiety, depression, and LDs first may substantially improve CD behaviors (Encyclopedia of Children's Health, no date; Connor, 1998–2000). The clinician should initiate psychopharmacological treatment when symptoms develop.

Risperidone with or without psychostimulants may be effective in treating patients with ODD and CD who exhibit severe aggressive behaviors (Turgay, 2009). Mood-stabilizing drugs, such as lithium and carbamazepine, may be helpful in controlling severe aggressive behavior (Encyclopedia of Children's Health, no date). However, placing youth in a treatment program or structured setting may be just as effective as drug treatment for severe aggressive behaviors.

Prognosis

Children with CD are at risk for developing a variety of problems as adults, including ASP, affective disorders, and engaging in persistent criminal activities (Biederman et al., 2008a; Biederman et al., 2008b; Encyclopedia of Children's Health, no date). Based on a longitudinal study of the course of ODD and CD in boys with ADHD, Biederman et al. (2008a) showed that having ODD increased the likelihood that the boys would acquire ASP. However, CD was more likely to increase the likelihood of ASP than ODD. In addition, CD was more likely than ODD to predict the development of substance abuse disorders, smoking, and bipolar disorder.

In a 5-year longitudinal follow-up investigation of girls with ADHD, Biederman et al. (2008b) discovered that girls with both ADHD and ODD had a greater probability of having ODD and major depression at the time of follow-up than girls diagnosed with only ADHD. At follow-up, both groups of girls had an increased risk of having CD and bipolar disorder. Fortunately, early assessment and treatment and support over a long-term period can substantially reduce these risks (Encyclopedia of Children's Health, no date; Conner, 1998–2000).

The prognosis for CD is better if it begins during adolescence than during childhood (Encyclopedia of Children's Health, no date). Youth with adolescent-onset CD tend to have better interactions with peers and have a lower probability of having ASP as adults than youth with childhood-onset CD.

Among youth with adolescent-onset CD, there is less gender disparity (Encyclopedia of Children's Health, no date). In contrast, for youth with childhood-onset CD, the incidence of the disorder is higher for boys than girls.

Prevention

The best way to prevent CD is to offer youth a nurturing and structured home life (Encyclopedia of Children's Health, no date). Professionals should immediately identify and treat children with LDs. Early identification and treatment will provide academic help for these youth and help minimize frustration and threats to self-identity, which are precursors to CD-related behaviors.

Impact of CD on Family Functioning

Having a child with CD in the family can have major consequences for the social and emotional well-being of siblings and other members of the family (Encyclopedia of Children's Health, no date). Parents need to be aware of the social and emotional needs of their other children and modify family routines to adjust for the detrimental effects of having a child who exhibits antisocial behaviors. Parents should not leave the child with CD alone with other siblings, and if possible, they should get help with childcare. When the safety or the emotional well-being of family members is threatened, the parents may find it necessary to place the child with conduct-related problems in a residential or hospital-based therapy program for a while.

In Australia, Hazell et al. (2002) surveyed families who had one or more children with conduct-related disorders and comorbid conditions. The families rated mainstream community treatment which focused on counseling services as the highest priority. The families rated respite services and inpatient facilities as a lower priority. However, respite care, inpatient, and other out-of-the home services were ranked high in priority among low socioeconomic status families and those exposed to high stress. More research is needed regarding the ease with which families have access to community treatment services and the effectiveness of those services.

Case Study

The following case study illustrates the experiences of a male adolescent who was diagnosed with CD and substance dependence.

Josh is a 15-year-old adolescent, who resides in a residential treatment program for disturbed adolescents. His mother, a nurse, works full time and often works the night shift (11 p.m. to 7 a.m.). His father, an accountant, works traditional hours. He has two older sisters, both in college. Both sisters have had histories of drug and alcohol abuse and were hospitalized in the past. One sister has also had a history with the criminal justice system as an adolescent for the distribution of drugs.

Developmental milestones were all normal. When Josh began preschool, at age 3, he was seen as shy with peers and as cognitively in the low average range. In kindergarten, he was not seen as a problem. In first grade, he experienced some difficulty with reading, but no other problems were noted. In second grade, he began to receive assistance for reading. In third grade, his teacher perceived him as having attention problems and he was referred to the school psychologist for an evaluation. No evidence of ADHD was evident, but his reading problem was perceived to be significant, for he was still reading at a first-grade level. In fourth and fifth grades, Josh began to exhibit behavior problems. Specifically, he would disrupt the class. He was also suspected of stealing money from the teacher's purse, but there was no clear evidence and the accusation was dropped.

In middle school, Josh began to be friendly with older students who were perceived as troublemakers by staff. In sixth and seventh grades, he was twice caught shoplifting at local stores. In school, he was also caught stealing another student's hand-held game. During this time, his parents suspected that he was using marijuana, although he denied it. By eighth grade, he was threatening younger students and forcing them to pay him daily for "protection." He also had a physical fight with another student and was suspended for 5 days. At that time, his parents had him attend counseling on a weekly basis. He consistently missed appointments and the therapist reported that Josh had no investment in making changes. Counseling was terminated.

As a freshman in high school, he was arrested for breaking into a neighbor's home and stealing electronics. He was placed on supervision. Within 6 weeks, he was again arrested – for possession and distribution of marijuana at a local middle school. He was subsequently placed on house arrest for 2 months, placed on 2 years' probation, required to attend weekly counseling, and required to have random drug checks. When he failed a drug test, he was ordered to participate in an intensive outpatient drug treatment program. He was subsequently placed in a therapeutic school for children and adolescents with emotional and/or behavioral problems.

Josh was again arrested for breaking and entering and his house arrest was continued for another 6 months. He was then arrested for burglary. While awaiting trial, his parents placed him in a long-term residential facility in another state (on the advice of their attorney). At that time, he was diagnosed with CD, as well as substance dependence.

References

Alexander, J.F., Parsons, B.V. (1982). Short-term behavioral intervention with delinquent families: impact on family process and recidivism. J Abnorm Psychol, 81, 219–225.

Baker-Henningham, H., Walker, S.P., Powell, C., et al. (2009). Preventing behavior problems through a universal intervention in Jamaican basic schools: a pilot study. West Indian Med J, 58 (5), 460–464.

Biederman, J., Faraone, S., Chu, M., et al. (1999). Further evidence of a bi-directional overlap between juvenile mania and conduct disorder in children. J Am Acad Child Adolesc Psychiatr, 38 (4), 468–476.

Biederman, J., Petty, C.R., Dolan, C., et al. (2008a). The long-term longitudinal course of oppositional defiant disorder and conduct disorder in ADHD boys: findings from a controlled 10-year prospective longitudinal follow-up study. Psychol Med, 38 (7), 1027–1036.

Biederman, J., Petty, C.R., Monuteaux, M.C., et al. (2008b). The longitudinal course of comorbid oppositional defiant disorder in girls with attention-deficit/hyperactivity disorder: findings from a controlled 5-year prospective longitudinal follow-up study. J Dev Behav Pediatr, 29 (6), 501–507.

Boylan, K., Vaillancourt, T., Boyle, M., et al. (2007). Comorbidity of internalizing disorders in children with oppositional defiant disorder. Eur Child Adolesc Psychiatry, 16 (8), 484–494.

Burt, S.A. (2009). Rethinking environmental contributions to child and adolescent psychopathology: a meta-analysis of shared environmental influences. Psychol Bull, 135 (4), 608–637.

Byun, H., Yang, J., Lee, M., et al. (2006). Psychiatric comorbidity in Korean children and adolescents with attention-deficit hyperactivity disorder: psychopathology according to subtype. Yonsei Med J, 47 (1), 113–121.

Carlson, C., Tamm, L., Gaub, M. (1997). Gender differences in children with ADHD, oppositional defiant disorder, and co-occurring ADHD/oppositional defiant disorder identified within a school population. J Am Acad Child Adolesc Psychiatr, 36, 1706–1714.

Child Welfare Information Gateway (2007). Parent-child interaction therapy with at-risk families. Washington, DC: U.S. Department of Health and Human Services.

Chronis, A.M., Chacko, A., Fabiano, G.A., et al. (2004). Enhancements to the behavioral parent training paradigm for families of children with ADHD: review and future directions. Clin Child Fam Psychol Rev, 7 (1), 1–27.

Conner, M. (1998–2000). Understanding and dealing with conduct and oppositional disorders. Retrieved from http://www.CrisisCounseling.org

Connor, D.F., Barkley, R.A., Davis, H.T. (2000, January). A pilot study of methylphenidate, clonidine, or the combination in ADHD comorbid with aggressive oppositional defiant or conduct disorder. Clin Pediatr, 39 (1), 15–25.

Cowles, E.L., Castellano, T.C., Gransky, L.A. (1995). "Boot camp" drug treatment and aftercare interventions: an evaluation review, Research in Brief, U.S. DOJ. Washington, DC: National Institute of Justice. Retrieved March 3, 2010 from: http://www.druglibrary.org/SCHAFFER/GovPubs/btcamp.pdf

Cunningham, C.E., Boyle, M.H. (2002). Preschoolers at risk for attention-deficit hyperactivity disorder and oppositional defiant disorder: family, parenting, and behavioral correlates. J Abnorm Child Psychol, 30 (6), 555–569.

Daley, D., Jones, K., Hutchings, J., et al. (2009). Attention deficit hyperactivity disorder in preschool children: current findings, recommended interventions and future directions. Child Care Health Dev, 35 (6), 754–766.

Danforth, J.S., Harvey, E., Ulaszek, W.R., et al. (2006). The outcome of group parent training for families of children with attention-deficit hyperactivity disorder and defiant/aggressive behavior. J Behav Ther Exp Psychiatry, 37 (3), 188–205.

De Graaf, I., Speetjens, P., Smit, F., et al. (2008). Effectiveness of the Triple P Positive Parenting Program on behavioral problems in children: a meta-analysis. Behav Modif, 32 (5), 714–735.

Dishion, T.J., Andrews, D.W. (1995). Prevention escalation in problem behaviors with high-risk young adolescents: immediate and one-year outcome. J Consult Clin Psychol, 63 (4), 538–548.

Donovan, S., Steart, J., Nunes, E., et al. (2000). Am J Psychiatry, 157, 818–820.

Ehringer, M.A., Rhee, S.H., Young, S., et al. (2006). Genetic and environmental contributions to common psychopathologies of childhood and adolescence: a study of twins and their siblings. J Abnorm Child Psychol, 34 (1), 1–17.

Encyclopedia of Children's Health. (no date). Conduct disorder. Retrieved from http://www.healthofchildren.com

Feldman, R.A. (1992). The St. Louis experiment: effective treatment of antisocial youths in prosocial peer groups. In J. McCord, R.E. Tremblay (Eds.), Preventing antisocial behavior. New York, NY: Guilford Press, pp. 233–252.

Gallagher, N. (2003). Effects of parent-child interaction therapy on young children with disruptive behavior disorders. Bridges: Pract-Based Res Synthesis, 1, 1–17.

Goldstein, R.B., Grant, B.F., Ruan, W.J., et al. (2006). Antisocial personality disorder with childhood- vs. adolescence-onset conduct disorder: results from the National Epidemiologic Survey on Alcohol and Related Conditions. J Nerv Ment Dis, 194 (9), 667–675.

Grizenko, N. (1997). Outcome of multimodal day treatment for children with severe behavior problems: a five-year follow-up. J Am Acad Child Adol Psychiatry, 36, 989–997.

Hahlweg, K., Heinrichs, N., Kuschel, A., et al. (2010). Long-term outcome of a randomized controlled universal prevention trial through a positive parenting program: is it worth the effort? Child Adolesc Psychiatry Ment Health, 4, 14.

Hart, E.L., Lahey, B.B., Loeber, R., et al. (1994). Criterion validity of informants in the diagnosis of disruptive behavior disorders in children: a preliminary study. J Consult Clin Psychol, 62 (2), 410–414.

Hazell, P.L., Tarren-Sweeney, M., Vimpani, G.V., et al. (2002). Children with disruptive behaviours II: clinical and community service needs. J Paediatr Child Health, 38 (1), 32–40.

Henggeler, S., Rowland, M., Randall, J., et al. (1999). Home-based multi-systemic therapy as an alternative to the hospitalization of youths in psychiatric crisis: clinical outcomes. J Am Acad Child Adol Psychiatry, 38, 1331–1339.

Jacob, T. (Ed.) (1987). Family interaction and psychopathology: theories, methods, and findings. New York, NY: Plenum Press.

Jones, K., Daley, D., Hutchings, J., et al. (2007). Efficacy of the Incredible Years Basic parent training programme as an early intervention for children with conduct problems and ADHD. Child Care Health Dev, 33 (6), 749–756.

Jones, K., Daley, D., Hutchings, J., et al. (2008). Efficacy of the Incredible Years Programme as an early intervention for children with conduct problems and ADHD: long-term follow-up. Child Care Health Dev, 34 (3), 380–390.

Kazdin, A.E. (1985). Treatment of antisocial behavior in children and adolescents. Homewood, IL: Dorsey Press.

Kazdin, A.E. (1987). Conduct disorder in childhood and adolescence. Newbury Park, CA: Sage.

Kazdin, A.E. (1994). Interventions for aggressive and antisocial children. In L.D. Eron, J.H. Gentry, P. Schlegel (Eds.), Reason to hope: a psychological perspective on violence and youth. Washington, DC: American Psychological Association, pp. 341–382.

Kazdin, A., Wassell, G. (2000). Therapeutic changes in children, parents, and families resulting from treatment of children with conduct problems. J Am Acad Child Adol Psychiatry, 39, 414–420.

Kilic, B.G., Sener, S. (2005). Family functioning and psychosocial characteristics in children with attention deficit hyperactivity disorder with comorbid oppositional defiant disorder or conduct disorder. Turk Psikiyatri Derg, 16 (1), 21–28.

Klassen, A.F., Miller, A., Fine, S. (2004, November). Health-related quality of life in children and adolescents who have a diagnosis of attention-deficit/hyperactivity disorder. Pediatrics, 114 (5), e541–547.

Koegl, C.J., Farrington, D.P., Augimeri, L.K., et al. (2008, July). Evaluation of a targeted cognitive-behavioral program for children with conduct problems—the SNAP Under 12 Outreach Project: service intensity, age and gender effects on short- and long-term outcomes. Clin Child Psychol Psychiatry, 13 (3), 419–434.

Kolko, D., Bukstein, O., Barron, J. (1999). Methylphenidate and behavior modification in children with ADHD and comorbid Oppositional Defiant Disorder or Conduct Disorder: main and incremental effects across settings. J Am Acad Child Adolesc Psychiatry, 38 (5), 578–586.

Kutcher, S., Aman, M., Brooks, S.J., et al. (2004). International consensus statement on attention deficit/hyperactivity disorder (ADHD) and disruptive behaviour disorders (DBDs): clinical implications and treatment practice suggestions. Eur Neuropsychopharmacol, 14 (1), 11–28.

Lahey, B., Loeber, R., Hart, E., et al. (1995). Four-year longitudinal study of conduct disorder in boys: patterns of predictors of persistence. J Abnorm Psychol, 104, 93.

Loeber, R., Lahey, B., Thomas, C. (1991). Diagnostic conundrum of oppositional defiant disorder and conduct disorder. J Abnorm Psychol, 100 (3), 379–390.

Lorber, T. (1981). Parental tracking of childhood behavior as a function of family stress. Unpublished doctoral dissertation, University of Oregon, Eugene.

Maughan, B., Rowe, R., Messer, J., et al. (2004). Conduct disorder and oppositional defiant disorder in a national sample: developmental epidemiology. J Child Psychol Psychiatry, 45 (3), 609–621.

Moffitt, T. (1993). The neuropsychology of conduct disorder. Dev Psychopath, 5, 135–151.

Munoz-Solomando, A., Kendall, T., Whittington, C.J. (2008). Cognitive behavioural therapy for children and adolescents. Curr Opin Psychiatry, 21 (4), 332–337.

Office of Child and Family Policy. (2008). A clinical information guide: conduct disorder and oppositional defiant disorder.

Patterson, G.R., Reid, J.B., Dishion, T.J. (1992). Antisocial boys. Eugene, OR: Castalia.

Reid, J.B., Kavanagh, K., Baldwin, D.V. (1987). Abusive parents' perceptions of child problem behaviors: an example of parental bias. J Abn Child Psychol, 15, 457–466.

Riggs, P., Leon, S., Mikulich, S. (1998). An open trial of bupropion for ADHD in adolescents with substance abuse disorders and conduct disorder. J Am Acad Child Adol Psychiatry, 37 (12), 1271–1278.

Robins, L.N. (1981). Epidemiological approaches to natural history research: antisocial disorders in children. J Am Acad Child Psychiatry, 20, 566–580.

Sanders, M.R. (1999, June). Triple P-Positive Parenting Program: towards an empirically validated multilevel parenting and family support strategy for the prevention of behavior and emotional problems in children. Clin Child Fam Psychol Rev, 2 (2), 71–90.

Sanders, M.R., Markie-Dadds, C., Tully, L.A., et al. (2000). The triple P-positive parenting program: a comparison of enhanced, standard, and self-directed behavioral family intervention for parents of children with early onset problems. J Consult Clin Psychol, 68 (4), 624–640.

Scahill, L., Sukhodolsky, D.G., Bearss, K., et al. (2006). Randomized trial of parent management training in children with tic disorders and disruptive behavior. J Child Neurol, 21 (8), 650–656.

Schoenwald, S., Henggeler, S. (1999). Treatment of oppositional defiant disorder and conduct disorder in home and community settings. In H. Quay, A. Hogan, et al. (Eds.), Handbook of disruptive behavior disorders. New York: Kluwer Academic/Plenum Publishers, pp. 475–493.

Siminoff, E., Pickles, A., Meyer, J., et al. (1997). The Virginia twin study of adolescent behavioral development: influences of age, sex, and impairment on rates of disorder. Arch Gen Psychiatry, 54 (9), 801–808.

Speltz, M.L. (1990). The treatment of preschool conduct problems: An integration of behavioral and attachment concepts. In M.T. Greenberg, D. Cicchetti, M. Cummings (Eds.), Attachment in the preschool years: theory, research, and intervention. Chicago: University of Chicago Press, pp. 399–426.

Steiner, H. (1997). Practice parameters for the assessment and treatment of children and adolescents with conduct disorder. J Am Acad Child Adol Psychiatry, 36 (10 Suppl), 122S–139S.

Thomas, R., Zimmer-Gembeck, M.J. (2007). Behavioral outcomes of Parent-Child Interaction Therapy and Triple P-Positive Parenting Program: a review and meta-analysis. J Abnorm Child Psychol, 35 (3), 475–495.

Turgay, A. (2005). Treatment of comorbidity in conduct disorder with attention-deficit hyperactivity disorder (ADHD). Essent Psychopharmacol, 6 (5), 277–290.

Turgay, A. (2009). Psychopharmacological treatment of oppositional defiant disorder. CNS Drugs, 23 (1), 1–17.

Turner, W., Macdonald, G.M., Dennis, J.A. (2005). Cognitive-behavioural training interventions for assisting foster carers in the management of difficult behaviour. Cochrane Database Syst Rev, 18 (2), CD003760.

van de Wiel, N., Matthys, W., Cohen-Kettenis, P.C., et al. (2002). Effective treatments of school-aged conduct disordered children: recommendations for changing clinical and research practices. Eur Child Adolesc Psychiatry, 11 (2), 79–84.

Webster-Stratton, C., Hammond, M. (1997). Treating children with early-onset conduct problems a comparison of child and parent training interventions. J Consulting Clin Psychology, 65, 93–109.

Webster-Stratton, C., Jamila Reid, M., Stoolmiller, M. (2008). Preventing conduct problems and improving school readiness: evaluation of the Incredible Years Teacher and Child Training Programs in high-risk schools. J Child Psychol Psychiatry, 49 (5), 471–488.

Wrowley, T., Riggs, P. (1995). Adolescent substance use disorders with conduct disorder, comorbid conditions. NIDA Res Monographs, 156, 49–111.

Young, S., Mikulich, S., Goodwin, M., et al. (1995). Treated delinquent boy' substance use: onset, pattern, relationship to conduct and mood disorders. Drug Alcohol Depend, 37 (2), 149–162.

Chapter 8
Depressive Disorders in Children and Adolescents

Depression in children and adolescents is not only widely recognized as a significant public health concern, but the prevalence rates are increasing. As with adult depression, there are numerous possible symptoms, including the cardinal symptoms of depressed mood and loss of pleasure in usual and customary activities (anhedonia). Sleep problems, appetite or weight changes, decreased motivation, and interference with memory and concentration may also be present. Other common symptoms include feelings of guilt or worthlessness, diminished ability to make decisions, and psychomotor agitation or retardation. Furthermore, depression in children and adolescents is typically associated with social withdrawal, interpersonal problems, decreased school performance, and increased school attendance issues. Depression also increases the risk of suicide in children and adolescents (Bhatia and Bhatia, 2007). Suicidal thoughts, ideation, rumination, plans, and attempts may be present, depending on the depth of the depression. Moreover, depression is linked to impairment in social and family functioning. There is also substantial comorbidity between depression and other psychiatric disorders, particularly anxiety disorders and substance use and abuse.

Epidemiology

Little is known about the prevalence of depression in preschoolers. According to research, major depressive disorders occur in about 1% of preschoolers. Based on a study of 796 four-year-old children, Lavigne et al. (2009) reported that depressive disorders and generalized anxiety disorder were identified in less than 1% of the sample. The investigators did not find any racial or ethnic differences in major depressive disorder. In addition, no gender differences were identified.

Mehler-Wex and Kolch (2008) note that depression in children and adolescents has prevalence rates of up to 8.9%. Other studies report that 3–5% of children and adolescents have major depression (Bhatia and Bhatia, 2007). Some investigations show that about 2% of children of school age and 5–8% of adolescents have depression (Jellinek and Synder, 1998; Birmaher et al., 1998). In successive generations, depression seems to be increasing in prevalence and the onset of the disorder is occurring at younger ages (Klerman et al., 1985; Gershon et al., 1987).

M.L. Goldstein, S. Morewitz, *Chronic Disorders in Children and Adolescents*,
DOI 10.1007/978-1-4419-9764-7_8, © Springer Science+Business Media, LLC 2011

In their review of the literature, Mehler-Wex and Kolch (2008) found that in childhood, there is a high rate of spontaneous remissions (33%). In addition, they discovered that 80% of cases of depression in childhood and adolescence persisted into adulthood.

Risk Factors

A variety of risk factors for depression in children and adolescents have been identified (Bouma et al., 2008; Greszta, 2006; Son and Kirchner, 2000). Youth who experience demoralization or subclinical symptoms of depression may have an elevated risk of depression (Purper-Ouakil et al., 2002). In addition, those children and adolescents who have had prior depressive episodes have an increased probability of depression. Youth with comorbid conditions, such as dysthymic disorder (depressed/irritable mood for most of the day, for more days than not, for 1 year) and substance abuse, are at increased risk of developing depression (Purper-Ouakil et al., 2002; Son and Kirchner, 2000).

Anxiety also predicts the subsequent development of depression in children and adolescents. In a 3-year longitudinal study of elementary school students and their parents, Cole et al. (1998) discovered that high levels of anxiety increased the risk of depression during later time periods. Stressful life events also increase the risk of depression in early adolescence. Stressful life events, such as difficulties in academic performance, are a risk factor for the disorder (Bouma et al., 2008). Based on a longitudinal cohort study of pre-adolescents, Bouma et al. (2008) found that adolescents with parents who had a lifetime depressive episode were more sensitive to the depression-causing impact of stressful life events than adolescents who did not have depressed parents. They discovered that girls were more sensitive to these depression-triggering influences than boys.

Youth who have a family history of depression are at increased risk for the disorder. Family characteristics, such as family violence, child abuse, neglect, marital conflict, difficulties in family communication, and inappropriate parenting, e.g., harsh discipline, lack of parental emotional warmth, overprotection, rejection, and lack of supportive behavior, may increase the vulnerability to depression and other types of psychosocial morbidity in children and adolescents (Greszta, 2006; Oldehinkel et al., 2006; Purper-Ouakil et al., 2002; Morewitz, 2004).

McFarlane et al. (2003) examined the behaviors of children who were exposed and not exposed to intimate partner violence and found that children of abused mothers were more likely to exhibit internalizing behaviors, such as depression, anxiety, and withdrawal, and externalizing behaviors, such as aggressive behaviors and attention difficulties, than children of non-abused mothers. Other studies suggest that symptoms of depression among adolescents are less likely to occur in families that have characteristics such as warm parenting, firm control, and democratic discipline (Greszta, 2006).

Family risk for depression may be due to psychological, social, and genetic causes (Purper-Ouakil et al., 2002). The extent to which pathological parenting leads to depression in adolescence is probably influenced by the interaction of psychosocial, genetic, and family factors (Greszta, 2006).

Insecure attachment also may be linked to depressive symptoms. Based on a sample of 350 adolescents, in grades six through ten, Lee and Hankin (2009) noted that anxious and avoidant attachment each predicted internalizing conditions, such as depressive and anxiety symptoms.

Research has also shown that divorce may contribute to the onset of depressive symptoms (Greszta, 2006). In addition, low self-esteem and lack of intimate relationships among the adolescents from divorced families may contribute to the depression. Drawing on a sample of 1,656 adolescents, aged 16–22, Palosaari and Aro (1995) showed that depression was highest among adolescents from divorced families who had low self-esteem at age 16 and who did not have intimate relationships in young adulthood. Palosaari et al. (1996) also demonstrated that the long-term effects of divorce on depression were mediated by a lack of a close relationship to the father. Girls from divorced families did not have a high rate of depression when they had a close relationship with their father. This association was not found among boys. A longitudinal study also reported that women of divorced parents had high levels of depression, while men did not have this problem (Rodgers, 1994).

The degree of social support also may play a role in the development of depression. One investigation reported that adolescents with levels of positive emotionality and low social support were more likely to experience an increase in anhedonic symptoms of depression (Wetter and Hankin, 2009).

Other studies have demonstrated that temperament traits may place youth at an elevated risk for depression (Oldehinkel et al., 2006; Purper-Ouakil et al., 2002). For example, getting upset easily and intensely has been linked to an elevated risk of depression (Purper Ouakil et al., 2002). Temperament traits may influence the impact of perceived or actual parenting practices. Based on a sample of 2,230 children, aged 10–12, in the North of The Netherlands, Oldehinkel et al. (2006) discovered that feelings of frustration increased the depression-triggering impact of parental overprotection. They also showed that among girls, the feelings of fearfulness increased the impact of parental rejection, but not among boys.

Low self-esteem, low levels of social competence, and other aspects of cognitive style may increase the probability of depression in children and adolescents (Purper-Ouakil et al., 2002).

Problems in sexual orientation along with at-school victimization may increase the chances of depression, suicidality, substance abuse, and risky sexual behaviors in children and adolescents. Based on a sample of 7,376 seventh and eighth grade students from a large Midwestern county, Birkett et al. (2009) found that students who were questioning their sexual orientation reported the highest levels of bullying, the most homophobic victimization, the highest levels of drug use, the most feelings of depression and suicidality, and more truancy than either heterosexual students or lesbian, gay, and bisexual (LGB) students.

Using data from the 1995 Youth Risk Behavior Survey, Bontempo and D'Augelli (2002) discovered that the combined impacts of LGB status and a high degree of victimization at school were related to LGB students' increased levels of substance use, suicidality, and sexual risk behaviors than heterosexual peers who reported high levels of at-school victimization. Based on a literature review and meta-analysis, King et al. (2008) also have shown that LGB persons are at higher risk of mental disorders, suicidal ideation, substance abuse, and deliberate self-harm than heterosexual individuals.

Children and adolescents who are the victims of bullying and other forms of violence in the schools and community are at increased risk of depression, anxiety, suicide, and other problems, such as eating disorders and somatic symptoms (Brunstein Klomek et al., 2007; Sansone and Sansone, 2008; Kaltiala-Heino et al., 1999). Based on a self-report survey of 2,342 students in the ninth through twelfth grades, Brunstein Klomek et al. (2007) discovered that students who were frequently bullied or who bullied others had a high risk of depression, suicide ideation, and suicide attempts relative to those not involved in bullying. The researchers also reported that adolescents who were infrequently involved in bullying behavior had an elevated risk for depression and suicidal ideation and attempts, especially among girls. In a school-based survey of Finnish adolescents, Kaltiala-Heino et al. (1999) found that adolescents who had been bullied at school as well as those who were bullies were more likely to have depression and severe suicide ideation. In their investigation, depression was equally prevalent among both groups.

Childhood sexual abuse also may increase the risk of depression in adulthood (Morewitz, 2004). A number of researchers suggest that depression related to childhood sexual abuse is due to posttraumatic stress disorder.

In addition, youth who have conduct disorders (CD) and other disruptive problems are at elevated risk for depression (Purper-Ouakil et al., 2002). These results are consistent with the findings that children and adolescents with oppositional defiant disorder (ODD) often have comorbid psychiatric disorders, such as depressive and anxiety disorders (Boylan et al., 2007).

The victims of violence are not only at elevated risk for depression, but they also may be more predisposed to commit violence against others. For example, studies show that many youth who have been bullied subsequently become bullies themselves. Kaltiala-Heino et al. (1999) found that depression was most prevalent among adolescents who were bullied by others and who also were bullies themselves.

Types of Depression

Children and adolescents can develop a variety of depressive disorders, ranging from sadness variation and bereavement to a major depressive disorder (MDD) (Son and Kirchner, 2000), as well as dysthymic disorder, adjustment disorder with depressed mood, cyclothymic disorder, and bipolar disorder.

Sadness Variation

Youth who experience sadness variation have temporary, normal depressive responses or mood alterations in response to stressors.

Bereavement Disorder

Like adults, children and adolescents experience sadness associated with a major loss, e.g., the death of a family member. Bereavement disorder refers to sadness that lasts less than 2 months after suffering the loss. The disorder does not include feelings of guilt about issues other than survivor behavior at the time of death. A child or adolescent who experiences the bereavement disorder typically has thoughts of death and has a pathological preoccupation with feelings of worthlessness.

Sadness Problem

A sadness problem is classified as sadness or irritability that starts to resemble a milder form of major depressive disorders. This milder form is not severe enough to meet the criteria for a depressive disorder. In these cases, the child or adolescent has symptoms of sadness or irritability that are more than temporary symptoms. Moreover, these symptoms often have an impact on the individual's functioning. A child or adolescent who experiences bereavement for more than 2 months may meet the criteria for sadness problem.

Adjustment Disorder with Depressed Mood

Adjustment disorder with depressed mood occurs when a child or adolescent develops behavioral or emotional problems in response to a known stressor (e.g., divorce, changing schools, loss of relationship, and economic change in the household) and the symptoms take place within 3 months of the stressor. The child or adolescent typically suffers substantial disruption in social, family, and/or school activities. The person may suffer depressed mood, tearfulness, and hopelessness. These feelings are excessive compared to what an individual would normally experience after responding to this type of stressor. The symptoms of the adjustment disorder with depressed mood usually go away within 6 months after the stressor or its impact has been successfully handled. Acute episodes of the disorder are of less than 6 months duration, while chronic episodes of the condition are of 6 months duration.

Major Depressive Disorder (MDD)

Children or adolescents can experience a MDD, which is characterized by substantial distress and impairment in social, family, educational, and work functioning. The individual suffers from a number of emotional and social difficulties, including feeling depressed and/or irritable, having recurrent thoughts of death and suicidal ideation, reduced interest or pleasure, fatigue, weight loss or gain, and insomnia. To meet the classification of a MDD, children or adolescents experience these disabling problems almost daily for 2 weeks. They must exhibit symptoms of a depressed and/or irritable mood or reduced interest or pleasure and must show an alteration in previous functional status.

Dysthymic Disorder

Dysthymic disorder is characterized by a depressed and/or irritable mood for the majority of the day and for more days than not for at least 1 year. From 0.6 to 4.6% of children and 1.6 to 8.0% of adolescents develop this chronic depressive condition (Nobile et al., 2003). Children or adolescents with this disorder suffer from two of the following problems: little appetite or overeating, problems sleeping or excessive sleeping, poor energy or fatigue, difficulty in concentrating and making decisions, and feeling hopeless. In contrast to a MDD, the symptoms of a dysthymic disorder are less severe but last longer. The condition can last 3 years, while the duration of a MDD can last 7–9 months (Birmaher et al., 1998; Kovacs et al., 1984). Dysthymic disorder has more adverse outcomes than MDD and often is associated with comorbid conditions (Nobile et al., 2003).

Cyclothymic Disorder

Cyclothymic disorder is characterized by the presence of hypomanic symptoms and numerous periods with depressive symptoms for at least 1 year. During this time, the child or adolescent has not been without the symptoms for more than 2 months at a time. However, the individual does not meet the criterion for MDD. After the initial first year, there may be superimposed manic or mixed episodes or MDD episodes. The symptoms are not due to the direct physiological effects of drug abuse, a medication, or a medical condition such as hyperthyroidism, and this condition is not better accounted for by schizoaffective disorder, schizophreniform disorder, delusional disorder, or psychotic disorder NOS. The symptoms of cyclothymic disorder cause significant distress or impairment in social and/or school functioning.

Bipolar I Disorder

Youth who suffer from this disorder are currently suffering from a major depressive episode and have a history of one manic episode or one that consists of both depressive and manic symptoms. These mood episodes cannot be better explained by a schizoaffective disorder and are not part of schizophrenia, schizophreniform disorder, delusional disorder, or a psychotic disorder that is not otherwise classified.

Children and adolescents with bipolar disorder are at increased risk of engaging in suicidal behavior (Jolin et al., 2007). Most of the studies in this area have focused on suicidal behavior in older adolescents and adults with bipolar disorder. These investigations are limited due to their retrospective design.

Preliminary research indicates that early onset of bipolar disorder increases the risk of suicide (Jolin et al., 2007). However, only a limited number of investigations prospectively analyze the impact of previous suicidal behavior, clinical course, comorbid psychiatric problems, family suicidality, and psychosocial issues on suicidal behavior in young people with bipolar disorders.

Bipolar II Disorder

Persons with this condition have one major depressive episode or a history of such a disorder and one episode of hypomania. This hypomanic episode is similar to a manic episode but differs in that a hypomanic episode only lasts a few days and does not cause a severe disruption in social, family, educational, and work functioning. The child or adolescent has never suffered from a manic episode or one that involved both depressed and manic symptoms. These mood episodes cannot be better explained by schizoaffective disorder, delusional disorder, schizophrenia, or psychotic disorder. Overall, these symptoms cause the children and adolescents marked distress and substantial impairment in functional status.

Depressive Disorder Not Otherwise Specified (NOS)

A large percentage of adolescents who suffer depressive symptoms and significant distress or disruption in functioning do not meet the criteria for a MDD (Sihvola et al., 2007; Gonzalez-Tejera et al., 2005). Many of these individuals may fulfill the criteria for depressive disorder not otherwise specified (DDNOS). Minor depression (mDEP) is one type of DDNOS. Adolescents who suffer from mDEP may be underdiagnosed and untreated (Sihvola et al., 2007). They have not been considered serious enough to warrant treatment and the risk factors for this disorder have not been studied extensively. In mDEP, the individual does not experience the five symptoms required for a MDD (Gonzalez-Tejera et al., 2005).

Minor depression in adolescence is poorly understood due to the scarcity of research in this area. Nevertheless, some studies reveal the traumatic impact of this condition. Based on a sample of 909 girls and 945 boys (mean age of 14 years), Sihvola et al. (2007) discovered that mDEP was linked to suicidal thoughts, plans and attempts, recurrences, and a greater number of comorbid conditions. Fourteen percent of adolescents younger than age 15 years had depressive symptoms with severe potential. However, a majority of them did not fulfill the criteria for MDD. Only 1.7% of the adolescents had been in any type of psychiatric therapy. Forty percent of the depressed adolescents who had made a suicide attempt had no contact with the mental health system.

In a study of mDEP among Puerto Rican adolescents, aged 11–17, Gonzalez-Tejera et al. (2005) reported that youth with minor depression suffered substantial impairment, and compared to those with a MDD, they used more mental health services. Both adolescents with minor depression and MDD had similar comorbidities and correlates.

Youth who suffer minor depression may be at elevated risk for a major depressive disorder and associated impairment. Using data from the Pittsburgh Girls Study,

Keenan et al. (2008) showed that girls who did not have a MDD at age 9 years had an elevated risk of developing a MDD and suffering related impairment at age 10 or 11 years, as the number of their depressive symptoms increased. The authors noted that these results highlight the stability in minor depression among pre-adolescent girls. They recommend secondary prevention of depression in girls by treating minor depression as it emerges.

Assessment

The diagnostic criteria for depression in children and adolescents are basically the same as those for adults (Bhatia and Bhatia, 2007). However, the expression of symptoms of depressive disorders varies by age (Son and Kirchner, 2000). Extensive research has evaluated school-aged children and adolescents; however, investigators know less about the extent to which preschoolers develop depression (Luby et al., 2009; Curtis and Luby, 2008).

Using a sample of 305 preschoolers, aged 3–6 years, Luby et al. (2009) showed that functional impairment was linked to depression in this sample. These functional impairments were observed in different domains and contexts. Guilt-related symptoms and severe fatigue were very specific for depression in these preschoolers. However, the investigators did not find that depression was related to developmental delays in preschoolers. The authors suggest that there is a window of opportunity to intervene early in preschoolers since depressed preschoolers were not developmentally delayed.

In another study of preschoolers, Curtis and Luby (2008) reported that chronic medical conditions were linked to the early onset of depressive symptoms and impaired social functioning in several areas. Chronic health problems were associated with more severe depression, an increased frequency of asocial behavior, impaired behaviors toward others, and poor cooperation with daycare roles. Preschoolers with at least one chronic health problem were more likely to suffer more frequent peer rejection and bullying relative to peers who do not have chronic health problems.

For the most part, infants and preschoolers are unable to use language to express sadness (Son and Kirchner, 2000). As a result, clinicians have to infer symptoms of sadness from actual behavior, such as evidence of apathy, social withdrawal, a failure to meet developmental milestones or a regression of milestones, and a failure to thrive that cannot be explained by medical causes (Jellinek and Synder, 1998; Wolraich et al., 1996). Providers need to rely on different data sources to help make the diagnosis, such as parental history, interactions between parent and child, and play interviews (Lewis, 1996).

As children reach school age, they develop the ability to internalize various stressors, such as family conflict and difficulties in school, and as a consequence develop problems, such as low self-esteem and feeling guilty (Son and Kirchner, 2000). School-aged children often express these problems by having somatic complaints such as stomachaches and headaches. They may also exhibit their problems by experiencing school phobia, separation anxiety, and other types of anxiety-related conditions. Moreover, these children demonstrate their turmoil in the form of irritability, such as temper tantrums, and other behavioral difficulties.

Using longitudinal data on 232 nine-year-old girls from the Pittsburgh Girls Study, Keenan et al. (2008) discovered that early developing depressive symptoms in girls are stable. Moreover, they found that these early emerging symptoms of depression predict depressive disorders and impairment in functioning. The investigators recommend interventions for girls who are suffering these emerging symptoms to achieve secondary prevention of depression in this vulnerable population.

Teachers should be consulted and involved in the assessment process because during school hours they spend a considerable amount of time with these children (Son and Kirchner, 2000). Depressive symptoms may go undetected since depressed children may try to make up for their low self-esteem by performing well in school in order to please their teachers (Jellinek and Synder, 1998).

During the storm and stress of adolescence, young people are especially vulnerable to feelings of depression (Son and Kirchner, 2000). They can develop depressive symptoms as they have difficulties becoming independent and forming their self-identity. Compared to depressed school-aged children, depressed adolescents suffer more intense feelings of hopelessness. Moreover, they have greater capacity to kill themselves than younger children. Depressed adolescents show less interest in pleasurable activities, sleep excessively, experience more changes in their weight, and experience substance abuse compared to depressed school-aged children. Given the problems of adolescence, e.g., the tendency of adolescents to challenge authority, clinicians need to establish a trusting relationship with their adolescent patients and should inform them about when information will be divulged to parents or others (Lewis, 1996).

Although differences have been identified between depressed school-aged children and depressed adolescents, both have similar symptoms with regard to major depressive disorder (Son and Kirchner, 2000). The frequency and severity of their symptoms, including depressed mood, feelings of guilt, irritability, and low self-esteem, overlap among both groups (Ryan et al., 1987).

Clinicians should consider the possibility that the child or adolescent has dysthymic disorder, which has milder symptoms but lasts longer than major depressive disorder. The persistence of dysthymic disorder can impair the individuals' acquisition of social skills that can help them deal with these difficulties (Son and Kirchner, 2000).

MDD and dysthymic disorder can have substantial comorbidity, especially comorbid psychiatric conditions (Treatment for Adolescents with Depression Study (TADS), 2005; Son and Kirchner, 2000; Birmaher et al., 1998). Based on a study of 439 adolescents, in the 12–17 year age group, the researchers reported that the most prevalent comorbid conditions were generalized anxiety disorder (15.3%), attention-deficit hyperactivity disorder (13.7%), ODD (13.2%), social phobia (10.7%), and dysthymic disorder (10.5%).

Youth can also suffer so-called double depression when one condition becomes superimposed on the other. Young people with comorbid conditions have a more negative prognosis because comorbidity is linked to increased duration and severity of MDD symptoms. Moreover, comorbid conditions increase the likelihood that a MDD will reoccur as well as suicidal risks (Jellinek and Synder, 1998; Birmaher et al., 1996; Ryan et al., 1987; Kovacs et al., 1984).

Diagnosis

Most psychosocial conditions are missed by health-care providers (Son and Kirchner, 2000). Some investigations have found that only one-third of parents who were worried about their children's psychosocial functioning indicated that they were going to share their concerns with their pediatrician. Furthermore, only 40% of the pediatricians responded when the parents actually did discuss their children's psychosocial issues with their pediatrician. Research indicates that the pediatrician's response rate was even lower if the parents had lower levels of educational attainment (Cassidy and Jellinek, 1998; Jellinek et al., 1995).

The failure of health-care clinicians to diagnose and treat depression in children and adolescents is especially serious since effective assessment and treatment can reduce the substantial morbidity and mortality associated with these disorders (Son and Kirchner, 2000). Screening measures, such as the Pediatric Symptom Checklist, should be used. The Pediatric Symptom Checklist is a 35-item instrument, which is completed by parents of children aged 6–12 years (Jellinek et al., 1995, 1988). This protocol has been found to have good specificity and sensitivity and is easy to administer. Therefore, the tool can help physicians improve their assessment of patients in busy health-care settings.

After a patient has been identified, the clinician should obtain a thorough psychosocial history to determine if the patient should receive treatment or a referral (Son and Kirchner, 2000; Hack and Jellinek, 1998). To diagnose depressive disorders, the provider must complete a complete medical and psychiatric assessment. Clinicians should order laboratory studies based on the patient's history and physical examination.

Clinicians should assess the possibility that various medical conditions are causing depressed symptoms in children and adolescents (Son and Kirchner, 2000). Infections, neurologic disorders, endocrine disorders, medications, and other conditions, such as substance abuse, electrolyte abnormality, hypokalemia, anemia, and Wilson's disease, may cause depression. Laboratory studies include complete blood cell count with differential, determination of electrolytes, creatinine level, BUN, liver function studies, thyroid function tests, and electroencephalogram.

A psychiatric assessment involves taking a history that details the onset, duration, frequency, intensity, and severity of symptoms (Son and Kirchner, 2000). The provider also should consider if the patient's symptoms occur in different settings such as home and school. Various medical and psychiatric conditions should be ruled out since depression is associated with chronic medical conditions in young people and many psychiatric comorbid disorders. In addition, the practitioner should take a developmental history, social history, and family history regarding psychiatric conditions. It is also essential that the clinician elicit possible stressors in the patient's home, school, and community (Lewis, 1996; Cassidy and Jellinek, 1998).

The clinician should conduct a clinical interview that is tailored to the patient's age and developmental stage (Son and Kirchner, 2000). For infants and toddlers, unstructured play interviews and observation of child–parent behaviors are recommended. For children of school age, play interviews along with open-ended questioning is suggested. For adolescents, in-depth interviews are suggested. Neuropsychologic testing can help determine if the patient has neurologic or learning problems and developmental stage (Lewis, 1996).

When the pediatrician perceives possible depression, referral to an appropriate mental health practitioner should be considered. However, many physicians treat mild to moderate depression in children and adolescents and do not feel the need to make a referral. In instances when counseling appears to be needed, or in more severe depressions when psychotropic medication appears to be needed, a referral may be necessary.

Treatment

The best treatment for depression in children and adolescents is multidisciplinary in nature and includes different forms of psychotherapy, psychosocial interventions, educating the patient and family, and using medications (Kapornai and Vetro, 2008; Mehler-Wex and Kolch, 2008; Michael and Crowley, 2002; Son and Kirchner, 2000).

The treatment of child and adolescent depression has been classified into three phases: acute, continuation, and maintenance (Emslie et al., 2005). In the acute phase, the young person responds to treatment and has a remission of symptoms. Prevention of symptom relapse occurs in the continuation phase. In the maintenance phase, the young person does not develop new episodes or recurrences of depression.

Use of selective serotonin reuptake inhibitors (SSRIs) is thought to be the first-line therapy for the acute treatment of depression in children and adolescents (Emslie et al., 2005). Non-specific psychotherapy may be utilized as an adjunctive strategy in the management of depressive symptoms, but non-specific psychotherapy has not been shown to be as effective as medications or specific psychotherapies alone. By contrast, cognitive behavior therapy (CBT) and interpersonal therapy have been found to be effective in the treatment of early-onset depression. However, severe symptoms of depression, comorbid conditions, family conflict, and increased disability are obstacles to remission and promote non-compliance.

For children and adolescents with mild to moderate depression, psychotherapy can be an effective, initial treatment strategy (Son and Kirchner, 2000). For children with more severe symptoms, psychotherapy should be used as an adjunct to medications (Birmaher et al., 1998). Practitioners should consider a range of psychotherapeutic approaches, including play therapy, supportive therapy, family therapy, and CBT. The choice of approaches depends on the patient's cognitive and emotional development. For depressed children of pre-school age, play therapy and parental education would be recommended. In contrast, older children and adolescents would benefit from psychodynamic therapy or CBT (Weller et al., 1996).

Most research suggests that CBT appears to be the psychotherapy modality of choice for the treatment of child and adolescent depression. CBT has been found to be useful for patients 10 years and older (Son and Kirchner, 2000). This strategy helps patients change their negative views about themselves and the environment. Reinecke et al. (1998), in their meta-analysis, found that for adolescents with depressed or dysphoric mood, CBT was effective on a short-term and long-term basis. CBT has been shown to be more useful than nondirective supportive therapy and systemic-behavioral family therapy because CBT seems to deal with the distorted cognitions that are prevalent in this age group (Brent et al., 1998). However, Kapornai and Vetro (2008) report that recent research on psychotherapies reveals a different picture regarding effectiveness.

Other reports reveal that different types of psychotherapy are effective in treating moderate to severe depression in children and young adolescents. For example, Trowell et al. (2007) reported that both individual therapy and family therapy resolved depressive symptoms in patients aged 9–15 years.

For the treatment of dysthymic disorder, multiple interventions may be effective since this condition is frequently associated with different psychosocial problems. The goals of treating dysthymic disorder are to eliminate the depressive symptoms, reduce the risk of other mood disorders, and enhance the functional status (Nobile et al., 2003). Individual psychotherapy, family therapy, family education, and medication can be helpful. In children and adolescents with moderate to severe depression who have either dysthymic disorder or double depression, CBT and interpersonal therapy have been shown to be effective. SSRIs are the first-line medical treatment for children and adolescents with dysthymia because of their safety and ease of administration. However, it is essential for parents and other caregivers to receive psychoeducational interventions and psychosocial support during the acute treatment phase. These interventions and support will help the parents and caregivers cope with their child's irritable mood and help ensure patient compliance. Both acute and continuation treatment approaches should be emphasized.

For children and adolescents with bipolar disorder, research indicates that medication plays a primary role in treatment. However, adjunctive psychosocial treatment also plays an important role (West and Pavuluri, 2009). Preliminary evidence suggests that multi-family psychoeducational groups and child- and family-centered CBT are effective for the treatment of bipolar disorder in school-aged children. For adolescents with bipolar disorder, interpersonal and social therapy produces positive outcomes.

The use of selective serotonin reuptake inhibitors (SSRIs) to treat depressive symptoms in children and adolescents can be effective (Brent et al., 2008; March et al., 2007). The side effects of SSRIs include mild gastrointestinal upset and sleepiness (Son and Kirchner, 2000). However, the US Food and Drug Administration issued warnings that using antidepressants can result in a small but significant risk of suicidal ideation and suicide attempts among children and adolescents (Bridge et al., 2007). Once children are placed on an antidepressant, family members should watch them closely for any alterations in behavior, especially increased suicidal ideation (Brock et al., 2005). Any changes in behavior should be reported to the primary health-care provider immediately for assessment.

Based on a review of 27 trials of antidepressant treatment for pediatric patients with MDDs, obsessive–compulsive disorder (OCD), and non-OCD anxiety disorders, Bridge et al. (2007) showed that the benefits of antidepressants seem to be much greater than the risks of suicidal ideation or suicide attempts. However, the risk–benefit analysis depends on the indication for antidepressants, the patient's age, the chronic nature of the disorder, and the experimental conditions of the different trials.

Reports on adults have not found differences in the risk of suicide for patients treated with antidepressants and those in the placebo group (Hjalmarsson et al., 2005; Hammad et al., 2006). In these trials, the few numbers of suicides and the subsequent lack of statistical power make it impossible to determine whether drug or placebo treatment increases the risk of suicide (Hammad et al., 2006).

Using results from the Treatment for Adolescents with Depression Study (TADS), Vitiello et al. (2009) analyzed suicidal events during a 36-week randomized, controlled clinical trial with 439 youths receiving medications and psychotherapy. Forty-four patients experienced at least one suicidal event (attempt or ideation) and no completed suicides occurred. Suicide attempts or ideation took place on average 0.4–31.1 weeks after initiating treatment. Patients who received medication did not differ between those who did receive medications with regard to the timing of these suicide events. The results indicated that the severity of baseline suicidal ideation and symptoms of depression increased the probability of suicidal ideation and attempts during treatment. Patients who suffered suicide events were more likely to have moderate illness before the event and showed only minimal improvement. The authors suggest that a majority of suicidal attempts and ideation took place because of chronic depressive symptoms and inadequate improvement rather than in response to medications.

Researchers have been investigating the effectiveness of SSRIs, alone or combined with CBT. Brent et al. (2008) noted that only approximately 60% of depressed adolescents will improve with an initial trial of a SSRI. They conducted a randomized, controlled trial using 334 patients with major depressive disorder, aged 12–18, who had not responded to a 2-month initial treatment with an SSRI. The researchers showed that for these patients, combining CBT and changing to another antidepressant produced greater improvements than just switching to another drug alone. However, changing to another SSRI was just as effective as changing to venlafaxine and produced fewer side effects.

Based on data from TADS, a randomized, controlled trial in 13 academic and community settings, March et al. (2007) revealed that the SSRI, fluoxetine, alone or combined with CBT, accelerated improvements in adolescents with moderate to severe depression. The investigators also found that the safety of the drug was improved by adding CBT.

In a related investigation using the TADS data, Emslie et al. (2006) showed that depressed adolescents had high rates of physical symptoms at the start of clinical trial, which improved as their depressive symptoms improved. In at least 2% of those depressed adolescents treated with fluoxetine and/or in combination with CBT, patients experienced sedation, insomnia, vomiting, and upper abdominal pain. These side effects were twice the rate of those in the placebo group. In the group treated with fluoxetine, the rate of psychiatric adverse events was 11%, 5.6% in the combined treatment group, 4.5% in the placebo group, and 0.9% in the CBT group. Overall, suicide ideation improved, and patients in the combined treatment group experienced the largest improvement in suicide ideation. During the 12-week study period, 24 suicide-related incidents took place. Ten adolescents who were treated with fluoxetine had suicide-associated events, 5 in the combined treatment group, 5 in the CBT group and 3 in the placebo group. The investigators reported only five suicide attempts and no completed suicides. Emslie et al. (2006) concluded that combining CBT and fluoxetine may be safer than the drug alone in treating depression in adolescents.

Not all investigators have found that the combination of CBT and SSRI is superior to monotherapy. Based on a sample of 208 British adolescents, aged 11–17, with moderate to severe major depression who had not responded to a brief initial intervention, Goodyer et al. (2007) and Goodyer et al. (2008) showed that combining CBT with SSRI in the context of routine clinical care did not produce better results. The authors recommend that for adolescents with moderate depression (six to eight symptoms) to severe depression (more than eight symptoms) and those who exhibit overt risk of suicide or substantial functional impairment, clinicians should not allow responses to brief psychosocial interventions to exceed 2–4 weeks. After that time, they recommend treatment with fluoxetine.

A variety of factors may affect treatment outcomes. Lewis et al. (2009) assessed the role of readiness to change in response to treatment of depressed adolescents. Based on a sample of 332 adolescents with major depressive disorder who were participating in the TADS, the investigators showed that treatment response was not affected by any of the readiness scores from an abbreviated Stages of Change Questionnaire. However, they discovered that higher action scores from the Stages of Change Questionnaire predicted better treatment outcomes regardless of therapeutic modality. In addition, the researchers demonstrated that alterations in action scores during the first 6 weeks of therapy mediated treatment outcomes. Specifically, they found that increases in action scores were associated with more improvement in depressive symptoms.

Finally, it should be noted that children and adolescents with a history of childhood abuse may have more severe depressive symptoms and may respond differently to treatment than non-abused children and adolescents. Based on a sample of 90 young persons who had recently engaged in deliberate self-harm (DSH) behaviors, Spinhoven et al. (2009) discovered that those with a history of childhood sexual abuse had more Axis I disorders and reported more severe DSH behaviors, depressive symptoms, suicidal ideation, anxiety, and dissociative behaviors. Individuals treated with CBT had lower risk of repeated DSH behaviors than those receiving usual treatment, after controlling for baseline differences in DSH behaviors and associated disorders.

Impact on Social, Family, and School Functioning

Depression in children and adolescents can impair social, family, educational, and work functioning and can result in an elevated risk of recurrent episodes, increased suicidal risks, and/or lead to the development of bipolar disorder (Purper-Ouakil et al., 2002). Depression in childhood can produce a variety of adverse consequences, including violence and use of addictive substances.

In a study of 603 predominantly Hispanic children, aged 10–14 years, Ferguson et al. (2009) reported that depression, along with the influence of delinquent peers, antisocial personality, and parents or guardians who employ psychosocial abuse in intimate relations, increases the risk for youth violence.

Based on a longitudinal investigation of 1,545 adolescent twins in Finland, Sihvola et al. (2008) discovered that onset of depression at age 14 increased the risk of smoking, use of smokeless tobacco, frequent use of illicit drugs, frequent consumption of alcohol and recurring intoxication 3 years later. As noted previously, comorbid disorders worsen the prognosis for depressed children and adolescents.

Children and adolescents may continue to show adverse effects after recovering from MDD (Son and Kirchner, 2000). They may continue to experience difficulties in relationships, have low self-esteem, participate in risky behaviors, and suffer disruption in their overall functioning (Birmaher et al., 1996). Primary care providers should assess for MDDs as well as their sequelae throughout the individual's life (Son and Kirchner, 2000).

Case Study

The following case study describes a girl with depression. Melissa is a 12-year-old Caucasian female, who lives with her mother in an upper middle class suburb. Her parents were divorced 2 years ago. She has two older siblings, a 19-year-old sister who is a freshman in college and a 17-year-old brother, who is a junior in high school. Her mother is an attorney at a large law firm. Her father is also an attorney. She has visitation with her father on alternate weekends, as well as one dinner per week. Her father rarely exercises his midweek dinner visits and typically picks Melissa up on Saturday at noon, rather than Friday night. He lives in an adjoining suburb.

Melissa's school performance decreased dramatically in fifth grade. Prior to that time, she had been a superior student, performing at the 95th percentile or higher in all academic areas and was placed in the gifted program for both reading and math. In fifth grade, homework completion became a problem and her performance on tests significantly decreased. She was eventually removed from the gifted program.

In sixth grade, she completed homework only half the time, despite two conferences between the school and her parents.

Melissa had participated in figure skating since she was 4 years old and she had been identified as having a special talent. She took private lessons 4 days per week and was also on the synchronized skating team. In addition, she competed in local, regional, and national competitions. Through figure skating, she had a number of friends, although she also had friends at school. Melissa also participated in competitive gymnastics, although she did not experience as much success in this endeavor. Coaches described her as energetic, hard working, friendly, and "sweet." In the past year, she had become increasingly irritable, easily frustrated, and short-tempered. This behavior was also noted at school and home. In particular, she and her mother began to have almost daily conflict. Most of her old friends avoided her and stopped calling her. Melissa began to associate with a new peer group, consisting primarily of outcasts and/or children with behavior problems. Her parents suspected drugs, but disagreed whether she should be evaluated. They consulted the school social worker, who spoke with Melissa. It was the social worker's perception that the problems stemmed from the divorce. Melissa's father questioned whether depression was a possibility, but the social worker related that adjustment disorder was more likely, because Melissa was not having appetite or sleep problems.

When she was found intoxicated by her mother 6 weeks later, she was referred to a clinical psychologist for an evaluation. She was interviewed and administered the Personality Assessment Inventory – Adolescent and the Rorschach Inkblot Test and diagnosed with depression. The psychologist explained to the parents that the absence of appetite and sleep issues was not that atypical for depression in adolescents. She was subsequently referred to a psychiatrist and placed on an antidepressant medication (Zoloft) and began individual counseling. Melissa also had some conjoint sessions with her parents. Her depression responded to treatment and there was a noticeable change in behavior, particularly increased motivation regarding school work and decreased irritability and anger. She continues in therapy.

References

Bhatia, S.K., Bhatia, S.C. (2007). Childhood and adolescent depression. Am Fam Physician, 75 (1), 73–80.

Birkett, M., Espelage, D.L., Koenig, B. (2009). LGB and questioning students in schools: the moderating effects homophobic bullying and school climate on negative outcomes. J Youth Adolesc, 38 (7), 989–1000.

Birmaher, B., Brent, D.A., Benson, R.S. (1998, November). Summary of the practice parameters for the assessment and treatment of children and adolescents with depressive disorders. Amer Acad Child Adol Psychiatry, 37 (11), 1234–1238.

Birmaher, B., Ryan, N.D., Williamson, D.E., et al. (1996). Childhood and adolescent depression: a review of the past 10 years. Part 1. J Am Acad Child Adolesc Psychiatry, 35, 1427–1439.

Bontempo, D.E., D'Augelli, A.R. (2002). Effects of at-school victimization and sexual orientation on lesbian, gay, or bisexual youths' health risk behaviors. J Adolesc Health, 5, 364–374.

Bouma, E.M., Ormel, J., Verhulst, F.C., et al. (2008). Stressful life events and depressive symptoms in early adolescent boys and girls: the influence of parental depression, temperament, and family environment. J Affect Disord, 105 (1–3), 185–193.

Boylan, K., Vaillancourt, T., Boyle, M., et al. (2007). Comorbidity of internalizing disorders in children with oppositional defiant disorder. Eur Child Adolesc Psychiatry, 16 (8), 484–494.

Brent, D., Emslie, G., Clarke, G., et al. (2008). Switching to another SSRI or to venlafaxine with or without cognitive behavioral therapy for adolescents with SSRI-resistant depression: the TORDIA randomized controlled trial. J Am Med Assoc, 299 (8), 901–913.

Brent, D.A., Kolko, D.J., Birmaher, B., et al. (1998). Predictors of treatment efficacy in a clinical trial of three psychosocial treatments for adolescent depression. J Am Acad Child Adolesc Psychiatry, 37, 906–914.

Bridge, J.A., Ivengar, S., Salary, C.B., et al. (2007). Clinical response and risk for reported suicidal ideation and suicide attempts in pediatric antidepressant treatment: a meta-analysis of randomized controlled trials. J Am Med Assoc, 297 (15), 1683–1696.

Brock, K., Nguyen, B., Liu, N., et al. (2005). The use of antidepressants in school-age children. J Sch Nurs, 21 (6), 318–322.

Brunstein Klomek, A., Marrocco, F., Kleinman, M., et al. (2007). Bullying, depression, and suicidality in adolescents. J Am Acad Child Adolesc Psychiatry, 46 (1), 40–49.

Cassidy, L.J., Jellinek, M.S. (1998). Approaches to recognition and management of childhood psychiatric disorders in pediatric primary care. Pediatr Clin North Am, 45, 1037–1052.

Cole, D.A., Peeke, L.G., Martin, J.M., et al. (1998). A longitudinal look at the relation between depression and anxiety in children and adolescents. J Consult Clin Psychol, 66 (3), 451–460.

Curtis, C.E., Luby, J.L. (2008). Depression and social functioning in preschool children with chronic medical conditions. J Pediatr, 153 (3), 408–413.

Emslie, G., Kratochvil, C., Vitiello, B., et al. (2006). Treatment for Adolescents with Depression Study (TADS): safety result. J Am Acad Child Adolesc Psychiatry, 45 (12), 1440–1455.

Emslie, G.J., Mayes, T.L., Ruberu, M. (2005). Continuation and maintenance therapy of early-onset major depressive disorder. Paediatr Drugs, 7 (4), 203–217.

Ferguson, C.J., San Miguel, C., Hartley, R.D. (2009, December). A multivariate analysis of youth violence and aggression: the influence of family, peers, depression, and media violence. J Pediatr, 155 (6), 904–908.

Gershon, E.S., Hamovit, J.H., Guroff, J.J., et al. (1987, April). Birth-cohort changes in manic and depressive disorders in relatives of bipolar and schizoaffective patients. Arch Gen Psychiatry, 44 (4), 314–319.

Gonzalez-Tejera, G., Canino, G., Ramirez, R., et al. (2005). Examining minor and major depression in adolescents. J Child Psychol Psychiatry, 46 (8), 888–899.

Goodyer, I., Dubicka, B., Wilkinson, P., et al. (2007). Selective serotonin reuptake inhibitors (SSRIs) and routine specialist care with and without cognitive behaviour therapy in adolescents with major depression: randomized controlled trial. BMJ, 335 (7611), 142.

Goodyer, I.M., Dubicka, B., Wilkinson, P., et al. (2008). A randomized controlled trial of cognitive behaviour therapy in adolescents with major depression treated by selective serotonin reuptake inhibitors. The ADAPT trial. Health Technol Assess, 12 (14), iii–iv, ix–60.

Greszta, E. (2006). Family environment risk factors of depression in adolescence. Psychiatr Pol, 40 (4), 719–730.

Hack, S., Jellinek, M.S. (1998). Historical clues to the diagnosis of the dysfunctional child and other psychiatric disorders in children. Pediatr Clin North Am, 45, 25–48.

Hammad, T.A., Laughren, T.P., Racoosin, J.A. (2006). Suicide rates in short-term randomized controlled trials of newer antidepressants. J Clin Psychopharmacol, Apr 26 (2), 203–207.

Hjalmarsson, L., Corcos, M., Jeammet, P. (2005). Selective serotonin reuptake inhibitors in major depressive disorder in children and adolescents (ratio of benefits/risks). Encephale, 31 (3), 309–316.

Jellinek, M., Little, M., Murphy, J.M., et al. (1995). The Pediatric Symptom Checklist. Support for a role in a managed care environment. Arch Pediatr Adolesc Med, 149, 740–746.

Jellinek, M.S., Synder, J.B. (1998, August). Depression and suicide in children and adolescents. Pediatr Rev, 19 (8), 255–264.

Jolin, E.M., Weller, E.B., Weller, R.A. (2007). Suicide risk factors in children and adolescents with bipolar disorder. Curr Psychiatry Rep, 9 (2), 122–128.

Kaltiala-Heino, R., Rimpela, M., Marttunen, M., et al. (1999). Bullying, depression, and suicidal ideation in Finnish adolescents: school survey. BMJ, 319 (7206), 348–351.

Kapornai, K., Vetro, A. (2008). Depression in children. Curr Opin Psychiatry, 21 (1), 1–7.

Keenan, K., Hipwell, A., Feng, X., et al. (2008). Subthreshold symptoms of depression in preadolescent girls are stable and predictive of depressive disorders. J Am Acad Child Adolesc Psychiatry, 47 (12), 1433–1442.

King, M., Semlyen, J., Tai, S.S., et al. (2008). A systematic review of mental disorder, suicide, and deliberate self harm in lesbian, gay, and bisexual people. BMC Psychiatry, 8, 70.

Klerman, G.L., Lavori, P.W., Rice, J., et al. (1985, July). Birth-cohort trends in rates of major depressive disorder among relatives of patients with affective disorder. Arch Gen Psychiatry, 42 (7), 689–693.

Kovacs, M., Feinberg, T.L., Crouse-Novak, M.A., et al. (1984). Depressive disorders in childhood. I. A longitudinal prospective study of characteristics and recovery. Arch Gen Psychiatry, 41, 229–237.

Lavigne, J.V., Lebailly, S.A., Hopkins, J., et al. (2009). The prevalence of ADHD, ODD, depression, and anxiety in a community sample of 4-year-olds. J Clin Child Adolesc Psychol, 38 (3), 315–328.

Lee, À., Hankin, B.L. (2009). Insecure attachment, dysfunctional attitudes, and low self-esteem predicting prospective symptoms of depression and anxiety during adolescence. J Clin Child Adolesc Psychol, 38 (2), 219–231.

Lewis, M. (1996). Psychiatric assessment of infant, children, and adolescents. In M. Lewis (Ed.), Child and adolescent psychiatry: a comprehensive textbook. Baltimore, MD: Williams & Wilkins, pp. 440–456.

Lewis, C.C., Simons, A.D., Silva, S.G., et al. (2009). The role of readiness to change in response to treatment of adolescent depression. J Consult Clin Psychol, 77 (3), 422–428.

Luby, J.L., Belden, A.C., Pautsch, J., et al. (2009). The clinical significance of preschool depression: impairment in functioning and clinical markers of the disorder. J Affect Disord, 112 (1–3), 111–119.

March, J.S., Silva, S., Petrycki, S., et al. (2007). The Treatment for Adolescents with Depression Study (TADS): long-term effectiveness and safety outcomes. Arch Gen Psychiatry, 64 (10), 1132–1143.

McFarlane, J.M., Groff, J.Y., O'Brien, J.A., et al. (2003). Behaviors of children who are exposed and not exposed to intimate partner violence: an analysis of 330 black, white, and Hispanic children. Pediatrics, 112 (3 Pt 1), e202–e207.

Mehler-Wex, C., Kolch, M. (2008). Depression in children and adolescents. Dtsch Arztebl Int, 105 (9), 149–155.

Michael, K.D., Crowley, S.L. (2002). How effective are treatments for child and adolescent depression? A meta-analytic review. Clin Psychol Rev, 22 (2), 247–269.

Morewitz, S. (2004). Domestic violence and maternal and child health. New York, NY: Kluwer/Plenum.

Nobile, M., Cataldo, G.M., Marino, C., et al. (2003). Diagnosis and treatment of dysthymia in children and adolescents. CNS Drugs, 17 (13), 927–946.

Oldehinkel, A.J., Veenstra, R., Ormel, J., et al. (2006). Temperament, parenting, and depressive symptoms in a population sample of preadolescents. J Child Psychol Psychiatry, 47 (7), 684–695.

Palosaari, U.K., Aro, H.M. (1995). Parental divorce, self-esteem and depression: an intimate relationship as a protective factor in young adulthood. J Affect Disord, 35 (3), 91–96.

Palosaari, U.K., Aro, H.M., Laippala, P. (1996). Parental divorce and depression in young adulthood: adolescents' closeness to parents and self-esteem as mediating factor. Acta Psychiatr Scand, 93 (1), 20–26.

Purper-Ouakil, D., Michel, G., Mouren-Simeoni, M.C. (2002). Vulnerability to depression in children and adolescents: update and perspectives. Encephale, 28 (3 Pt 1), 234–240.

Reinecke, M.A., Ryan, N.E., DuBois, D.L. (1998). Cognitive-behavioral therapy of depression and depressive symptoms during adolescence: a review and meta-analysis. J Am Acad Child Adolesc Psychiatry, 37, 26–34.

Rodgers, B. (1994). Pathways between parental divorce and adult depression. J Child Psychol Psychiatry, 35 (7), 1289–1308.

Ryan, N.D., Puig-Antich, J., Ambrosini, P., et al. (1987). The clinical picture of major depression in children and adolescents. Arch Gen Psychiatry, 44, 854–861.

Sansone, R.A., Sansone, L.A. (2008). Bully victims: psychological and somatic aftermaths. Psychiatry (Edgmont), 5 (6), 62–64.

Sihvola, E., Keski-Rahkonen, A., Dick, D.M., et al. (2007). Minor depression in adolescence: phenomenology and clinical correlates. J Affect Disord, 97 (1–3), 211–218.

Sihvola, E., Rose, R.J., Dick, D.M., et al. (2008). Early-onset depressive disorders predict the use of addictive substances in adolescence: a prospective study of adolescent Finnish twins. Addiction, 103 (12), 2045–2053.

Son, S.E., Kirchner, J.T. (2000). Depression in children and adolescents. Am Fam Physician, Nov 15, 1–13.

Spinhoven, P., Slee, N., Garnefski, N., et al. (2009). Childhood sexual abuse differentially predict outcome of cognitive-behavioral therapy for deliberate self-harm. J Nerv Ment Dis, 197 (6), 455–457.

Treatment for Adolescents with Depression Study (TADS) (2005). The Treatment for Adolescents with Depression Study (TADS): demographic and clinical characteristics. J Am Acad Child Adolesc Psychiatry, 44 (1), 28–40.

Trowell, J., Joffe, I., Campbell, J., et al. (2007). Childhood depression: a place for psychotherapy. An outcome study comparing individual psychodynamic psychotherapy and family therapy. Eur Child Adolesc Psychiatry, 16 (3), 157–167.

Vitiello, B., Silva, S.G., Rohde, P., et al. (2009). Suicidal events in the Treatment for Adolescents with Depression Study (TADS). J Clin Psychiatry, 70 (5), 741–747.

Weller, E.B., Weller, R.A., Svadjian, H. (1996). Mood disorders. In M. Lewis (Ed.), Child and adolescent psychiatry: A comprehensive textbook. Baltimore, MD: Williams & Wilkins, pp. 650–655.

West, A.E., Pavuluri, M.N. (2009). Psychosocial treatments for childhood and adolescent bipolar disorder. Child Adolesc Psychiatr Clin N Am, 18 (2), 471–482, x–xi.

Wetter, E.K., Hankin, B.L. (2009). Mediational pathways through which positive and negative emotionality contribute to anhedonic symptoms of depression: a prospective study of adolescents. J Abnorm Child Psychol, 37 (4), 507–520.

Wolraich, M., Felice, M.E., Drotar, D. (1996). The classification of child and adolescent mental diagnoses in primary care: diagnostic and statistical manual for primary care (DSM-PC) child and adolescent version. Elk Grove Village, IL: American Academy of Pediatrics.

References

[illegible], R. [illegible] and [illegible], R.M. [illegible] (1995) [illegible] and depression in [illegible] children [illegible] to parental [illegible] self [illegible]. [illegible] and [illegible] 25, [illegible]

[illegible] Morgan [illegible] [illegible] (1989) [illegible] [illegible] [illegible] [illegible] [illegible] [illegible] [illegible] depressive [illegible] [illegible]

R[illegible], M. [illegible], Ryan, N.D., Dahl [illegible] (1998) Comorbid [illegible] and [illegible] and depressive symptoms [illegible] [illegible] [illegible] [illegible] Adolesc. Psychiatry, 37, [illegible]

[illegible] [illegible] [illegible] [illegible] [illegible] [illegible] [illegible] [illegible] [illegible] [illegible]

[illegible] [illegible] [illegible] Adolesc. [illegible] [illegible] [illegible] [illegible] [illegible] [illegible]

[illegible] [illegible] [illegible] [illegible] [illegible] [illegible] psychopath[illegible] [illegible] [illegible]

[illegible]

Chapter 9
Eating Disorders

Eating disorders cause substantial morbidity and mortality in children, adolescents, and adults.

Individuals with AN refuse to keep a minimally normal body weight. They fear gaining weight and have a severely disturbed perception of their body shape or size. Postmenarcheal females with AN are amenorrheic. Persons with the disorder maintain a body weight that is below minimally normal standards for age and height. Children and younger adolescents who develop AN may fail to reach expected weight gains and therefore may not lose weight. Persons with the condition can be classified as having a restricting type, e.g., the persons lose weight by dieting, fasting, or excessive exercise, or binge eating (BE)/purging type, e.g., the individual regularly participates in BE or purging or both.

Individuals with AN who are severely underweight may suffer symptoms of depression such as depressed mood, social withdrawal, irritability, inability to sleep, and reduced libido (American Psychiatric Association, DSM-IV-TR). Many of the symptoms of depression are due to the physiological effects of starvation.

Persons with AN regularly engage in obsessive–compulsive behaviors, which may or may not be associated with food (American Psychiatric Association, DSM-IV-TR). They may collect recipes and hoard food. Their obsessions and compulsions associated with food may be triggered or worsened by malnutrition. Persons with AN who do not have food-related obsessions and compulsions may meet the criteria for obsessive–compulsive disorder.

People with the disorder often are concerned about eating in public (American Psychiatric Association, DSM-IV-TR). They may feel ineffective and have a strong desire to control their environment. They often exhibit inflexibility in thinking and have reduced social spontaneity. Moreover, they are perfectionistic and have very limited initiative and emotional expression.

Persons with AN often also have a personality disorder. Compared to those with the restricting type, those persons with AN who have the BE/purging type often experience problems with impulse control, are more likely to have a substance disorder, be sexually active, have more suicide attempts, and have a borderline personality disorder.

Persons with BN engage in BE and use inappropriate compensatory methods to prevent weight gain (American Psychiatric Association, DSM-IV-TR). Individuals

M.L. Goldstein, S. Morewitz, *Chronic Disorders in Children and Adolescents*,
DOI 10.1007/978-1-4419-9764-7_9,

with BN excessively emphasize body shape and weight and base their self-evaluations on body shape and weight. BE refers to eating in a specific period of time an amount of food that is much more than a majority of people would eat in a similar situation. Their BE and inappropriate compensatory methods occur at least two times a week for 3 months.

Individuals with BN can be classified as having a purging type, e.g., the individual regularly participates in self-induced vomiting or misuses laxatives, diuretics, or enemas or nonpurging type, e.g., the person engages in other inappropriate compensatory activities, such as fasting or excessive exercise, but does not regularly engage in purging behaviors.

Those with BN may have normal weight, but some may be slightly overweight or underweight (American Psychiatric Association, DSM-IV-TR). BN is not prevalent among obese individuals. Between BE episodes, the persons often limit their total caloric intake and select low-calorie and low-fat foods or foods that they think will trigger their BE episodes.

Persons with BN have an increased likelihood of depressive symptoms or mood disorders, particularly dysthymic disorder and major depressive disorder (American Psychiatric Association, DSM-IV-TR). The disturbance of mood often starts at the same time that BN develops or after the disorder emerges. Individuals with BN also frequently develop anxiety symptoms or anxiety disorders. Following effective therapy for BN, the individuals' mood and anxiety disorders are controlled. About 30% of persons with BN have a lifetime prevalence of substance abuse or dependence. These persons are particularly at risk for abusing alcohol or stimulants. Persons begin to use stimulants as a way to control their appetite and weight.

Among women, the lifetime prevalence of BN is about 1–3%, whereas males have a lifetime prevalence that is one-tenth of that in females (American Psychiatric Association, DSM-IV-TR). The disorder often starts in late adolescence or early adulthood.

Persons with binge eating disorder (BED) lose control of their eating but do not engage in compensatory behaviors, such as purging that are typical of persons with BN (American Psychiatric Association, DSM-IV-TR; Bak-Sosnowska, 2009). Individuals with the condition may eat quickly, eat until feeling uncomfortably full, and eat large quantities of food when not hungry. They may eat alone because they feel embarrassed about how much they are eating and may feel disgust, guilt, or depressed after eating too much. BE episodes occur at least 2 days per week for at least 6 months. Persons with the disorder report that their eating behaviors or weight disrupts their social, family, and occupational functioning. Some persons with the disorder report that feeling depressed or anxious triggers their BE episodes. Other people are not able to pinpoint any specific trigger but instead report general feelings of tension that are reduced by BE.

In samples obtained from weight control programs, the prevalence of BED varies from about 15 to 50%. Females are about 1.5 times more likely to have BED than males. The disorder often begins in late adolescence or in early adulthood and develops soon after dieting-related weight loss.

Research into the etiology, risk factors, screening, assessment, and treatment of these conditions will help prevent the conditions and improve assessment and management.

Etiology and Risk Factors

Researchers suggest that a variety of social, cultural, environmental, psychological, organizational, physiological, and genetic factors may contribute to the development of EDs (Westerberg et al., 2008; Dupont and Corcos, 2008; Rome et al., 2003). Nations that emphasize thinness for women as an indicator of beauty have higher prevalence of EDs than nations that do not have such a cultural and social emphasis. For example, in a study of AN among Greek and Turkish adolescents, Fichter et al. (1988) showed that AN prevalence was two times the rate for female Greek adolescents residing in Germany than for those living in Greece and Turkey. The authors suggest that compared to Germany, girls living in Greece and Turkey are subjected to less cultural and social pressures to be thin and therefore have lower rates of EDs.

Individuals with body dysmorphic disorder (BDD) frequently have a comorbid ED (Ruffolo et al., 2006). An investigation of persons with BDD by Ruffolo et al. (2006) revealed that 32.5% of the BDD persons had a comorbid lifetime ED. Nine percent of the sample had AN, 6.5% had BN, and 17.5% had an ED that was not otherwise specified. Compared to BDD persons without a comorbid ED, those with a comorbid lifetime ED were more likely to be female, have more comorbidities, show greater body dissatisfaction and disturbance, and were less likely to be African-American. Although both groups exhibited poor functioning and impaired quality of life, BDD persons with a comorbid lifetime ED were more likely to be hospitalized for psychiatric conditions, had more psychotherapy sessions, and had more use of psychotropic drugs.

Overvaluation or the excessive influence of body shape or weight perceptions and beliefs on self-evaluation is a major risk factor for EDs (Hrabosky et al., 2007). Based on a sample of persons with BED, investigators analyzed overvaluation of body shape and weight using semi-structured interviews, including the eating disorder examination, and several self-report measures. The authors found that body shape and weight overvaluation correlated with psychopathology associated with eating and psychosocial problems such as depression and low self-esteem. However, overvaluation of body shape and weight was not correlated with body mass index (BMI). According to the investigators, people who have body shape and weight overvaluation are not just concerned about being overweight. Instead, their overvaluation of body weight and shape is correlated with psychopathology associated with eating and impaired psychological status. The authors believe that overvaluation should be considered a diagnostic feature of BED.

Other studies have shown that BMI may be a risk factor for EDs. A longitudinal investigation of Swedish adolescent girls revealed that having a higher BMI than their peers was one of the factors that predicted dysfunctional eating attitudes 2 years later (Westerberg et al., 2008).

Children and adolescent who are dissatisfied with their body image or who have body image distortion are at increased risk for developing an ED (Zoletic and Durakovic-Belko, 2009; Lukacs-Marton et al., 2008; Dupont and Corcos, 2008; Rome et al., 2003). In a study of women with AN, Pike et al. (2008) demonstrated that concerns about weight and body shape were most important in the year before onset of the ED. Dupont and Corcos (2008) suggest that individuals' body dissatisfaction and responses to food and eating are incorporated into their patterns of unstable relationships with their parents. These relationships alternate between feelings of merging and rejection and feelings of being engulfed and remote.

Children and adolescents who are teased, bullied, or sexually harassed about their body weight, size, and shape by their friends, acquaintances, and others may be more likely to develop dysfunctional weight control behaviors and weight-associated attitudes and acquire EDs (Eisenberg and Neumark-Sztainer, 2008; Neumark-Sztainer et al., 2002; U.S. DHHS, 2000). Using data from a population-based study of weight issues and eating patterns among teens, Neumark-Sztainer et al. (2002) demonstrated that perceived weight-teasing was significantly correlated with disordered eating among both overweight and non-overweight girls and boys. Girls and boys who experienced frequent weight-teasing were more likely to report binge eating (BE) (29 and 18%, respectively) than by girls and boys who did not report weight-teasing (16 and 7%, respectively).

In an investigation of male and female adolescents by Libbey et al. (2008), frequent teasing by family members and peers was related to more disordered eating thoughts and behaviors, symptoms of depression, anxiety, anger, and lower self-esteem. Adolescents who disliked being teased about their weight were more likely to value thinness, and their self-evaluation was affected by their body weight and shape. Victims who were teased frequently and negatively responded to such harassment were more likely to favor severe forms of BE and have symptoms of depression.

Peer harassment, including bullying and teasing, increases the chances that the victims will acquire other forms of dysfunctional weight-related attitudes. For example, victims of peer harassment are more likely to be dissatisfied with their body weight and shape (Eisenberg and Neumark-Sztainer, 2008).

Body-image dissatisfaction may increase the probability of suicidal ideation during adolescence (Kim and Kim, 2009; Rodriguez-Cano et al., 2006). Drawing on longitudinal data from the Korea Youth Panel, Kim and Kim (2009) demonstrated that body-image dissatisfaction was associated with an increased risk of suicidal ideation in early-adolescent girls and mid-adolescent boys. The authors suggest that interventions should be tailored to the gender and adolescent stage to reduce risk of suicide in these populations.

A community-longitudinal investigation by Rodriguez-Cano et al. (2006) showed that prior suicidal thinking and scores on the Body Shape Questionnaire increased the probability of reported suicide attempts in the next 2 years.

Children and adolescents who have a history of excessive dieting and frequently miss meals and engage in compulsive exercise may be at increased risk of developing EDs (Rome et al., 2003).

In terms of other psychosocial factors, various dysfunctional eating attitudes, low self-esteem, the inability to develop a well-developed identity, problems with attachment, and dependency resulting from poorly internalized relationships are thought to cause EDs (Westerberg et al., 2008; Rome et al., 2003; Dupont and Corcos, 2008; Cozzi and Ostuzzi, 2007; Stein and Corte, 2007). AN and BN may represent attempts to cope with the failure of defense mechanisms and problems with psychological organization (Dupont and Corcos, 2008).

A longitudinal investigation of disturbed eating attitudes in adolescent girls revealed that children's eating attitudes was on the conditions that predicted disturbed eating attitudes 2 years later (Westerberg et al., 2008). The frequency of dysfunctional eating attitudes increased with increased age in the adolescent girls.

Perfectionism and obsessive–compulsive (OC) personality traits may increase the risk of ED in childhood and adolescence (Zoletic and Durakovic-Belko, 2009; Halmi et al., 2005; Anderluh et al., 2003; Rome et al., 2003). Using a case–control study design, Anderluh et al. (2003) showed that childhood obsessive personality traits predicted the subsequent onset of EDs. The investigators discovered that individuals with EDs who exhibited perfectionism and rigidity during childhood were more likely to develop obsessive–compulsive personality disorder (OCPD) and obsessive–compulsive disorder (OCD) later in life than those persons with an EDs who did not have those traits.

Participation in various sports, such as ballet, gymnastics, fashion modeling, and horse racing, are risk factors for acquiring EDs (Lukacs-Marton et al., 2008; Zoletic and Durakovic-Belko, 2009). Based on a sample of fashion models from Transylvania, Lukacs-Marton et al. (2008) discovered that fashion models used more weight-reducing methods, scored higher on Dieting and Bulimia subscales of the Eating Behaviour Severity Scale, and exhibited more body dissatisfaction than control groups.

Another investigation of female ballet dancers and models by Zoletic and Durakovic-Belko (2009) found that female ballet dancers and models showed more body image distortion, eating disorder behaviors, and symptoms of neurotic perfectionism than a control group of students from the University of Sarajevo.

Halmi et al. (2005) evaluated the relation among perfectionism, OCPD, and OCD in persons with EDs. They discovered that perfectionism is more closely related to OCPD symptoms than OCD among individuals with AN and BN. They suggest that the pairing of perfectionism and OCPD increases one's risk for EDs.

Affective disorders are linked to EDs (Fernandez-Aranda et al., 2007). Researchers have found that major depression is a risk factor for EDs among adolescents (Rome et al., 2003; Strober and Katz, 1988; Patton et al., 1999).

Researchers have analyzed the symptoms of major depressive disorder (MDD) in women with EDs. Almost 73% of the women had a lifetime prevalence of MDD. Almost 35% of those women with a lifetime prevalence of MDD reported the onset of MDD before the onset of ED. Women who reported the onset of MDD before the onset of ED exhibited more psychomotor agitation and thoughts about their own death (but not suicide attempts or ideation). Among the women who had MDD onset before ED onset, 26.5% had the MDD onset in the year prior to ED onset.

Children and adolescents with anxiety disorders appear to be at increased risk of developing EDs. Kaye et al. (2004) found that among persons with AN and BN, the rates of anxiety disorders in general and OCD in particular was significantly higher than in a non-clinical community sample of women. The authors reported that among persons with EDs, approximately two-thirds had one or more lifetime anxiety disorders, with the most prevalent ones were OCD and social phobia. Most of those studied developed OCD, social phobia, specific phobia, and generalized anxiety disorder in childhood before acquiring an ED.

Children and adolescents with a history of childhood trauma, such as childhood abuse (e.g., sexual, physical, and emotional abuse, and neglect), may be at increased risk of developing an ED (Rome et al., 2003; Corstorphine et al., 2007; Svirko and Hawton, 2007; Rayworth et al., 2004). In a study of persons with an ED, Corstorphine et al. (2007) showed that those with a history of childhood trauma were more likely to report impulsive behaviors. Those individuals with ED with a history of childhood sexual abuse had a higher probability of engaging in self-cutting, alcohol abuse, and other substance abuse, including amphetamines, cocaine, cannabis, and ketamine, than those without a history of childhood sexual abuse.

In addition to childhood abuse in the family setting, family conflict may be a risk factor for the development of certain types of EDs (Skarderud and Sommerfeldt, 2009; Pike et al., 2008). Pike et al. (2008) discovered that women with AN had a higher rate of family conflict compared to women with non-EDs. A high degree of family conflict and other factors, such as impulsivity, OC symptoms, and dissociative states, may be more likely to predict the onset of self-harm among patients with BN and AN binge type than among patients with the AN restrictive type (Skarderud and Sommerfeldt, 2009).

Other investigators have found a strong positive association between self-harm behaviors and EDs, indicating that self-harm may be a risk factor for EDs (Skarderud and Sommerfeldt, 2009; Corstorphine et al., 2007). According to Skarderud and Sommerfeldt (2009), the reported prevalence of self-harm among patients with EDs has ranged from 13 to 68%. Patients with BN and the binge-type AN have had higher rates of self-harm than patients with AN restrictive type. Common factors related to both self-harm behaviors and these EDs may include impulsiveness, OC traits, dissociation, trauma, and substantial family conflict.

Childhood abuse may increase the risk of body dissatisfaction, depression, low self-esteem in persons, alcohol and drug abuse, and self-harm with EDs (Corstorphine et al., 2007; Grilo and Masheb, 2001). In one study of outpatients with BED, different types of childhood maltreatment were linked to different psychosocial problems (Grilo and Masheb, 2001). Among men and women with BED, a history of childhood emotional abuse was associated with increased body dissatisfaction, higher depression, and lower self-esteem. Childhood sexual abuse was related to increased body dissatisfaction among men with BED. However, the authors did not find an association between any form of childhood maltreatment and age of onset of overweight, dieting, or BE behaviors in this sample of men and women with BED.

Other family characteristics, behaviors, and dynamics may increase the risk of developing EDS (Rome et al., 2003). Children and adolescents who are teased about their body by their family members may be at increased risk of developing EDs. In a study of middle school girls, Keery et al. (2005) discovered that girls who reported that they had been teased about their body appearance by at least one sibling experienced greater body dissatisfaction, internalization of the thin ideal, restriction, bulimic behaviors, depressive symptoms, and lower self-esteem compared to girls who had not reported being teased by their siblings. Increased frequency of teasing was related to worse outcomes.

Higher parental demands may increase the likelihood of AN and other EDs. In a case–control study of women with AN, Pike et al. (2008) identified higher parental demands as a possible risk factor for the onset of AN.

In a Swedish study, Ahren-Moonga et al. (2009) demonstrated that the higher levels of parental and grandparental education and higher academic performance may result in an increased risk of hospitalization for EDs among female offspring. The authors suggest that female offspring may be at increased risk because of high internal and external demands.

Research offers evidence of familial transmission of risk for EDs (Wagner et al., 2008; Rome et al., 2003; Strober et al., 2000). Case–control investigations reveal a higher prevalence of AN among relatives of probands who have AN. Moreover, rate of BN is higher among relatives of AN probands. Strober et al. (2000) suggest that the increased rates of AN and BN among families may be due to several factors, including the co-occurrence of BE and AN, similar patterns of gender and personality characteristics among persons who have both disorders, and the fact that persons with AN and BN often suffer from mood and anxiety disorders.

The risk of acquiring AN is different from that of other affective disorders even though AN and major depression may have shared origins (Rome et al., 2003). An important caveat is that depression occurs because of starvation, and many symptoms can be improved when weight is restored.

In a German study, Wagner et al. (2008) showed that the rates of AN and MDD were higher among first- and second-degree relatives of AN and bulimic individuals, compared to the relatives of healthy controls. The trends were more evident among the relatives of bulimic patients.

A family history of an ED or obesity is a risk factor for ED (Rome et al., 2003). In addition, parental eating behavior, weight, and eating-related attitudes may help to predict the onset of EDs in children and adolescents (Canals et al., 2009; Westerberg et al., 2008; Rome et al., 2003).

Canals et al. (2009) evaluated the influence of parent's eating attitudes on EDs in school adolescents and showed that the mother's body dissatisfaction, drive for thinness, and the father's drive for thinness and perfectionism were positively associated with the adolescent's long-term ED.

In a 2-year longitudinal investigation, Westerberg et al. (2008) discovered that fathers' eating attitude was one of the factors that predicted disturbed eating attitudes among adolescent children 2 years later.

Substance use disorders are common among individuals with EDs and their families. For example, among women with BN and their family members, substance use disorders are prevalent (Kaye et al., 1996). Studies have found that affective disorder, substance dependence, including alcoholism, in first-degree relatives is a risk factor for EDs (Redgrave et al., 2007; Rome et al., 2003; Kaye et al., 1996). Based on an investigation of female inpatients at a specialty ED service, Redgrave et al. (2007) discovered that inpatients with alcoholic first-degree relatives had more ED-related psychopathology, substance use, vulnerable personality characteristics, compared to those without alcoholic first-degree relatives.

Parent–child communications may play a role in the onset of EDs (Kim and Yang, 2008). A study of the relationship between EDs and parent–adolescent communication revealed that EDs were more likely in adolescents who had reduced parent–adolescent communication (Kim and Yang, 2008).

Characteristics of school experiences may increase the risk of EDS and other problems among certain individuals. Boujut and Bruchon-Schweitzer (2009) developed a college freshman stress questionnaire and discovered that EDs, symptoms of depression, somatic symptoms, and life satisfaction were correlated with academic stress, university functioning, feeling lonely, and having difficulties with primary relations.

The characteristics of certain occupations and industries, such as fashion modeling, ballet, and sports, may increase the likelihood that those working in these occupations and industries will acquire EDs (Lukacs-Marton et al., 2008; Zoletic and Durakovic-Belko, 2009).

Some scientists suggest that physiologic factors cause EDS. Some theorize that dysfunctional pituitary, hypothalamus, and different neurotransmitters lead to the onset of EDs (Rome et al., 2003). However, functional imaging studies show that these physiological processes are corrected when the persons achieve normal weight, suggesting that these physiological processes are not primary etiological factors.

Other investigations have evaluated the role of serotonin in the etiology of EDs since the neurotransmitter serotonin influences the control of appetite, sexual and social interactions, and responses to stress and mood (Rome et al., 2003). A reduction in brain serotonin function is linked to psychosocial problems, such as depression, impulsive behavior, and aggression. In persons with AN who are underweight, the serotonin metabolite, 5-hydroxyindoleacetic acid, is at a low level. However, after these individuals have returned to long-term normal functioning, the metabolite increases to above normal levels.

Research has led to the speculation that impaired serotonergic function may increase the risk of AN and BN (Rome et al., 2003). An allelic association between the B1438 A/G promoter polymorphism of the 5-HT2A gene and AN has been found, but the findings have not been replicated consistently.

Leptin, a hormone which is secreted by fat cells, is not likely an etiological factor in AN even though leptin plays a role in the regulation of body fat (Rome et al., 2003). Low weight or AN is related to low levels of serum leptin, which is associated with a reduction of fat tissue. Serum leptin levels increase when the person gains weight (Grinspoon et al., 1996; Mantzoros et al., 1997). Serum leptin levels appear to return to normal before body weight is normalized. This trend helps to explain why persons with AN have difficulty reaching and maintaining normal weight.

Various PET, magnetic resonance, and imaging scans show that the brains of girls with AN have some changes in the function and structure of their brains. However, these investigations have not provided clues as to the etiology of AN (Katzman et al., 1996; Katzman et al., 1997; Gordon et al., 2000).

Screening and Assessment

Different ED screening instruments are available. However, clinicians do not usually rely on these tools (Rome et al., 2003). Clinicians should ask a number of questions in screening for EDs. They should ask the patient about the history of their present illness, weight history, desired weight, frequency that they weigh themselves, when they began to lose weight, their weight control methods, and their diet history. Primary care providers should inquire about their patient's current dietary practices, including amounts of food, food groups, restrictions in fluid intake, binge and purging behaviors, abuse of diuretics, laxatives, diet pills, history of exercise, and menstrual history.

Clinicians should perform a review of systems, noting the presence of symptoms, such as dizziness and blackouts, easy bruising, cold intolerance, hair loss, vomiting, diarrhea, constipation, bloating, chest pain, and menstrual irregularities. In addition, primary care providers should assess for symptoms of hyperthyroidism, DM, malignancy, infection, inflammatory bowel disease, psychosocial symptoms, past medical history, family history, and social history, including history of sexual abuse and substance abuse.

If symptoms of disordered eating are detected, practitioners should perform a diagnostic interview to determine if formal criteria for EDs are met (Rome et al., 2003). Earlier identification of an ED generally results in a more favorable prognosis. Primary care providers should determine if the patient has lost weight, is afraid to gain weight, has a fat phobia, is preoccupied with food, and has restrictive patterns of eating. Moreover, the practitioner should find out if the patient engages in purging and binging behaviors, has a distorted body image, exhibits uncontrollable eating, and has menstrual irregularity.

Assessment is often difficult because a patient with disordered eating or EDs will not answer the clinician's questions truthfully or with accuracy (Rome et al., 2003). Data about the patient obtained from family, friends, and school personnel can be very useful. Other information, such as whether the patient prefers to eat alone, has very restricted choices of food, prefers to eat with only a certain bowl or plate, eats food in a particular order, chews gum or ice excessively, and has excessive intake of fluids, helps the provider make a presumptive diagnosis of an ED.

If the practitioner suspects that the patient has an ED, then the patient should be screened for risk of suicide (Rome et al., 2003).

Patients who present with ED symptoms, such as appetite loss, weight loss, menstrual irregularities, or unexplained vomiting, could actually be suffering from a variety of medical disorders (Rome et al., 2003). Providers should consider medical and psychiatric diagnoses when they suspect that the patient has an ED, but common aspects of the disorder are not present. At the same time, clinicians should consider the possibility that the patient is in denial or is intentionally deceiving them. Sometimes, clinicians will mistakenly diagnose an ED when the patient actually has such conditions as inflammatory bowel disease, cancer, thyroid disease, diabetes mellitus, and diseases of the central nervous system. Moreover, practitioners may mistakenly diagnose an ED when the patient is actually suffering from psychiatric conditions. For example, clinicians may mistakenly diagnose an ED when the patient's loss of appetite and subsequent weight loss is actually due to major depression. In addition, symptoms of an ED may mimic OCD, alcohol and drug abuse, and psychosis.

Afflicted individuals will rarely admit to having an ED (Rome et al., 2003). A parent, teacher, coach, or school nurse may become suspicious and then refer the child. It is more frequent that the child will seek medical attention for symptoms, such as dizziness, constipation, heartburn, headaches, or menstrual irregularities, which are due to weight loss or disordered eating.

Health-care providers should work with the patient and family. If parents have concerns about their child's eating problems, the clinician should ascertain parental concerns in the patient's presence (Rome et al., 2003). The patient should then be interviewed alone. The clinician should conduct the patient interview with empathy and should be nonjudgmental to find out whether the patient has an ED. The physical examination may be inconclusive. However, a number of clues may indicate that the patient is suffering from an ED. For example, the patient with ED may exhibit the following symptoms: emaciation, sunken eyes, loss of shine or brittle hair, atrophy of the breasts, the loss of tooth enamel, edema of the extremities, and diminished deep tendon reflexes.

Treatment

If possible, the primary care provider should assemble a team consisting of a registered dietitian and therapist who have experience working with children and adolescents with EDs (Rome et al., 2003). Parents should be involved early in the treatment and management plans. In addition, a psychiatric consultation is sometimes important to assess the ED and comorbid conditions, such as depression, suicidal risks, OCD, anxiety disorder, and psychiatric medications.

In some cases, clinicians should discuss the patient's calorie and fat gram needs, while for other patients, it is not useful. Parents with younger children may be taught to prepare and plate their child's food and oversee their food consumption to ensure that the child is eating sufficient food portions.

Rome et al. (2003) suggest that the treatment should vary depending on the severity of the condition. For patients with mild or early ED (85–95% of ideal body weight and stable vital signs), the clinician should begin a food plan consisting of three meals and three snacks with a minimum of 1,200–1,500 calories per day, depending on the patient's recent caloric intake. The food plan should be increased once or two times per week. The clinician should refer the patient to a dietitian and therapist.

For patients with mild or early ED, the provider should establish a patient contract for expected rate of weight gain, target weight goal, hospitalization weight goal, and what will happen if the patient fails to reach her/his weight. The clinician can draw a target weight line, and this graph can be shown to the patient to provide feedback on treatment progress. The patient should see the health-care provider every 2 weeks until she/he is gaining weight on a consistent basis. Once consistent weight gain has been achieved, the patient should be seen at least once a month until the patient achieves target the weight range. For patients with mild or early ED, the clinician should communicate weight, vital signs, and other issues to the therapist and dietitian every few weeks.

For children and adolescents with mild or early ED who do not gain weight adequately, the provider should add liquid supplements and/or restrict the patient's activity. If the patient is bradycardic, the patient's activity should be restricted. In addition, if the patient does not gain weight, parental supervision of patient food consumption should be added to the treatment plan.

Patients with moderate or established ED are 75–85% of ideal body weight (Rome et al., 2003). Their vital signs may be going downhill or they may have minor laboratory abnormalities. For these patients, referral to a dietitian and therapist should be required.

These patients should have their physical activity restricted until they have a weight gaining trend and their vital signs continue to be stable (Rome et al., 2003). A short-term goal for these patients is to achieve a weight at which they can exercise safely.

The provider should establish a contract with the patient, specifying expected rate of weight gain, the patient's target weight, hospitalization weight, and what will happen if the patient fails to gain her/his target weight. A target line also should be drawn. The clinician should see the patient weekly until the patient is gaining weight on a consistent basis. Afterward, the provider should see the patient every 2 weeks until the target weight range is reached. On a regular basis, the provider should communicate weight, vital signs, and other relevant information to other members of the team. In addition, the clinician should consider liquid supplements to increase caloric intake. The provider should discuss the need for hospitalization if the patient cannot reach her/his weight goals.

Patients with a severe ED are less than 75% of ideal body weight, are medically unstable, have a pulse less than 50, and may be dehydrated (Rome et al., 2003). These patients should be hospitalized immediately. The hospital nursing staff should participate in the treatment plan. They should be both firm and supportive. They should not bargain with the patient and should keep other members of health team updated on all relevant information.

In the hospital setting, the goal is to restore nutrition, which is planned by a dietitian (Rome et al., 2003). The dietitian plans the patient's food trays with the expectation that the patient will follow the prescribed nutritional plan. The patient will be given an oral or nasogastric supplement which is equivalent to any uneaten food portion. Over the course of the day, the patient will receive three meals and three snacks. The provider should set the minimum calorie level range at 1,200–1,500 per day and increase it by 200 kcal per day until the patient is gaining weight. Once the patient is gaining weight, the provider should increase it by 200 kcal per day every 2–3 days until the patient is consuming the recommended calories. Patients should be monitored for acute medical complications, such as the re-feeding syndrome, shifts in fluid, and cardiac arrhythmias.

To ensure patient compliance and support, the patient should be monitored closely while eating and 1 h afterward (Rome et al., 2003). To prevent purging or exercise and prevent injuries associated with orthostatic hypotension, the staff should supervise bathroom time.

Another important component of hospital treatment is to provide the patient with psychological support several times per week (Rome et al., 2003). The patient's cognitive functioning is frequently impaired at this time. As a result, supportive therapy is recommended until the patient's nutritional and cognitive functioning improves. Once this is accomplished, the therapist can begin to offer therapy. During therapy, one strategy is to ask the patient to write a list of positive messages that she/he can rely on when she is having difficulty overcoming the ED. Moreover, the patient can learn to use relaxation methods before and after meals to help reduce the stress associated with these time periods.

How long should the hospitalization last? The patient should be hospitalized for a long enough period so that the patient stops losing weight, is able to develop a weight-gaining trend, and has normal vital signs and laboratory values (Rome et al., 2003). In addition, the hospitalization should be long enough to enable the patient to eat independently so that she/he continues to gain weight on an outpatient basis.

Clinicians set higher weight goals for patients who have been hospitalized more than once (Rome et al., 2003). With improved health status, providers should give the patient more autonomy in selecting their meals. Patients can choose meals from the hospital menu in collaboration with her/his family. Moreover, the patient can have some unsupervised meals.

The treatment plan should be evaluated and, modified, if necessary, on a continuous basis by the primary care provider, other members of the treatment team, and the patient's parents to ensure that progress is being made.

Patients frequently drop out of inpatient treatment for AN, and dropout from inpatient treatment is associated with worse outcomes. Using a French sample of 601 consecutive female patients with AN, restrictive (AN-R) or AN, binge/purging (AN-B/P) subtypes, Huas et al. (2011) evaluated dropout rates and predictors of dropout. They showed that 50.0% of the AN-R patients and 56.2% of the AN-B/P patients dropped out of AN inpatient treatment between 1988 and 2004. Factors that predicted dropout were as follows: having one or more children, low desired BMI, a low minimum BMI, paranoid ideation, pathological eating behaviors, and low educational attainment. Patients who dropped out early were more likely to have lower desired BMI, paranoid ideation, and more impulsive behaviors, e.g., use alcohol and have suicide attempts. The authors suggest that certain factors reflect illness severity and should be warning signs for clinicians, e.g., pathological eating behaviors and low minimum BMI, while other factors could be targeted before hospitalization, such as patients who have one or more children and low desired BMI.

Treatment guidelines and clinical pathways for treating AN in adolescents have become popular (Rome et al., 2003). The American Psychiatric Association and the Society for Adolescent Medicine have published guidelines for AN treatment. Health-care providers at Stanford developed the first clinical pathway for treating AN in adolescents.

Investigators have evaluated the effectiveness of psychological treatments for individuals with different EDs (Eisler et al., 2007; Lock et al., 2006; Loeb et al., 2007). Family-based therapy (FBT) can be effective in treating adolescent AN. Based on 86 persons who had been previously treated in a randomized clinical trial using FBT, Lock et al. (2006) discovered that short-term FBT was just as effective as longer term FBT in improving the participants' ideal body weight. Eighty-nine percent of the research subjects were above 90% ideal body weight at follow-up. Seventy-four percent had eating disorder examination scores in the normal range. In addition, 91% of the postmenarcheal females who were not on birth control had normal menstruation.

Clinicians have developed a manual-based form of cognitive behavior therapy to treat BN (CBT-BN). In a review of the literature, Hay et al. (2009) evaluated the effectiveness of cognitive behavior therapy (CBT), CBT-BN, and other psychotherapies. Based on a review of 48 studies involving 3,054 participants, the authors found that CBT is effective, especially CBT-BN in treating persons with BN and associated ED conditions. The literature review also showed that other psychotherapies were effective, especially interpersonal psychotherapy (IPT) in treating persons with BN and related syndromes in the long term. The trials revealed that self-help therapies that used very structured CBT models had potential. However, the literature showed that exposure and response prevention approaches did not improve the effectiveness of CBT.

CBT has been shown to be effective in treating individuals who have core symptoms of BED (Striegel-Moore et al., 2010; Wilson et al., 2010). Based on a sample of 123 persons, including 10% with BN, 48% with BED, and 41.4% with recurrent BE without BN or BED, Striegel-Moore et al. (2010) tested whether a manual-based guided self-help type of CBT (CBT-GSH) that was given in 8 sessions at a health maintenance organization over a 12-week period was more effective than usual care. The authors discovered that CBT-GSH produced greater avoidance of BE than usual care at 12-month follow-up. Participation in CBT-GSH also was associated with improvements in dietary restraint, eating, concerns about shape and weight, depression symptoms, and social adjustment. However, CBT-GSH did not lead to significant weight change. The authors suggest that CBT-GSH is useful as a first-line therapy for most patients with recurrent BE without BN or AN.

Wilson et al. (2010) report that behavioral weight loss treatment (BWL) and CBT-GSH have produced short-term reductions in BE in obese patients with BED. The authors compared both BWL and CBT-GSH with IPT using a sample of 205 women and men with BMI between 27 and 45 who met the DSM-IV criteria for BED. At 2-year follow-up, IPT and CBT-GSH were more effective than BWL in curing BE. The investigators conclude that CBT-GSH should be the first-line therapy for a majority of patients with BED. IPT or a complete form of CBT should be undertaken to treat patients with low self-esteem and severe ED symptoms.

Complications

The duration, severity, number of instances of nutritional restriction, and the timing of those episodes of food restriction in relationship to normal growth and physical development influence the outcomes of nutritional deprivation (Rome et al., 2003). All body tissues and organ may be impacted by acute and severe malnutrition. Among adolescents with AN, damage to brain and bone tissues may or may not be fully restored even with nutritional replenishment. Severe nutritional problems may be associated with diagnoses of EDs and disordered eating. Adolescents also may suffer from substantial nutritional dysfunction that occurs because of stressful life events and their need to make their own food selections without effective knowledge or supervision. As part of normal adolescent life or experimentation during this life stage, adolescents engage in risky behaviors. Children in competitive sports, fashion modeling, and dance are especially vulnerable to nutritional risk-taking. In addition, those with chronic diseases are susceptible.

The Impact of EDs on Family Functioning

Families of children and adolescents with EDs can experience significant stress. An investigation by Sim et al. (2009) analyzed family functioning of adolescent girls with AN to those with a chronic health condition, insulin-dependent diabetes mellitus (IDDM), and girls without a health problem. They found that the families of adolescent girls with AN had more family conflict, impaired parental alliance, and increased depressive symptoms, compared to the mothers of daughters with IDDM. However, after statistically controlling for the psychosocial impact of the health problem on the mothers, group differences were eliminated.

A 2-year longitudinal investigation revealed that adolescent girls who evaluated their relation to their family as less healthy were more likely to experience dysfunctional eating attitudes 2 years later (Westerberg et al., 2008).

Family members of relatives with EDs can experience substantial distress because of the problems in performing their caregiving role (Sepulveda et al., 2008;

Whitney et al., 2007). Based on a sample of persons caring for an individual with an ED, Whitney et al. (2007) discovered that 36% of the caregivers had mental health problems and 17% reported high levels of psychological distress. Caregivers who had negative experiences as caregivers were more likely to report psychological distress. Negative evaluations of caregiving were related to shorter illness duration, less support, and perceptions that the illness had major consequences.

Sepulveda et al. (2008) developed an Eating Disorders Symptom Impact Scale for caregivers of people with EDs. This scale may be used to evaluate the effects of ED symptoms on family caregivers to determine their needs and assess therapeutic outcomes.

To what extent do children with EDs agree with their parents' perception of family functioning? Using a sample of females at an outpatient ED program, Dancyger et al. (2005) showed that mothers evaluated family functioning healthier and less dysfunctional than their daughters who were ED patients. However, fathers did not rate family functioning differently than their daughters. The authors assert that differences in perceptions between daughters and their mothers can lead to the maintenance of impaired family interactions, EDs, and adverse treatment outcomes.

What may cause these differing perceptions of family functioning between mothers and their adolescent daughters? Dancyger et al. (2006) discovered that the daughters' general distrust of people explained differences between mothers and daughters' scores in problem solving, communication, affective responsiveness, and general functioning.

Psychosocial Adjustment in Young Adulthood of Individuals Who Had an ED During Adolescence

How do young adults function if they had an ED as adolescent? Using a sample of high school girls, Striegel-Moore et al. (2003) discovered that individuals who had an ED during adolescence had substantial impairment in health, self-evaluation, and major areas of social functioning.

Persons with EDs are at risk for suicide and suicide attempts (Franko and Keel, 2006; Bulik et al., 2008; Foulon et al., 2007). Among AN patients, the standardized mortality ratio for suicide ranges from 1.0 to 5.3, whereas the suicide rates among BN patients are not elevated. However, with regard to suicide attempts, 3–20% of AN patients and 25–35% of BN patients attempt suicide.

Using a sample of individuals with current or lifetime AN from the Genetics of Anorexia Nervosa Collaborative Study, Bulik et al. (2008) found that about 16.9% of persons with AN attempted suicide. Only 7.4% of persons with the restricted subtype of AN reported at least one suicide attempt, while 26.1% of those with the purging AN subtype, 29.3% of the BE subtype, and 21.2% of the mixed type of AN and BN reported attempting suicide at least one time.

As noted previously, body image dissatisfaction is a risk factor for suicidal ideation (Kim and Kim, 2009). Other risk factors for suicidality in ED patients include purging behaviors, symptoms of depression, substance use disorders, and a history of childhood abuse (physical and/or sexual abuse) (Franko and Keel, 2006). Based on a sample of AN patients, Foulon et al. (2007) discovered having MDD and switching from the restrictive subtype of AN to the binging/purging subtype predicted an increase in the frequency of suicide attempts. Patients who had a substance-abuse problem, impulsive behaviors and traits, cluster B personality disorders, panic disorder, post-traumatic stress disorder, a low degree of self-directedness, and severe ED were more likely to make suicide attempts.

Clinicians should regularly assess for suicidal ideation in ED patients, especially those who have comorbid conditions, regardless of the severity of the ED or symptoms of depression (Franko and Keel, 2006).

Case Study

The following case describes a female adolescent with AN. Alyson is a 16-year-old Caucasian female, who is currently in her sophomore year at a public suburban high school. She lives with her parents and three younger siblings. Her father owns a chain of furniture stores, while her mother is a homemaker. Both parents are very weight-conscious and work out with their personal trainer at least four times per week. Her mother also plays tennis several times per week at the local country club.

Alyson has always been an excellent student, typically receiving all A's on her report card. She has participated in competitive gymnastics since she was 5 years old and also participates in dance. She currently takes three dance classes each week and has gymnastics practice approximately 10 h per week.

She began dating in eighth grade, with encouragement from both parents, especially her mother. Alyson became sexually active this year with a boyfriend, but he broke up with her recently. She immediately became involved with another boy, but has yet to have intercourse with him. Her mother put her on birth control pills at the beginning of her freshman year of high school.

Although Alyson was always on the thin side, her weight was within normal limits for her age and stature. Approximately, 6 months ago, she decided that she was "fat," and made a conscious decision to lose weight. Initially, she began to increase her exercise regimen, often exercising 2 or more hours per day in addition to her dance and gymnastics. She began to take laxatives 4 months ago and would also force herself to vomit if she ate high caloric foods. When she forced herself to vomit at a friend's house and was caught by her friend, she feigned illness.

When her father became concerned about her weight loss, she was taken to the family physician, who diagnosed her with an eating disorder. He referred the family to a nutritionist, who subsequently met with Alyson and her mother. However, her weight loss continued and she developed amenorrhea. One of Alyson's friends then called Alyson's mother and informed her of Alyson's forced vomiting. At that point, the parents consulted with the family physician, which referred Alyson to a clinical psychologist who specialized in eating disorders. Alyson was diagnosed with AN. She was resistant to therapy, and subsequently lost more weight. She was then placed in an inpatient eating disorder program, which included individual and group therapy, family therapy, and work with a nutritionist. Alyson was subsequently released from the hospital, but continues with individual counseling, family counseling, and work with a nutritionist.

References

Ahren-Moonga, J., Silverwood, R., Klinteberg, B.A. et al. (2009). Association of higher parental and grandparental education and higher school grades with risk of hospitalization for eating disorders in females: the Uppsala birth cohort multigenerational study. Am J Epidemiol, 170 (5), 566–575.

Anderluh, M.B., Tchanturia, K., Rabe-Hesketh, S. et al. (2003). Childhood obsessive-compulsive personality traits in adult women with eating disorders: defining a broader eating disorder phenotype. Am J Psychiatry, 160 (2), 242–247.

Bak-Sosnowska, M. (2009, July–August). Psychological intervention in binge eating disorder. Psychiatr Pol, 43 (4), 445–455.

Boujut, E., Bruchon-Schweitzer, M. (2009). A construction and validation of a Freshman Stress Questionnaire: an exploration study. Psychol Rep, 104 (2), 680–692.

Bulik, C.M., Thornton, L., Pinheiro, A.P. et al. (2008). Suicide attempts in anorexia nervosa. Psychosom Med, 70 (3), 378–383.

Canals, J., Sancho, C., Arija, M.V. (2009). Influence of parent's eating attitudes on eating disorders in school adolescents. Eur Child Adolesc Psychiatry, 18 (6), 353–359.

Corstorphine, E., Waller, G., Lawson, R. et al. (2007). Trauma and multi-impulsivity in the eating disorders. Eat Behav, 8 (1), 23–30.

Cozzi, F., Ostuzzi, R. (2007). Relational competence and eating disorders. Eat Weight Disord, 12 (2), 101–107.

Dancyger, I., Fornari, V., Scionti, L. et al. (2005). Do daughters with eating disorders agree with their parents' perception of family functioning? Compr Psychiatry, 46 (2), 135–139.

Dancyger, I., Fornari, V., Sunday, S. (2006). What may underlie differing perceptions of family functioning between mothers and their adolescent daughters with eating disorders? Int J Adolesc Med Health, 18 (2), 281–286.

Dupont, M.E., Corcos, M. (2008). Psychopathology in eating disorders: new trends. Rev Prat, 58 (2), 141–143, 145–146, 148–149.

Eisenberg, M., Neumark-Sztainer, D. (2008). Peer harassment and disordered eating. Int J Adolesc Med Health, 20 (2), 155–164.

Eisler, I., Simic, M., Russell, G.F. (2007). A randomized controlled treatment trial of two forms of family therapy in adolescent anorexia nervosa: a five-year follow-up. J Child Psychol Psychiatry, 48 (6), 552–560.

Fernandez-Aranda, F., Pinheiro, A.P., Tozzi, F. et al. (2007). Symptom profile of major depressive disorder in women with eating disorders. Aust N Z J Psychiatry, 41 (1), 24–31.

Fichter, M.M., Elton, M., Sourdi, L. et al. (1988). Anorexia nervosa in Greek and Turkish adolescents. Eur Arch Psychiatry Neurol Sci, 237, 200–208.

Foulon, C., Guelfi, J.D., Kipman, A. et al. (2007). Switching to the bingeing/purging subtype of anorexia nervosa is frequently associated with suicidal attempts. Eur Psychiatry, 22 (8), 513–519.

Franko, D.L., Keel, P.K. (2006). Suicidality in eating disorders: occurrence, correlates, and clinical implications. Clin Psychol Rev, 26 (6), 769–782.

Gordon, C.M., Dougherty, D.D., Rauch, S.L., et al. (2000, March). Neuroanatomy of human appetitive function: a positron emission tomography investigation. Int J Eat Disord, 27 (2), 163–171.

Grilo, C.M., Masheb, R.M. (2001). Childhood psychological, physical, and sexual maltreatment in outpatients with binge eating disorder: frequency and associations with gender, obesity, and eating-related psychopathology. Obes Res, 9 (5), 320–325.

Grinspoon, S., Gulick, T., Askari, H., et al. (1996, November). Serum leptin levels in women with anorexia nervosa. J Clin Endocrinol Metab, 81 (11), 3861–3863.

Halmi, K.A., Tozzi, F., Thornton, L.M. et al. (2005). The relation among perfectionism, obsessive-compulsive personality disorder and obsessive-compulsive disorder in individuals with eating disorders. Int J Disord, 38 (4), 371–374.

Hay, P.P., Bacaltchuk, J., Stefano, S., et al. (2009, October 7). Psychological treatments for bulimia nervosa and binging. Cochrane Database Syst Rev, Issue 4, Art. No.: CD000562.

Hrabosky, J.I., Masheb, R.M., White, M.A. et al. (2007). Overvaluation of shape and weight in binge eating disorder. J Consult Clin Psychol, 75 (1), 175–180.

Huas, C., Godart, N., Foulon, C., et al. (2011, February 28). Predictors of dropout from inpatient treatment for anorexia nervosa: data from a large French sample. Psychiatry Res, 185 (3), 421–426.

Katzman, D.K., Lambe, E.K., Mikulis, D.J., et al. (1996, December). Cerebral gray matter and white matter volume deficits in adolescent girls with anorexia nervosa. J Pediatr, 129 (6), 794–803.

Katzman, D.K., Zipursky, R.B., Lambe, E.K., et al. (1997, August). A longitudinal magnetic resonance imaging study of brain changes in adolescents with anorexia nervosa. Arch Pediatr Adolesc Med, 151 (8), 793–797.

Kaye, W.H., Bulik, C.M., Thornton, L. et al. (2004). Comorbidity of anxiety disorders with anorexia and bulimia nervosa. Am J Psychiatry, 161 (12), 2215–2221.

Kaye, W.H., Lilenfeld, L.R., Plotnicov, K. et al. (1996). Bulimia nervosa and substance dependence: association and family transmission. Alcohol Clin Exp Res, 20 (5), 878–881.

Keery, H., Boutelle, K., van den Berg, P. et al. (2005). The impact of appearance-related teasing by family members. J Adolesc Health, 37 (2), 120–127.

Kim, D.S., Kim, H.S. (2009). Body-image dissatisfaction as a predictor of suicidal ideation among Korean boys and girls in different stages of adolescence: a two-year longitudinal study. J Adolesc Health, 45 (1), 47–54.

Kim, K.H., Yang, K.M. (2008). The relationship between eating disorders and parent-adolescent communication in middle school students in rural areas. Taehan Kanho Hakoe Chi, 38 (1), 55–63.

Libbey, H.P., Story, M.T., Neumark-Sztainer, D.R. et al. (2008). Teasing, disordered eating behaviors, and psychological morbidities among overweight adolescents. Obesity, 16 (Suppl 2), S24–S29.

Lock, J., Couturier, J., Agras, W.S. (2006). Comparison of long-term outcomes in adolescents with anorexia nervosa treated with family therapy. J Am Acad Child Adolesc Psychiatry, 45 (6), 666–672.

Loeb, K.L., Walsh, B.T., Lock, J. et al. (2007). Open trial of family-based treatment for full and partial anorexia nervosa in adolescence: evidence of successful dissemination. J Am Acad Child Adolesc Psychiatry, 46 (7), 792–800.

Lukacs-Marton, R., Vasarhelyi, E., Szabo, P. (2008). Entrapped by the beauty industry: eating and body attitudes of those working in the beauty industry. Psychiatr Hung, 23 (6), 455–463.

Mantzoros, C., Flier, J.S., Lesem, M.D., et al. (1997, June). Cerebrospinal fluid leptin in anorexia nervosa: correlation with nutritional status and potential role in resistance to weight gain. J Clin Endocrinol Metab, 82 (6), 1845–1851.

Neumark-Sztainer, D., Falkner, N., Story, M. et al. (2002). Weight-teasing among adolescents: correlations with weight status and disordered eating behaviors. Int J Obes Relat Metab Disord, 26 (1), 123–131.

Patton, G.C., Selzer, R., Coffey, C. et al. (1999). Onset of eating disorders: population based cohort over 3 years. BMJ, 318, 765–768.

Pike, K.M., Hilbert, A., Wilfley, D.E. et al. (2008). Toward an understanding of risk factors for anorexia nervosa: a case-control study. Psychol Med, 38 (10), 1443–1453.

Rayworth, B.B., Wise, L.A., Harlow, B.L. (2004). Childhood abuse and risk of eating disorders in women. Epidemiol, 15 (3), 271–278.

Redgrave, G.W., Coughlin, J.W., Heinberg, L.J. et al. (2007). First-degree relative history of alcoholism in eating disorder inpatients: relationship to eating and substance use psychopathology. Eat Behav, 8 (1), 15–22.

Rodriguez-Cano, T., Beato-Fernandez, L., Llario, A.B. (2006). Body dissatisfaction as a predictor of self-reported suicide attempts in adolescents: a Spanish community prospective study. J Adolesc Health, 38 (6), 684–688.

Rome, E.S., Ammerman, S., Rosen, D.S. et al. (2003). Children and adolescents with eating disorders: the state of the art. Pediatrics, 111 (1), e98–e108.

Ruffolo, J.S., Phillips, K.A., Menard, W. et al. (2006). Comorbidity of body dysmorphic disorder and eating disorders: severity of psychopathology and body image disturbance. Int J Eat Disord, 39 (1), 11–19.

Sepulveda, A.R., Whitney, J., Hankins, M. et al. (2008). Development and validation of an Eating Disorders Symptom Impact Scale (EDSIS) for carers of people with eating disorders. Health Qual Life Outcomes, 6, 28.

Sim, L.A., Homme, J.H., Lteif, A.N. et al. (2009). Family functioning and maternal distress in adolescent girls with anorexia nervosa. Int J Eat Disord, 42 (6), 531–539.

Skarderud, F., Sommerfeldt, B. (2009). Self-harm and eating disorders. Tidsskr Nor Laegeforen, 129 (9), 877–881.

Stein, K.F., Corte, C. (2007). Identity impairment and the eating disorders: content and organization of the self-concept in women with anorexia nervosa and bulimia nervosa. Eur Eat Disorder Rev, 15 (1), 58–69.

Striegel-Moore, R.H., Seeley, J.R., Lewinsohn, P.M. (2003). Psychosocial adjustment in young adulthood of women who experienced an eating disorder during adolescence. J Am Acad Child Adolesc Psychiatry, 42 (5), 587–593.

Striegel-Moore, R.H., Wilson, G.T., DeBar, L. et al. (2010). Cognitive behavioral guided self-help for the treatment of recurrent binge eating. J Consult Clin Psychol, 78 (3), 312–321.

Strober, M., Freeman, R., Lampert, C. et al. (2000). Controlled family study of anorexia nervosa and bulimia nervosa: evidence of shared liability and transmission of partial syndromes. Am J Psychiatry, 157, 393–401.

Strober, M., Katz, J.L. (1988). Depression in the eating disorders: a review and analysis of descriptive family and biological findings. In D.M. Garner, P.E. Garfinkel (Eds.), Diagnostic issues in anorexia nervosa and bulimia nervosa. New York, NY: Brunner/Mazel, pp. 80–111.

Svirko, E., Hawton, K. (2007). Self-injurious behavior and eating disorders: the extent and nature of the association. Suicide Life Threat Behav, 37 (4), 409–421.

U.S.DHHS (2000). Bodywise handbook (2nd ed.). Washington, DC: Office on Women's Health, U.S. DHHS. Retrieved March 1, 2010 from: http://www.mandometerusa.com/pdf/BodyWise.pdf.

Wagner, A., Wockel, L., Bolte, S. et al. (2008). Mental disorders among relatives of patients with anorexia nervosa and bulimia nervosa. Z Kinder Jugendpsychiatr Psychother, 36 (3), 177–184.

Westerberg, J., Edlund, B., Ghaderi, A. (2008). A 2-year longitudinal study of eating attitudes, BMI, perfectionism, asceticism, and family climate in adolescent girls and their parents. Eat Weight Disord, 13 (2), 64–72.

Whitney, J., Haigh, R., Weinman, J. et al. (2007). Caring for people with eating disorders: factors associated with psychological distress and negative caregiving appraisals in carers of people with eating disorders. Br J Clin Psychol, 46 (Pt 4), 413–428.

Wilson, G.T., Wilfley, D.E., Agras, W.S. et al. (2010). Psychological treatments of binge eating disorder. Arch Gen Psychiatry, 67 (1), 94–101.

Zoletic, E., Durakovic-Belko, E. (2009). Body image distortion perfectionism and eating disorder symptoms in risk group of female ballet dancers and models and in control group of female students. Psychiatr Danub, 21 (3), 302–309.

Chapter 10
Childhood and Adolescent Obesity

Between 10 and 15% of children and teens are overweight. According to the Center for Disease Control, "overweight" is defined as at or above the 95th percentile on the CDC's body mass index (BMI) for age growth charts.

Many factors, often in combination, increase a child or adolescent's risk of becoming overweight and obese. Genetics, unhealthy nutrition, sedentary lifestyle, cognitive factors, family patterns, ethnic and cultural traditions, community conditions, and school factors can increase the risk of obesity and its complications (Mayo Clinic Staff, 2006).

Socioeconomic Status and Demographic Factors

A variety of socioeconomic status (SES) and demographic activity factors have been linked to high rates of sedentary behavior and overweight and obesity. Lower SES groups have the highest rates of obesity and diabetes mellitus (DM) (Drewnowski and Darmon, 2005). The highest rates of obesity occur in populations with the lowest educational attainment and the lowest income (Drewnowski and Specter, 2004).

Lower SES groups may be more likely than higher SES groups to consume energy-dense foods consisting of refined grains, added sugars, and added fat, which are some of the cheapest forms of dietary energy (Drewnowski and Darmon, 2005). There are lower daily food consumptions costs associated with these energy-dense foods, so lower SES groups can save money by having this type of diet. In contrast, higher SES groups are more likely to consume more expensive, nutrient-dense foods, e.g., fresh fruits and vegetables, lean meats, and fish. Laboratory research indicates that energy-dense foods are less able to satiate one's appetite and may lead to overeating and weight gain. Energy-dense food is also less nutritious than nutrient-dense foods.

Increases in the rate of overweight and obesity among children and adolescents in the USA are not linked to any one ethnic, gender, or age group (Crawford et al., 2001). A wide range of environmental factors contribute to the obesity epidemic. Nevertheless, ethnic and cultural conditions influence individual and family food-associated beliefs, attitudes, and behaviors, which can affect the risk of obesity

M.L. Goldstein, S. Morewitz, *Chronic Disorders in Children and Adolescents*,
DOI 10.1007/978-1-4419-9764-7_10, © Springer Science+Business Media, LLC 2011

in children and adolescents (Kumanyika, 2007; GAO Congressional Briefing, 2006, http://www.gao.gov).

Ethnic and cultural influences, along with SES factors, are reflected by the fact that African-American and Hispanic children are at higher risk for overweight than white children (Crawford et al., 2001).

Using data from the National Longitudinal Survey of Youth, Strauss and Pollack (2001) found that overweight increased among African-American, Hispanic, and white children during the period, 1986–1998. By 1998, Hispanics and African-Americans had the largest rates of overweight among Hispanic (21.8%) and African-American children (21.5%), compared to non-Hispanic whites (12.3%). The fastest increases in overweight occurred among children from minority groups and southern states.

Thorpe et al. (2004) assessed racial and ethnic disparities in childhood overweight and obesity in New York City and showed that the highest rates of obesity were in Latino (31%) and African-American children, compared to 15% for white and Asian children.

With regard to Native American and Asian-Americans, few national studies have been conducted on the prevalence of overweight (Crawford et al., 2001). Moreover, studies that aggregate diverse ethnic/cultural populations, such as Asians and Pacific Islanders, into one category do not provide reliable and valid data.

SES and gender factors may influence the prevalence of overweight among certain ethnic and racial groups (Gordon-Larsen et al., 2003; Crawford et al., 2001). Among whites, parents' SES seems to be a protective factor since it is inversely associated with childhood obesity (Crawford et al., 2001). However, higher parental SES is not protective against obesity for African-American and Hispanic children. Parental income and education are not related to childhood obesity in these two minority groups.

Based on a data from the National Longitudinal Study of Adolescent Health, Gordon-Larsen et al. (2003) showed that among white adolescent females, the prevalence of overweight decreased as parental SES increased. In contrast, among African-American adolescent females, the prevalence of overweight remained high and actually increased among African-American adolescent females with higher SES. The African-American/white differences in the prevalence of overweight increased at the highest level of parental SES. However, among white, Hispanic, and Asian adolescent females, differences were reduced at the highest level of SES. In terms of males, differences in overweight prevalence were reduced the most at the average level of parental SES.

Researchers have been exploring the extent to which ethnic and cultural beliefs and behaviors increase these risks of overweight and obesity for minority groups. Using the National Health and Nutrition Examination Survey III, Andersen et al. (1998) found lower levels of vigorous physical activity among non-Hispanic African-American and Mexican-American girls compared to all children in the survey. Eighty percent of the children indicated that they engaged in three or more instances of vigorous physical activity per week. However, only 69% of non-Hispanic African-American girls and 73% of Mexican girls reported such activities.

In the survey, 20% of children engaged in two or more instances of vigorous activity, and girls had a higher rate (26%) than boys (17%).

One investigation discovered that African-American eighth graders differed from white eighth graders in their participation in physical activities and leisure pursuits (Dowda et al., 2004). Based on a sample of 1,124 African-American and 1,068 white eighth graders from 31 middle schools, Dowda et al. (2004) showed that African-American girls had higher rates of participation in social dancing, basketball, watching television, and church attendance than white girls, but lower participation rates in calisthenics, ballet and other dance, jogging or sunning, rollerblading, soccer, softball or baseball, using an exercise machine, swimming, and homework.

Cognitive and Behavioral Factors

A variety of cognitive and behavioral factors have been linked to sedentary lifestyles and overweight and obesity in children and adolescents (Deforche et al., 2006; Robbins et al., 2003; Hesketh et al., 2005; Gordon-Larsen et al., 2003; Kimm et al., 2006; GAO Congressional Briefing, 2006, http://www.gao.gov). Children and adolescents who lack motivation, are self-conscious, and believe that they are not good enough are at increased risk of having reduced levels of physical activity. Some researchers have discovered that adolescents who were obese believed that they faced more barriers to physical activity than non-obese adolescents.

In a study of adolescent girls' who perceived barriers to physical activity, the top barriers were being self-conscious about their looks when they exercise and not being motivated to be active (Robbins et al., 2003).

Another report discovered that African-American girls were more accepting of their bodies than white girls (Mabry et al., 2003). These differences may increase the likelihood that African-American girls gain weight and maintain it, compared to white girls.

Social support can influence children's and adolescents' participation in physical activity. Mabry et al. (2003) showed that adolescents who were physically active indicated that social support was an important factor in motivating them to engage in physical activity.

Some, but not all investigations, have shown that increases in sedentary behavior are linked to a reduction in physical activity (GAO Congressional Briefing, 2006, http://www.gao.gov). Watching television, going to the movies, spending time on the Internet, playing video and computer games, and exposure to other media can increase the risk of obesity in children and adolescents (Powell et al., 2007; Salmon et al., 2005; Fleming-Moran and Thiagarajah, 2005; Stettler et al., 2004; Vandewater et al., 2004; Motl et al., 2006). Young persons who spend their time watching television, going to the movies, playing video games, and surfing the Internet are kept from participating in physical activity and exercise. They may snack while engaging in these sedentary activities. Moreover, they may be exposed to food advertising during some of these sedentary activities.

In a study of adolescents' exposure to food advertising on television, Powell et al. (2007) discovered that 26% of the advertising viewed by adolescents, aged 12–17 years, was food advertisements. With regard to race, African-American adolescents had a 14% greater exposure to food-associated advertising than white adolescents. The researchers found that total exposure to food advertising would be even greater for African-American youth since they spend more time watching television than white youth. The study revealed that fast food was the most frequently watched food product, making up 23% of all food advertisements viewed by adolescents.

Andersen et al. (1998) showed that non-Hispanic African-American children had the highest rates of watching four or more hours of television daily relative to all children in the survey. Those boys and girls who watched four or more hours of television daily had more body fat and a higher BMI than those who watched less than 2 h of television daily.

Some investigations have demonstrated that the children's sedentary behavior, such as video game playing and television watching, is affected by gender and the family's influence on children's television viewing patterns (GAO Congressional Briefing, 2006, http://www.gao.gov; Motl et al., 2006; Salmon et al., 2006).

Participation in physical activities can reduce the amount of time children and adolescents spend in front of the video or television. Using a sample of 4,594 adolescent boys and girls in a 2-year period, Motl et al. (2006) demonstrated that reduced time watching television was related to an increase in the frequency of leisure time physical activity.

Family and Maternal Characteristics

Family and maternal factors have an impact on the physical activity and weight problems of children and adolescents (GAO Congressional Briefing, 2006, http://www.gao.gov; Hesketh et al., 2005; Nichols-English et al., 2006; Davison et al., 2005). Parental and social support can encourage children and adolescents to pursue and maintain physical activity, healthy eating, and control weight problems. Likewise, family environments that promote television viewing increase sedentary patterns and the likelihood of overweight and obesity (Salmon et al., 2005).

Researchers have focused on other family and maternal characteristics to determine the extent to which they influence physical activity and weight problems in children and adolescents (Gibson et al., 2007). Bruch (1973) suggested that obese children were more likely to live in families that had a domineering, overprotective mother; and a father who was weak, not responsive, or supportive. Later investigations indicated that family conflict and disorganization, parental neglect, and families which lacked an interest in social and cultural activities were linked to an increased risk of childhood obesity (Banis et al., 1988; Beck and Terry, 1985; Lissau and Sorensen, 1994).

However, Kinston and Loader (1984) and Mendelson et al. (1995) did not find that obese children were more likely to live in dysfunctional families. Early studies suffered from methodological inadequacies, such as small sample sizes and single measures of family dysfunction (Gibson et al., 2007). In addition, earlier investigations did not formulate any underlying theory to describe the role of family characteristics in causing childhood obesity. About 20–30 years ago, obese children may have come from dysfunctional families. Since childhood obesity is more prevalent than in the past, the condition is not limited to dysfunctional families.

Using cross-sectional data from a population-based prospective study, Gibson et al. (2007) showed that children with an overweight mother and a single mother had an increased chance of being overweight or obese. However, the authors did not find that obesity was linked to negative maternal or family conditions, such as adverse life events, family dysfunction, maternal depression, or poor parenting.

In a study of African-American mothers and their daughters, Nichols-English et al. (2006) found mothers' BMI was positively correlated with their daughters' BMI. The BMI relationship was stronger when the spouse lived in the household. The daughters' BMI was lower and intent to be active was stronger when more individuals lived in the household. The authors also showed that both mothers and daughters believed that physical activity had beneficial outcomes. However, mothers' body fatness, physical activity beliefs and behaviors were not linked with their daughters' physical activity and physical outcome beliefs. Family income increased the relation of mothers' belief in the usefulness of physical activity and daughters' physical activity physical outcome beliefs.

Community Factors

A number of investigations have found that community and neighborhood characteristics can lead to reduced physical activity and increase the risk of overweight and obesity in children and adolescents (Nelson et al., 2006; Braza et al., 2004; Gómez et al., 2004; Gordon-Larsen et al., 2004; GAO Congressional Briefing, 2006, http://www.gao.gov). Using data from the Longitudinal Study of Adolescent Health, Nelson et al. (2006) discovered that adolescents in older suburban communities had a higher level of physical activity than those living in newer communities.

Unsafe communities may inhibit youth from engaging in physical activity. For example, based on a multi-level, longitudinal study of families and communities in Chicago, Molnar et al. (2004) found that lower neighborhood safety and social disorganization predicted less physical activity among children and adolescents.

Other investigations have examined characteristics of the built environment, e.g., land use patterns, the transportation system and design features that affect travel and physical activity and increase the risk of overweight and obesity in children and adolescents (Nelson et al., 2006; Gordon-Larsen et al., 2004; Jago et al., 2005; GAO Congressional Briefing, 2006, http://www.gao.gov). The lack of streetlights and having to cross busy streets reduced children's physical activity, such as walking and biking to school.

The availability of swimming pools and other recreational areas affects levels of physical activity and their risk of overweight and obesity among children and adolescents (Gordon-Larsen et al., 2004; GAO Congressional Briefing, 2006, http://www.gao.gov).

Community areas with low SES and disadvantaged ethnic/racial populations have fewer recreational resources than middle- and upper SES areas, leading to reduced physical activity and greater risk of overweight and obesity in these community areas (Powell et al., 2004; Gordon-Larsen et al., 2004; Janssen et al., 2004; Salmon et al., 2005; GAO Congressional Briefing, 2006, http://www.gao.gov). For example, using a sample of 6,684 students in grades 6 through 10 from 169 schools in Canada, Janssen et al. (2006) discovered that area-level measures (e.g., unemployment rate and percentage of adults with less than a high school education) were inversely related to obesity. Areas with the highest rates of employment and educational attainment had the lowest rates of obesity.

School Factors

School conditions contribute to the problems of sedentary patterns and increased risks of overweight and obesity in children and adolescents (Datar and Sturm, 2004; GAO Congressional Briefing, 2006, http://www.gao.gov). Schools that do not offer healthy foods and beverages and increased opportunities for frequent and intensive physical activity during and after school contribute to sedentary patterns and increase the likelihood of overweight and obesity in these school populations (Institute of Medicine, 2008). School programs that do not attempt to reduce screen time for children and adolescents and do not develop innovative programs for teaching health promotion also inhibit opportunities for physical activity and healthy eating.

School income and racial/ethnic composition of schools may predict ethnic/racial disparity in physical activity among adolescents, which increases the likelihood of overweight and obesity in these school populations (Richmond et al., 2006; GAO Congressional Briefing, 2006, http://www.gao.gov). Based on a cross-sectional sample of 17,007 adolescents from the National Longitudinal Study of Adolescents, Richmond et al. (2006) demonstrated that African-American and Hispanic adolescent girls were more likely to attend lower SES school with overall lower levels of physical activity than white adolescent girls. However, adolescent boys had more similar physical activity levels, with African-American boys having slightly higher physical activity levels.

One of the problems in reducing the overweight and obesity problem is that school-based physical education policies differ widely by state, school district, and school (GAO Congressional Briefing, 2006, http://www.gao.gov).

Being transported to and from school has been associated with increased sedentary behavior. Based on a sample of 219 fifth grade students from eight randomly selected urban and suburban elementary schools, Sirard et al. (2005) demonstrated that walking to school was linked to about 24 additional minutes of moderate-to-vigorous physical activity per day.

Industry and Media

Given the frequency and importance of screen time and television viewing among children and adolescents, it is not surprising that industry and the media impact their rates of physical activity and eating patterns (Institute of Medicine, 2008). The food and beverage industry should develop healthier products and packaging. The food and beverage industry should improve consumer nutrition information to enhance healthy eating. In addition, the media should offer clear and consistent media messages that promote healthy eating.

Complications and Comorbidities

In the past, obesity-related complications during childhood were viewed as fairly rare (Schwarz and Freemark, 2007). However, today, many minor and significant complications may develop from obesity during childhood and adolescence. A majority of these conditions adversely affect the quality of life (QOL) of children and adolescents, and some may lead to lower life expectancy.

The complications and comorbidities of obesity during childhood and adolescence are reflected in the perceived health of obese young persons. A cross-sectional school-based survey of 31,122 adolescents in grades 7–12 revealed that overweight adolescents had a greater likelihood of viewing their health as fair or poor than non-overweight adolescents (Neumark-Sztainer et al., 1997). A study of 182 children and adolescents from community pediatric clinics and a hospital obesity clinic by Pinhas-Hamiel et al. (2006) found that obese children reported having lower physical health compared to children with normal weight.

Wake et al. (2002), using a sample of 2,863 children, ages 5–13 years, from 24 primary schools in Victoria, Australia, showed that parents had a greater likelihood of reporting worse health and well-being for their obese and overweight children, especially obese boys. The parents' concern about their children's weight was strongly linked to their children's actual BMI.

The extent of impairment in obese children's QOL may vary depending on whether the parents or the children are making the assessment. Based on a clinical sample of 126 obese children and 71 controls, Hughes et al. (2007) discovered that parent-proxy's assessment of their obese children's health-related quality of life (HRQOL) was low for all domains. The parent-proxy's evaluations were lower than the children's self-report assessments for all domains except physical health and school functioning. Pinhas-Hamiel et al. (2006) also found that parents of obese children viewed their child's HRQOL was worse than the children's evaluation.

If a child or adolescent has any obesity-related complications and comorbidities, they should be used to motivate them to change their behaviors and lifestyle (Ponder and Anderson, 2007).

Glucose Tolerance

As body fat is accumulated, especially in a visceral distribution, sensitivity to insulin is reduced in skeletal muscle, liver tissue, and adipose tissue. As a result, obese children and adolescents are at increased risk of developing problems related to glucose tolerance and hypertriglyceridemia (Schwarz and Freemark, 2007). They face the possibility of acquiring hyperinsulinemia (Ponder and Anderson, 2007). Obesity during childhood and adolescence increases the risk of pre- and type 2 DM (Ponder and Anderson, 2007). The increasing prevalence of obesity among children and adolescents and associated insulin resistance seem to account for the increasing incidence of type 2 DM during adolescence, particular among minority teenagers (Schwarz and Freemark, 2007).

Clinicians may be concerned about an underlying insulin-resistant state among these at-risk patients and may order matching glucose and insulin levels during an oral glucose tolerance test (OGTT) or a random or fasting sample (Ponder and Anderson, 2007). However, confusion may occur when the patient's insulin responses are abnormal while the glucose level is normal. A referral to a pediatric endocrinologist may be helpful in interpreting OGTT measurements in children.

Normal blood glucose or normoglycemia along with hyperinsulinemia indicate that it is necessary to follow up children for type 2 DM on a periodic basis. These findings indicate that the children are at risk for type 2 DM, and these results may be used by health providers to encourage children and their families to change their behaviors and lifestyle. The American Diabetes Association (2007) recommends that children at risk for type 2 DM should start being tested for the condition at the age of 10 years or at puberty onset. The preferred measurement is fasting plasma glucose and it should be obtained every 2 years.

Obese children and adolescents face an increased risk of cardiometabolic complications (e.g., systolic and diastolic hypertension, low HDL cholesterol, and hypertriglyceridemia); orthopedic problems, such as genu valgum and slipped capital femoral epiphysis; pulmonary conditions (e.g., asthma and obstructive sleep apnea); and liver and gallbladder disease, such as fatty liver, hepatic steatosis, and cholecystitis (Schwarz and Freemark, 2007). They are at increased risk for dermatological conditions, including acanthosis nigricans, and reproductive health conditions, such as polycystic ovary syndrome and earlier menarche. Obese boys face the possibility of acquiring pseudo-micropenis.

Obesity and Psychosocial Functioning and Development

Psychosocial factors can be a cause and/or consequence of obesity for children and adolescents. Obese children and adolescents, like their adult counterparts, face widespread societal prejudice and discrimination which can take the form of bullying and teasing (Schwarz and Freemark, 2007). In other instances, overweight and obese persons may be left out of peer groups and activities. Some young people eat too much as a way to deal with these problems or to cope with stress, boredom, and other negative emotions (Mayo Clinic Staff, 2006). Likewise, the parents of these individuals may have similar coping patterns.

Obesity during childhood and adolescence is linked to emotional and psychosocial problems, including low self-esteem, feelings of hopelessness, depression, suicidal behaviors, anxiety, teasing and bullying, social isolation, behavior and learning problems, and eating disorders (Wake et al., 2002; Williams et al., 2005; Falkner et al., 2001; Schwarz and Freemark, 2007).

The relationship between self-esteem and obesity is complex. French et al. (1995) suggest that self-esteem is not consistently associated with obesity. The relationship between self-esteem and obesity may be global or it may be related to a child's physical appearance. The association between self-esteem and obesity may be influenced by a person's age, gender, race, or ethnicity.

In their review, French et al. (1995) found that 13 of 25 cross-sectional studies demonstrated that obese children and adolescents had lower self-esteem. In 5 of 6 cross-sectional investigations that included a body esteem measure, obese children and adolescents had lower body esteem relative to those with normal weight. Inconsistent findings were obtained in two prospective investigations that analyzed initial self-esteem and later obesity. In 6 of 8 obesity treatment evaluations, interventions appeared to improve the participants' self-esteem. However, it is not evident whether the enhanced self-esteem is due to the weight loss. Studies of self-esteem and obesity have been flawed because of small and select samples and inadequate control groups.

Investigations have found that obese children and adolescents experience a range of emotional and physical health problems. A study of 2,863 children, ages 5–13 years, in Victoria, Australia, revealed that obese boys were at increased risk of low self-esteem, poor mental health, and other physical and mental health problems (Wake et al., 2002). Troubled obese teenagers have reported that they have attempted suicide (Falkner et al., 2001).

Based on population-based sample of public school students in the 7th, 9th, and 11th grades, Falkner et al. (2001) showed that obese female adolescents had a greater likelihood of reporting serious emotional problems in the last year, feeling hopeless, and making a suicide attempt than average weight female adolescents. Obese boys were more likely than average weight boys to indicate that they had serious problems in the last year.

Compared to normal weight children and adolescents, obese youth tend to suffer higher levels of anxiety and have worse social skills and relations (Pearce et al.,

2002; Falkner et al., 2001). Obese young persons may respond to these difficulties by acting out and disrupting classes. Other obese youth may cope with these problems by withdrawing socially.

Researchers have evaluated different aspects of the relationships of obese children and adolescents relative to average weight peers (Griffiths et al., 2006; Pearce et al., 2002; Janssen et al., 2004). As noted above, obese children and adolescents can be both victims of different forms of teasing and bullying and perpetrators of bullying. These behaviors can have adverse psychosocial effects and may impede the psychosocial development of overweight and obese young people.

Investigators are evaluating the link between overweight and obesity and various types of bullying behaviors. Overweight and obese children and adolescents can experience relational victimization, e.g., withdrawing friendship or telling lies and rumors, and overt victimization, e.g., calling names, teasing, physical aggression, and sexual harassment (Falkner et al., 2001; Griffiths et al., 2006; Janssen et al., 2004; Pearce et al., 2002).

Because of weight status, obese young people may not want to socialize with their friends (Falkner et al., 2001). Moreover, they may feel that their friends do not really care about them. Based on a population-based sample of 4,742 male and 5,201 female public school students in grades 7, 9, and 11, Falkner et al. (2001) showed that obese boys were less likely to spend time with their friends in the previous week than boys with normal weight. Obese boys also had a greater likelihood of believing that their friends do not care about them. Obese girls also were less likely to hang out with their friends than their normal weight peers.

Using a representative sample of 5,749 Canadian boys and girls, ages 11–16 years, Janssen et al. (2004) discovered that BMI was related to different types of peer victimization in certain age and gender groups. Except for 15- to 16-year-old boys, overweight and obese young persons had a greater likelihood of being victimized than normal weight peers. Compared to normal weight young people, overweight and obese youth were more likely to experience both relational and overt forms of victimization, but not sexual harassment.

The researchers analyzed bullying perpetrator and found no association between BMI and being a bully perpetrator among 11- to 14-year olds, independent of gender (Janssen et al., 2004). However, they discovered that overweight and obese boys and girls, ages 15–16 years, had a greater likelihood of engaging in bullying behaviors than normal weight peers. Only overweight and obese boys were more likely to perpetrate relational types of bullying, while both boys and girls were more likely to engage in overt forms of bullying but not sexual harassment.

Investigators have evaluated possible gender differences in bullying victimization and perpetration among obese youth. In a study of 416 students in grades 9 through 12, Pearce et al. (2002) found that obese boys experienced more overt victimization, while obese girls were exposed to more relational victimization than average weight peers.

Based on a prospective cohort study of boys and girls at age 7.5 years, Griffiths et al. (2006) discovered that obese boys were 1.66 times more likely to engage in overt bullying and 1.54 times more likely to be overt victims of bullying. Obese girls were 1.53 times more likely to be overt victims of bullying. The authors suggest that because obese pre-adolescent vary from normal appearance, they have a greater chance of being the victims of bullying than their normal weight peers. Moreover, because of their physical prowess, obese pre-adolescent boys have a greater chance of being bullies than normal weight pre-adolescent boys.

Researchers have also analyzed dating patterns among obese and non-obese adolescents. In their study, Pearce et al. (2002) reported that obese female adolescents had a lower probability of dating than average weight peers. In addition, both obese girls and boys expressed more dissatisfaction with their dating situation than normal weight peers.

Young people involved in bullying as a victim and/or bully can develop physical health problems (Srabstein et al., 2006). Based on the USA data from the 1998 World Health Organization Health Behavior in School-aged Children Survey, Srabstein et al. (2006) evaluated morbidities related to bullying involvement in school-age children in grades 6 through 10. The researchers found that adolescents who reported experiencing one or more frequent physical symptoms (e.g., headaches, stomachaches, backaches, dizziness) or emotional symptoms (e.g., irritability, feeling nervous, and feeling low) several times weekly had a greater likelihood of being involved in bullying activities as a victim and/or as a bully relative to students who did not suffer these symptoms.

Teasing and bullying by peers and weight concerns can lead to social withdrawal and low self-esteem, which can produce overwhelming feelings of hopelessness. Those overweight and obese young people who lose hope that the quality of their lives will improve are at risk of suffering depression. Depressed children and adolescents may lose interest in normal activities. They may sleep more than normal or cry frequently. However, some depressed young people may cover up their depression and instead exhibit a flat affect. In any event, as in adults, depressive symptoms in children are a major concern. If parents suspect that their child is depressed, they should talk to her or him and express their concerns with her or his teacher and physician.

Among children and adolescents seen in obesity clinics, depression is prevalent (Ponder and Anderson, 2007). Different types of depression can limit the success of weight management interventions. In addition, children who are prescribed atypical anti-psychotics, such as olanzapine, risperidone, quetiapine, and clozapine, may be at increased risk of developing insulin resistance and type 2 DM.

Children and adolescents treated at obesity clinics often have eating disorders (EDs). Research has revealed that disordered eating starts around the age of 8 years, when children have or respond to complaints about body size or shape (U.S. DHHS, 2000). Youth of varying ethnic and cultural backgrounds are influenced by a dominant culture's emphasis on achieving a perfect body. As their bodies are developing, young people may be teased about their body size or shape. Some may be the victims of discrimination and harassment. As a result, they may feel shame, dissatisfaction, embarrassment, or even hatred toward their growing bodies.

In one study, the Harvard Eating Disorders Center discovered that among children, ages 8–10 years, about half of the girls and one-third of the boys were not happy with their body size (HEDC, 1999; Collins, 1991). A majority of these girls desired to be thinner. In contrast, approximately half of the discontented boys wanted to be heavier and/or more muscular.

Often people diagnosed with anorexia nervosa (AN) and bulimia nervosa (BN) have a memory of being teased about their body size or shape or remember that their difficulties started when they began to diet (U.S. DHHS, 2000). Based on a prospective investigation of a diverse sample of 2,516 adolescents, Haines et al. (2006) reported that about 25% of the respondents indicated that they had been teased about their weight at a minimum of a few times a year. Male adolescents who were teased about their weight were more likely to start binge eating with loss of control and unhealthy weight control activities 5 years later than their peers who were not teased. Five years later, girls who were teased about their weight were more likely to diet frequently than their peers who were not teased.

Many individuals remember being dissatisfied with their body and fearing being fat even though they were within the normal range. Although only a small proportion of persons who diet or are dissatisfied with body suffer EDs, the onset of these conditions frequently follow restrictive dieting, a type of disordered eating among young people.

Binge eating (BE) is an affliction affecting millions of people (NIDDK, 2004). Individuals with this condition have many episodes of eating a large amount of food and often feel that they cannot control their eating. BE can involves eating very quickly, eating until feeling too full, eating large amounts of food when not hungry, and eating alone because the individuals are embarrassed by how much they are eating (U.S. DHHS, 2000). Persons with this condition often suffer depression, guilt, or disgust following the BE.

BE may be the most prevalent ED; the condition afflicts approximately 2% of all US adults and approximately 10–15% of persons with mild obesity (NIDDK, 2004; U.S. DHHS, 2000). Most of these persons have a history of repeated dieting on their own or through weight loss programs and feel desperate about their problems in controlling their eating (U.S. DHHS, 2000).

BE, like other EDs, starts in childhood. Children and adolescents concerned about losing weight may initiate extreme weight control behaviors, such as taking diet medications, laxatives or diuretics, or vomiting. BE and extreme weight control behaviors may be prevalent among overweight young people. Using a cross-sectional school-based survey of 31,122 adolescents in grades 7–12, Neumark-Sztainer et al. (1997) found that overweight adolescents had a greater likelihood of reporting weight-related issues and engaging in long-term dieting and BE than non-overweight adolescents.

BE and extreme weight control methods may be especially prevalent among adolescent girls. Neumark-Sztainer et al. (2002), based on a sample of 4,746 adolescents, showed that a significant percentage of overweight teenagers, especially adolescent girls, engaged in unhealthy weight control behaviors and BE. Eighteen percent of very overweight adolescents girls reported participating in extreme weight control activities, compared to 6% of the very overweight adolescent boys.

Among adolescents, the use of unhealthy weight control methods may increase the risk of BE with feelings of loss of control and extreme weight control behaviors. Using a population-based 5-year longitudinal study of 2,516 adolescents, Neumark-Sztainer et al. (2006) found that adolescents who used unhealthy weight control methods were at increased risk of BE with loss of control and engaging in extreme weight control behaviors 5 years later. Adolescents who used unhealthy weight control behaviors were more likely to have increased their BMI by approximately one unit more and were about three times more likely to be overweight 5 years later than those not employing any weight control methods.

Therefore, clinicians should screen overweight and obese children for depression, EDs, unhealthy and extreme weight control behaviors, and other psychosocial problems (Ponder and Anderson, 2007; U.S. DHHS, 2000). Management of these problems can facilitate significant lifestyle changes. Practitioners should monitor weight during treatment using atypical antipsychotics.

School Performance and Developmental Functioning

Stress, anxiety, bullying, teasing, and social ostracizing related to obesity can disrupt learning and school performance. School-related performance problems can lead to a vicious cycle in which increasing anxiety triggers declining school achievement.

Researchers are beginning to evaluate the extent to which obese children and adolescents encounter more difficulties in achieving success in school and have more negative attitudes toward school. Falkner et al. (2001), using a population-based sample of public school students in the 7th, 9th, and 11th grades, discovered that obese female adolescents had a greater likelihood of being held back a grade and considering themselves poor students than average weight female adolescents. Obese boys in the sample were more likely to consider themselves as poor students and expect to drop out of school relative to normal weight boys. As noted earlier, obese girls and boys in the study reported more emotional difficulties compared to average weight peers.

Some investigations, using health-related quality of life (HRQOL) measures, have found that obese children and adolescents have lower school functioning relative to average weight children and adolescents (Hughes et al., 2007). Pinhas-Hamiel et al. (2006) showed that severely obese, but not moderately obese, children and adolescents had lower school functioning relative to normal weight children. In contrast, Williams et al. (2005), using a community-based sample, did not find a link between a child's body weight and school functioning. The authors note that the impact of child obesity on QOL is significant but less than in clinical samples.

Obesity may be linked to problems in developmental functioning in pre-school children. Based on nine consecutive cohorts of 9,415 male and female children, ages 4.4–8.6 years, in the Lower Bavaria area of Germany, Mond et al. (2007) discovered that obese male children had a higher rate of impairment in gross motor skills than male children with normal weight. Female children were more likely to be impaired in their ability to focus attention than female children with average weight.

Long-Term Complications

Obese children and adolescents have an increased probability of being obese as an adult, with its related long-term complications (Schwarz and Freemark, 2007). Adolescent males with moderate to severe obesity may have the highest risks for long-term health problems. However, obesity during infancy and early childhood is not as clearly linked to long-term complications. With increased age at the onset of obesity, individuals are more likely to be obese during adulthood. About 26–41% of pre-school children with obesity are obese as adults, while 42–63% of school-aged children are obese during adulthood. Moreover, individuals who are severely obese during childhood have a greater chance of being obese as adults. At age 18 years, persons with a BMI at or above the 95th percentile have a 66–78% risk of being overweight at age 35 years.

The epidemic of type 2 DM among obese children and adolescents will likely exacerbate the rise of type 2 DM and cardiovascular disease in early adulthood and produce a variety of diabetic complications in adulthood and reduced life expectancy (Schwarz and Freemark, 2007; James et al., 2004). Although limited, epidemiological studies reveal that adolescent obesity is linked to increased morbidity and mortality in adulthood.

One of the major long-term complications of obesity during childhood and adolescence is cardiovascular disease (Schwarz and Freemark, 2007). Low levels of high-density lipoprotein (HDL), which occur because of genetic factors and a lack of physical activity, may contribute to early coronary artery disease (CAD) among obese adults. Research has shown that males, but not females, who were obese during adolescence, have an increased risk of mortality from all causes and from CAD.

In terms of morbidity, follow-up data from the Harvard Growth Study revealed that among both men and women who were overweight (BMI greater than 75th percentile) during adolescence were at increased risk of suffering CAD- and atherosclerosis-related morbidity as adults. Men who were obese as teenagers had a greater probability of developing gout and colorectal cancer, while women who were obese during adolescence had an increased risk of developing arthritis. Many of these health problems seem to be independent of a person's weight during adulthood, which points to a direct link between adolescent obesity and morbidity and mortality during adulthood.

Obesity during childhood and adolescence is also associated with psychosocial difficulties in adulthood (Schwarz and Freemark, 2007). In a study of adolescents and young adults who were followed for 7 years, overweight females had completed fewer years of schools, were less likely to be married, and were poorer relative to normal weight females. Overweight males were less likely to be married compared to normal weight males.

Diagnosis, Treatment, and Rehabilitation Strategies

The child and the family are at the center of any effective prevention and treatment intervention (Ponder and Anderson, 2007). The behaviors of the child and his or her family ultimately will lead to the success or failure of the prevention and treatment strategies. It is necessary to determine who will be most amendable to lifestyle and behavior interventions. In considering who will benefit from these interventions it is important to realize that funding for weight loss therapy may be limited. Clinicians have limited cost reimbursement for obesity care and interventions. Moreover, there are various costs related to weight loss therapy, including the costs of health-care visits and expenses associated with food choices, exercise equipment, and sportswear.

In addition, families face a number of barriers in participating in obesity interventions. Family members may not be able to get off work to go to additional child health-care visits. The children must attend school and do not have time for health-care assessments. The families also may be geographically far away from their health-care providers and this limits their access to obesity interventions. Therefore, it is best to include obesity assessment in the health maintenance visits.

Treatment strategies should emphasize weight control while reducing BMI in a safe and effective manner. This weight control approach will help to prevent the long-term complications of obesity (Schwarz and Freemark, 2007). The first priority is managing any acute or chronic complications associated with obesity. In addition, it may be necessary to obtain a psychiatric consultation to treat youth who have EDs or substantial depressive symptoms. Clinicians should develop a treatment plan that stresses long-term nutrition and physical activity, a supportive family environment without major swings in body weight. An interdisciplinary team approach involving nurses, nutritionists, counselors, and exercise specialists can be very helpful. Positive behavioral change should be rewarded while a punishment-oriented approach should be avoided. In certain instances, family therapy can be very effective.

In regard to weight loss goals, adults who lose 5–20% of their total body weight can minimize many of the complications related to obesity (Schwarz and Freemark, 2007). However, for youth it is not known whether moderate weight loss or reductions in BMI can minimize obesity-related complications in children and adolescents or the long-term complications of obesity later in life. Instead of promoting a quick return to ideal body weight, counseling and treatment should stress realistic goals, consisting of gradual reductions in body fat and BMI and the maintenance of weight loss. This is especially desirable since both obese youth and adults have great problems in reducing their BMI. Youth who reduce their body weight will have equivalent losses in the expenditure of energy. As a consequence, obese children and adolescents who maintain a lower body weight will require less energy intake than those who have never been obese.

Smoking tobacco curbs appetite, and to inhibit or minimize weight gain, some youth and a large number of adults will smoke tobacco (Schwarz and Freemark, 2007). Smoking should be discouraged in all populations since the adverse effects of smoking clearly outweigh any benefits related to weight control. For obese children and adolescents who stop smoking, strategies should be followed to prevent weight gain.

Obese youth should be encouraged to participate in exercise and physical activity and follow a safe and effective diet (Schwarz and Freemark, 2007). Parents, teachers, and clinicians should encourage young people to engage in exercise and vigorous physical activity as a lifetime lifestyle. The youth should be discouraged from devoting too much time to sedentary activities, especially television, videos, and computer games. It is important to note that walking for 20–30 min daily can help achieve weight control. Through expenditure of energy, exercise inhibits weight gain. Exercise enhances cardiovascular functioning, reduces body fat and total cholesterol levels, increases lean body mass and HDL levels, and improves psychosocial functioning.

For children and adolescents, clinical trials have revealed that lifestyle-related exercise and physical activity programs, in conjunction with diet, are effective in achieving long-term weight control (Schwarz and Freemark, 2007). In children and adolescents with mild or moderate obesity, weight gain can be limited with an energy-restricted balanced diet, along with family education, family behavior modification, and exercise. The most effective programs are those that alter the eating patterns of families. Young people who eat large amounts of high fat and packaged fast food, including pizza, French fries, and crackers should reduce their intake of total and saturated fat.

For US youth, the typical diet consists of about 35% fat (Schwarz and Freemark, 2007). The World Health Organization recommends lowering fat intake to 30% of total energy consumed. However, studies indicate that a diet, which is reduced in fat but is without other restrictions, does not lead to weight loss in obese persons. Young persons with prior obesity, particularly those whose families are susceptible to obesity, may benefit from a reduced fat diet to achieve primary secondary prevention of weight gain.

School-Based Interventions

Investigations have shown that school-based nutrition and physical activity interventions can improve the knowledge, attitudes, and behaviors of children and adolescents. Francis et al. (2010) evaluated the impact of a school-based intervention on dietary intakes and physical activity among 579 primary school children in Trinidad and Tobago. The researchers found that the intervention resulted in a significant decrease in the children's intake of fried foods; snack foods high in fat, sugar, and salt; sodas and an increase in knowledge scores. These findings were independent of age, gender, BMI, ethnicity. However, the intervention did not produce changes in the children's physical activity.

Using a 2-year, school-based intervention in Chile, involving 1759 children from three schools and 671 children from a control school, Kain et al. (2009) discovered that obesity was reduced only in boys during the first year of the study.

Based on a nutrition intervention for 191 students, aged 12–13 years, in an urban area of Athens, Greece, Mihas et al. (2010) showed that 12 months after the intervention, students in the nutrition program had lower BMI, daily energy intake, and total fat intake.

Other investigations have focused on the impact of school-based physical activity programs on fitness and adiposity in children and adolescents. In a cluster randomized controlled trial in Switzerland, Kriemler et al. (2010) compared 297 children who participated in three existing physical education lessons per week and two additional lessons per week, daily short activity breaks, and physical activity homework with 205 children and parents in a control group. They demonstrated that children in the intervention had improved physical activity and fitness and lower adiposity than children in the control group.

Researchers also have assessed the impact of after-school physical activity on preventing obesity in children. Martinez Vizcaino et al. (2008) assessed the effects of three 90-min sessions of recreational, non-competitive physical activity among children in Spain, using a cluster-randomized controlled trial with 10 intervention and 10 control schools. Participation in the after-school program recreational physical activity resulted in children having lower adiposity, increased apo A-I, and reduced apo B.

Peer-Based Approaches

Because peers can be especially important to children and adolescents, researchers have begun to develop peer-based weight control programs. Using a sample of 76 adolescents, aged 13–16 years, Jelalian et al. (2006) compared the impact of peer-related activities plus cognitive-behavioral therapy (CBT) with that of a program that involved CBT plus aerobic exercise. Adolescents in the combined peer activities and CBT intervention maintained greater weight loss (10 pounds) than those in the CBT plus aerobic exercise intervention 10 months after being randomized to either treatment (35% vs. 12%). At the end of the intervention, older adolescents in the peer activities plus CBT intervention had more than four times the weight loss of older adolescents randomized to the CBT and aerobic exercise treatment.

Family–Child Interventions

Parent–child treatments have been shown to be effective in treating childhood obesity. Based on a sample of 56 obese children and their families randomized to 16 sessions of CBT for only parents or for a combined treatment of children and their parents, Munsch et al. (2008) demonstrated that both interventions significantly reduced the children's percent overweight equally at 6-month follow-up. In addition, both treatments had similar results in reducing the children's behavioral problems, anxiety, and depression.

Family-based therapies may be helpful in treating severe obesity in children and adolescents. Kalarchian et al. (2009) tested the effectiveness of a family-based weight control approach using a sample of 192 children, aged 8–12 years, and their families. Compared to children in the usual care intervention, children who participated in the family-based weight control treatment had small significant improvements in medical outcomes 6 and 12 months after the start of the study. Children in the family-based weight control therapy who participated in 75% or more of the treatment sessions maintained reductions in child percent overweight after 18 months after the start of the trial.

Clinic-Based and Inpatient Treatment

Intensive interventions may be warranted for children with severe obesity (Schwarz and Freemark, 2007). Anecdotal data have revealed that these young people may attempt suicide and develop manic depression or other mental disorders that necessitate hospital admission or medications on a long-term basis. Researchers are not sure whether these problems occur before, cause or are a consequence of the obesity, or its therapy. As with adults, young people who participate in obesity therapy intervention programs are at substantial risk of developing severe psychosocial problems.

Therapy for psychosocial problems may worsen weight control efforts since many types of antidepressants, especially tricyclics, increase appetite and promote weight gain (Schwarz and Freemark, 2007). Obese children and adolescents should be given the opportunity for psychosocial support services. These youth should be referred for psychosocial or psychiatric assessment and intervention if evidence of severe problems or impairment is detected. Effective interventions with these troubled young people must actively involve all family members. Family therapy can be particularly helpful in instances in which the young person has resisted other treatments and in cases in which the patient's parents are obese.

A low-protein, very controlled energy diet, in conjunction with behavior modification and vigorous exercise, can help obese young people rapidly lose weight in the outpatient or inpatient context (Schwarz and Freemark, 2007). An investigation of 73 youth, ages 7–17 years, showed that this intervention reduced the percent overweight, total body fat, BMI, total and low-density lipoprotein cholesterol, triglycerides, and fasting serum insulin, but did not alter the percent of fat-free body mass. Researchers have difficulty in determining the impact of this type of diet on weight loss and control in obese youth since the intervention combined diet with behavior modification and vigorous exercise. Other studies have the same problem in determining the independent effects of diet alone in achieving weight loss and control.

A major difficulty with very controlled energy diet is that many people stop following the diet (Schwarz and Freemark, 2007). This diet has been linked to major complications, including loss of lean weight, gallstones, cardiac arrhythmias, and sudden death. In addition, research has found that after following a very controlled energy diet, individuals regain their weight, with excess weight occurring as a higher percentage of their body fat than before beginning this type of diet. Such weight cycling in adults has triggered concerns about its long-term cardiovascular hazards. However, it is unknown whether severe or cyclical weight changes during childhood and adolescence have potential risks.

Moreover, there is little information about the long-term impact of very controlled diets on growth and development, reproduction, and musculoskeletal formation in adolescents (Schwarz and Freemark, 2007). Likewise, the effects of very controlled diets on intermediary metabolism are not clear. Because of the above problems, a very controlled energy diet is not recommended for most youth.

Some investigators have assessed the effectiveness of clinic-based weight control interventions. Based on a sample of 204 children, aged 7–12 years, from a university-based weight control clinic, Wilfley et al. (2007) evaluated the effectiveness of clinic-based weight maintenance treatments. Weight maintenance interventions included behavioral skills maintenance, social facilitation maintenance, or a control group. The authors discovered that children in the weight maintenance treatments maintained weight better in the short-term than those in the control group. Children with fewer social problems at baseline who were in the social facilitiation maintenance had the best results compared to those in the control group.

Surgery

Bariatric surgery has been used in some adolescents. In most surgical centers, patient are 15 years and older with a BMI of greater than 40 or weight more than 100% of ideal body weight (Schwarz and Freemark, 2007). Gastric restriction is involved in most of these bariatric surgical procedures. A pouch of 15- to 30 mL capacity is constructed in the vertical-banded gastroplasty (VBG). This technique substantially limits the amount of food that can be consumed at any time.

In contrast to the VBG, the gastric bypass involves having a larger pouch that empties into the jejunum (Schwarz and Freemark, 2007). In this procedure, nutrients bypass the duodenum and a majority of the stomach. This technique frequently causes a dumping syndrome. The procedure produces substantial weight loss, reduces obesity-related complications, and increases life expectancy. However, 1% mortality occurs among adults, and surgical complications, including encephalopathy, nephrolithiasis, cholelithiasis, protein-losing enteropathy, and other nutritional problems, can develop.

VBG has been replaced by the laparoscopic placement of an adjustable gastric ban (LAGB) since the latter technique is safer and reversible (Schwarz and Freemark, 2007). In the LAGB, a collar with an internal saline-filled balloon is placed around the upper stomach, 1–2 cm below the esophagogastric junction. This technique produces a 30 mL upper gastric pouch which can be altered with small saline injections into a subcutaneous port connected to the balloon. The LAGB has been shown to yield better outcomes with fewer complications than VBG. Given its reversibility, LABG is considered a good alternative therapy for adolescents.

However, any surgical procedure should only be used for adolescents who face the most serious complications from obesity.

Medications

Sibutramine (Meridia), a selective serotonin norepinephrine reuptake inhibitor, and a pancreatic lipase inhibitor, orlistat (Alli, Xenical), are drugs approved for the long-term management of obesity in adults (Schwarz and Freemark, 2007). Sibutramine is classified as an anorectic drug, whereas orlistat induces lipid maldigestion. Long-term research has demonstrated that both of these drugs produce weight loss. However, Sibutramine has been found to be effective only when combined with a safe diet and exercise regimen.

These medications have only a modest impact on total body weight and individual responses to drug treatment vary widely. Obese adults who take these drugs lose only 2–10 kg of weight losses on a long-term basis (Schwarz and Freemark, 2007). Within the first 6 months of treatment is the time in which a majority of the weight loss is attained. This period is followed by the stabilizing of weight or by a slight weight increase. Patients who terminate drug treatment usually experience rebound weight gain and lose their advantage over patients in a placebo group unless they make substantial changes in their lifestyle.

All of the obesity medications have major side effects that can result in limited use (Schwarz and Freemark, 2007). For example, nausea, bloating, and discomfort from steatorrhea frequently occur when taking orlistat. Dry mouth, insomnia, nervousness, diaphoresis, hypertension, nausea, and constipation are side effects of sibutramine. Within 2 weeks of continuous therapy, patients develop tolerance to a majority of the side effects.

Research has been underway to assess the effectiveness of medications in achieving weight loss in obese adolescents (Schwarz and Freemark, 2007). Dunican et al. (2007), in a randomized trial, showed that orlistat stabilized weight and reduced body fat in obese adolescents, while patients receiving a placebo experienced weight gain. However, Bray and Ryan (2007) did not find any beneficial effects from using orlistat. In a 12-month, randomized trial of sibutramine, Daniels et al. (2007) noted a significant drug-related drop in BMI without any adverse effects on cardiovascular status.

Despite these encouraging results, these medications are not routinely indicated for preventing or treating obese children or adolescents (Schwarz and Freemark, 2007). Until carefully conducted randomized controlled trials are undertaken to assess drug safety and efficacy, these medications should not be used for prepubertal children. For post-pubertal adolescents, anorectic agents may be used only after vigorous behavior modification, diet, and family support have failed. All post-pubertal adolescents treated with anorectic drugs should also participate in nutritional and family treatment and should participate in a regimen of exercise and physical activity.

A variety of consultations should be considered in managing obese children and adolescents. Consultations in nutrition, exercise physiology, psychosocial assessment and management, sleep medicine, orthopedics, and gastroenterology may be needed (Schwarz and Freemark, 2007).

Coping Strategies

Coping, locus of control and problem-solving strategies in young people may affect the extent to which they can achieve weight loss and overall improved psychosocial functioning and health. Coping skills can help children and adolescents deal with the stigma of being overweight. Puhl and Brownell (2003) note that overweight and obese individuals can cope with weight stigma in different ways. They may try to change the stigmatizing condition by losing weight. Another coping technique is for the persons to take pride in their condition and participate in social, political, and legal action to fight discrimination.

Moreover, coping mechanisms can help young people achieve attitudinal and behavioral modification goals (e.g., better react to being exposed to food stimuli, improve responses to hunger, and enhance one's ability to respond to social pressure to eat unhealthy food and eat excessively). In addition, enhancing the coping, locus of control, and problem-solving strategies of the parents of overweight and obese children and adolescents also may be effective in achieving desired weight loss and behavioral change goals for the family. Social buffers and coping processes may limit the adverse psychological impact of obesity bias (Rukavina and Li, 2008).

References

American Diabetes Association (2007). Standards of medical care in diabetes – 2007. Diab Care, 30 (Suppl. 1), S4–S41.

Andersen, R.E., Crespo, C.J., Bartlett, S.J., et al. (1998). Relationship of physical activity and television watching with body weight and level of fatness among children: results from the Third National Health and Nutrition Examination Survey. J Am Med Assoc, 279 (12), 938–942.

Banis, H.T., Varni, J.W., Wallander, J.L., et al. (1988). Psychological and social adjustment of obese children and their families. Child Care Health Dev, 14, 157–173.

Beck, S., Terry, K.A. (1985). A comparison of obese and normal-weight families' psychological consequences. Am J Fam Ther, 13, 55–59.

Bray, G.A., Ryan, D.H. (2007). Drug treatment of the overweight patient. Gastroenterology, 132, 2239–2252.

Braza, M., Shoemaker, W., Seeley, A. (2004, November–December). Neighborhood design and rates of walking and biking to elementary school in 34 California communities. Am J Health Promot, 19 (2), 128–136.

Bruch, H. (1973). Eating disorders: obesity, anorexia nervosa, and the person within. New York, NY: Basic Books.

Collins, M.E. (1991). Body figure perceptions and preferences among preadolescent children. Int J Eating Disord, 10 (2), 199–208.

Crawford, P.B., Story, M., Wang, M.C., et al. (2001). Ethnic issues in the epidemiology of childhood obesity. Pediatr Clin North Am, 48 (4), 855–878.

Daniels, S.R., Long, B., Crow, S., et al. (2007). Cardiovascular effects of sibutramine in the treatment of obese adolescents: results of a randomized, double-blind, placebo-controlled study. Pediatrics, 120 (1), e147–e157.

Datar, A., Sturm, R. (2004, September). Physical education in elementary school and body mass index: evidence from the early childhood longitudinal study. Am J Public Health, 94 (9), 1501–1506.

Davison, K.K., Francis, L.A., Birch, L.L. (2005, October). Links between parents' and girls' television viewing behaviors: a longitudinal examination. J Pediatr, 147 (4), 436–442.

Deforche, B.I., De Bourdeaudhuij, I.M., Tanghe, A.P. (2006, May). Attitude toward physical activity in normal-weight, overweight and obese adolescents. J Adolesc Health, 38 (5), 560–568.

Dowda, M., Pate, R.R., Felton, G.M., et al. (2004, December). Physical activities and sedentary pursuits in African American and Caucasian girls. Res Q Exerc Sport, 75 (4), 352–360.

Drewnowski, A., Darmon, N. (2005, April). Food choices and diet costs: an economic analysis. J Nutr, 135 (4), 900–904.

Drewnowski, A., Specter, S.E. (2004, January). Poverty and obesity: the role of energy density and energy costs. Am J Clin Nutr, 79 (1), 6–16.

Dunican, K.C., Desilets, A.R., Montalbano, J.K. (2007). Pharmacotherapeutic options for overweight adolescents. Ann Pharmacother, 41 (9), 1445–1455.

Falkner, N.H., Neumark-Sztainer, D., Story, M., et al. (2001). Social, educational, and psychological correlates of weight status in adolescents. Obes Res, 9 (1), 32–42.

Fleming-Moran, M., Thiagarajah, K. (2005). Behavioral interventions and the role of television in the growing epidemic of adolescent obesity—data from the 2001 Youth Risk Behavioral Survey. Methods Inf Med, 44 (2), 303–309.

Francis, M., Nichols, S.S., Dalrymple, N. (2010). The effects of a school-based intervention programme on dietary intakes and physical activity among primary-school children in Trinidad and Tobago. Public Health Nutr, 13 (5), 738–747.

French, S.A., Story, M., Perry, C.L. (1995). Self-esteem and obesity in children and adolescents: a literature review. Obes Res, 3 (5), 479–490.

GAO letter to Senator Bill Frist, Majority Leader (2006) subject: Childhood obesity: factors affecting physical activity. Retrieved on February 20, 2010 from: http://www.gao.gov/new.items/d07260r.pdf.

Gibson, L.Y., Byrne, S.M., Davis, E.A., et al. (2007). The role of family and maternal factors in childhood obesity. Med J Austral, 186 (11), 591–595.

Gómez, J.E., Johnson, B.A., Selva, M., et al. (2004, November). Violent crime and outdoor physical activity among inner-city youth. Prev Med, 39 (5), 876–881.

Gordon-Larsen, P., Adair, L.S., Popkin, B.M. (2003). The relationship of ethnicity, socioeconomic factors, and overweight in US adolescents. Obes Res, 11 (1), 121–129.

Gordon-Larsen, P., Griffiths, P., Bentley, M.E., et al. (2004, October). Barriers to physical activity: qualitative data on caregiver-daughter perceptions and practices. Am J Prev Med, 27 (3), 218–223.

Griffiths, L.J., Wolke, D., Page, A.S., et al. (2006). Obesity and bullying: different effects for boys and girls. Arch Dis Child, 91 (2), 121–125.

Haines, J., Neumark-Sztainer, D., Eisenberg, M.E., et al. (2006). Weight teasing and disordered eating behaviors in adolescents: longitudinal findings from Project EAT (Eating Among Teens). Pediatrics, 117 (2), e209–15.

Harvard Eating Disorders Center (1999). Retrieved February 20, 2010 from: www.hedc.org

Hesketh, K., Waters, E., Green, J., et al. (2005, March). Healthy eating, activity and obesity prevention: a qualitative study of parent and child perceptions in Australia. Health Promot Int, 20 (1), 19–26.

Hughes, A.R., Farewell, K., Harris, D., et al. (2007). Quality of life in a clinical sample of obese children. Int J Obes (London), 31 (1), 39–44.

Institute of Medicine (2008). Focus on childhood obesity. Inst Med Nat Acad. Retrieved on February 30, 2010 from: http://www.iom.edu/CMS/22593.aspx.

Jago, R., Baranowski, T., Zakeri, I., et al. (2005, August). Observed environmental features and the physical activity of adolescent males. Am J Prev Med, 29 (2), 98–104.

James, P.T., Rigby, N., Leach, R., et al. (2004). The obesity epidemic, metabolic syndrome and future prevention strategies. Eur J Cardiovasc Prev Rehabil, 11 (1), 3–8.
Janssen, I., Craig, W.M., Boyce, W.F., et al. (2004). Associations between overweight and obesity with bullying behaviors in school-aged children. Pediatrics, 113 (5), 1187–1194.
Janssen, I., Boyce, W.F., Simpson, K., et al. (2006, January). Influence of individual- and area-level measures of socioeconomic status on obesity, unhealthy eating, and physical inactivity in Canadian adolescents. Am J Clin Nutr, 83 (1), 139–145.
Jelalian, E., Mehlenbeck, R., Lloyd-Richardson, E.E., et al. (2006). 'Adventure therapy' combined with cognitive-behavioral treatment for overweight adolescents. Int J Obes, 30 (1), 31–39.
Kain, J., Leyton, B., Cerda, R., et al. (2009). Two-year controlled effectiveness trial of a school-based intervention to prevent obesity in Chilean children. Public Health Nutr, 12 (9), 1451–1461.
Kalarchian, M.A., Levine, M.D., Arslanian, S.A., et al. (2009). Family-based treatment of severe pediatric obesity: randomized, controlled trial. Pediatrics, 124 (4), 1060–1068.
Kimm, S.Y., Glynn, N.W., McMahon, R.P., et al. (2006, March). Self-perceived barriers to activity participation among sedentary adolescent girls. Med Sci Sports Exerc, 38 (3), 534–540.
Kinston, W., Loader, P. (1984). Eliciting whole-family interaction with a standardized clinical interview. J Fam Ther, 6, 347–363.
Kriemler, S., Zahner, L., Schindler, C., et al. (2010). Effects of school based physical activity programme (KISS) on fitness and adiposity in primary schoolchildren: cluster randomized controlled trial. BMJ, 340, c785.
Kumanyika, S.K. (2007). Environmental influences on childhood obesity: ethnic and cultural influences in context. Physiol Behav, 94 (1), 61–70.
Lissau, I., Sorensen, T.I. (1994). Parental neglect during childhood and increased risk of obesity in young adulthood. Lancet, 343, 324–327.
Mabry, I.R., Young, D.R., Cooper, L.A., et al. (2003, November–December). Physical activity attitudes of African American and white adolescent girls. Ambul Pediatr, 3 (6), 312–316.
Martinez Vizcaino, V., Salcedo Aguilar, F., Franquelo Gutierrez, R., et al. (2008). Assessment of an after-school physical activity program to prevent obesity among 9- to 10-year-old children: a cluster randomized trial. Int J Obes, 32 (1), 12–22.
Mayo Clinic Staff (2006). Childhood obesity: complications. Retrieved February 20, 2010 from: http://www.mayoclinic.com/health/childhood obesity/DS00698/DSECTION=6.
Mendelson, B.K., White, D.R., Schliecker, E. (1995). Adolescents' weight, sex, and family functioning. Int J Eat Disorder, 17, 73–79.
Mihas, C., Mariolis, A., Manios, Y., et al. (2010). Evaluation of a nutrition intervention in adolescents of an urban area in Greece: short- and long-term effects of the VYRONAS study. Public Health Nutr, 13 (5), 712–719.
Molnar, B.E., Gortmaker, S.L., Bull, F.C., et al. (2004, May–June). Unsafe to play? Neighborhood disorder and lack of safety predict reduced physical activity among urban children and adolescents. Am J Health Promot, 18 (5), 378–386.
Mond, J.M., Stich, H., Hay, P.J., et al. (2007). Associations between obesity and developmental functioning in pre-school children: a population-based study. Int J Obes (London), 31 (7), 1068–1073.
Motl, R.W., McAuley, E., Birnbaum, A.S., et al. (2006, February). Naturally occurring changes in time spent watching television are inversely related to frequency of physical activity during early adolescence. J Adolesc, 29 (1), 19–32.
Munsch, S., Roth, B., Michael, T., et al. (2008). Randomized controlled comparison of two cognitive behavioral therapies for obese children: mother versus mother-child cognitive behavioral therapy. Psychother Psychosom, 77 (4), 235–246.
Nelson, M.C., Gordon-Larsen, P., Song, Y., et al. (2006, August). Built and social environments associations with adolescent overweight and activity. Am J Prev Med, 31 (2), 109–117.
Neumark-Sztainer, D., Falkner, N., Story, M., et al. (2002). Weight-teasing among adolescents: correlations with weight status and disordered eating behaviors. Int J Obes Relat Metab Disord, 26 (1), 123–131.

Neumark-Sztainer, D., Story, M., French, S.A., et al. (1997). Psychosocial concerns and health-compromising behaviors among overweight and non-overweight adolescents. Obes Res, 5 (3), 237–249.

Neumark-Sztainer, D., Wall, M., Guo, J., et al. (2006). Obesity, disordered eating, and eating disorders in a longitudinal study of adolescents: how do dieters fare 5 years later? J Am Diet Assoc, 106 (4), 559–568.

Nichols-English, G.J., Lemmon, C.R., Litaker, M.S., et al. (2006, Winter). Relations of black mothers' and daughters' body fatness, physical activity beliefs and behavior. Ethn Dis, 16 (1), 172–179.

NIDDK (2004). WIN Weight-Control Information Network. Binge eating disorder. USDHHS, NIH Publication No. 04-3589, September 2004. Retrieved February 20, 2010 from: http://win.niddk.nih.gov/publications/binge.htm

Pearce, M.J., Boergers, J., Prinstein, M.J. (2002). Adolescent obesity, overt and relational peer victimization, and romantic relationships. Obes Res, 10 (5), 386–393.

Pinhas-Hamiel, O., Singer, S., Pilpel, N., et al. (2006). Health-related quality of life among children and adolescents: associations with obesity. Int J Obes (London), 30 (2), 267–272.

Ponder, S.W., Anderson, M.A. (2007). Childhood obesity: practical considerations for prevention and management. Diab Spectrum, 20 (3), 148–153.

Powell, L.M., Szczypka, G., Chaloupka, F.J. (2007). Adolescent exposure to food advertising on television. Am J Prev Med, 33 (4), S251–S256.

Powell, C., Wedner, S., Hatt, S. (2004). Vision screening for correctable visual acuity deficits in school-age children and adolescents. Cochrane Database Syst Rev. (4). Art. No.: CD005023. DOI: 10.1002/14651858.CD005023.pub2.

Puhl, R., Brownell, K.D. (2003, March). Ways of coping with obesity stigma: review and conceptual analysis. Eat Behav, 4 (1), 53–78.

Richmond, T.K., Hayward, R.A., Gahagan, S., et al. (2006, June). Can school income and racial/ethnic composition explain the racial/ethnic disparity in adolescent physical activity participation? Pediatrics, 117 (6), 2158–2166.

Robbins, L.B., Pender, N.J., Kazanis, A.S. (2003, May–June). Barriers to physical activity perceived by adolescent girls. J Midwifery Womens Health, 48 (3), 206–212.

Rukavina, P.B., Li, W. (2008). School physical activity interventions: do not forget about obesity bias. Obes Rev, 9 (1), 67–75.

Salmon, J., Campbell, K.J., Crawford, D.A. (2006, January 16). Television viewing habits associated with obesity risk factors: a survey of Melbourne schoolchildren. Med J Aust, 184 (2), 64–67.

Salmon, J., Timperio, A., Cleland, V., et al. (2005, August). Trends in children's physical activity and weight status in high and low socio-economic status areas of Melbourne, Victoria, 1985–2001. Aust N Z J Public Health, 29 (4), 337–342.

Schwarz, S.M., Freemark, M. (2007). Obesity. Retrieved February 21, 2010 from: http://www.emedicine.com/ped/topic1699.htm

Sirard, J.R., Riner, W.F. Jr, McIver, K.L., et al. (2005, December). Physical activity and active commuting to elementary school. Med Sci Sports Exerc, 37 (12), 2062–2069.

Srabstein, J.C., McCarter, R.J., Shao, C., et al. (2006). Morbidities associated with bullying behaviors in adolescents. School based study of American adolescents. Int J Adolesc Med Health, 18 (4), 587–596.

Stettler, N., Signer, T.M., Suter, P.M. (2004, June). Electronic games and environmental factors associated with childhood obesity in Switzerland. Obes Res, 12 (6), 896–903.

Strauss, R.S., Pollack, H.A. (2001). Epidemic increase in childhood overweight, 1986–1998. J Am Med Assoc, 286 (22), 2845–2848.

Thorpe, L.E., List, D.G., Marx, T., et al. (2004). Childhood obesity in New York City elementary school students. Am J Public Health, 94, 1496–1500.

U.S.DHHS (2000). Bodywise handbook (2nd ed.). Washington, DC: Office on Women's Health, U.S. DHHS. Retrieved March 1, 2010 from: http://www.mandometerusa.com/pdf/BodyWise.pdf

Vandewater, E.A., Shim, M.S., Caplovitz, A.G. (2004, February). Linking obesity and activity level with children's television and video game use. J Adolesc, 27 (1), 71–85.

Wake, M., Salmon, L., Waters, E., et al. (2002). Parent-reported health status of overweight and obese Australian primary school children: a cross-sectional population survey. Int J Obes Relat Metab Disord, 26 (5), 717–724.

Wilfley, D.E., Stein, R.I., Saelens, B.E., et al. (2007). Efficacy of maintenance treatment approaches for childhood overweight: a randomized controlled trial. J Am Med Assoc, 298 (14), 1661–1673.

Williams, J., Wake, M., Hesketh, K., et al. (2005). Health-related quality of life of overweight and obese children. J Am Med Assoc, 293 (1), 70–76.

Chapter 11
Diabetes Mellitus

Diabetes mellitus (DM) is a group of diseases characterized by high levels of blood glucose resulting from defects in insulin production, insulin action, or both. Two types of DM, type 1 and type 2, are both associated with serious complications and premature death. In addition, there is a hybrid or mixed type of DM, as well as a secondary form of DM. Furthermore, another disease type, gestational diabetes mellitus (GDM) in pregnant women, creates an increased risk of the development of type 2 DM. Finally, another form of the disorder is maturity-onset DM of the young, which is a rare form of DM caused by a single gene defect that results in faulty insulin secretion.

DM is one of the most common chronic diseases in children and adolescents (Kelly et al., 2006; Ogden et al., 2002). In the United States, about 176,000 people under the age of 20 have the condition. Approximately 1 in every 400–600 children has type 1 DM (Centers for Disease Control & Prevention, 2005). Each year more than 13,000 children are diagnosed with type 1 DM (Libman et al., 1993). According to a study by Karvonen et al. (2000), the incidence of type 1 DM is about 7 per 100,000 in children ages 4 and under, 15 per 100,000 in children 5–9 years old, and about 22 per 100,000 in children 10–14 years old. Approximately 75% of all newly diagnosed cases of type 1 DM occur in those younger than 18 years of age.

A recent study by Ehehalt et al. (2008) discovered that in Germany, the number of children and adolescents with new onset type 1 DM has been rising at a faster pace than expected. Harjutsalo et al. (2008) also found that the incidence of type 1 DM in Finnish children has been increasing faster than before and that the number of new cases diagnosed at or before 14 years of age will double in the next 15 years.

Increasing numbers of children and adolescents have been diagnosed with type 2 DM. Both Fagot-Campagna et al. (2000) and Kaufman (2002) have related that the percentage of children newly diagnosed with type 2 DM has increased from less than 5% before 1994 to 30–50% in subsequent years. The number of overweight children and adolescents has doubled in the past two decades.

All ethnic groups have been affected by DM, but the disorder has disproportionately impacted American Indians, Mexican Americans, and Pacific Islanders (Acton et al., 2002; Fagot-Campagna et al., 2000). Among the Pima Indians, the incidence of the disease among 15–19 year olds has been found to be 5% (Fagot-Campagna et al., 2000).

M.L. Goldstein, S. Morewitz, *Chronic Disorders in Children and Adolescents*,
DOI 10.1007/978-1-4419-9764-7_11,

The role of race and ethnicity and their relationship to DM has been widely researched. Delameter et al. (1999) reported that lower income, black children with DM have an increased risk for glycemic control problems. Auslander et al. (1997) concluded that African-American children were at greater risk for poor glycemic control because of the prevalence of single parent families and lower adherence to diet and glucose testing in comparison to their Caucasian counterparts. Gallegos-Macias et al. (2003) indicated that Hispanic youth with type 1 DM was at greater risk for poor glycemic control due to their lower socioeconomic status rather than their ethnicity. Other researchers, including Egede et al. (2002) and Egede and Zheng (2003) have demonstrated a relationship between low income and DM.

Females have been found to have a higher risk for the development of DM as well. Blazer et al. (2002), Egede et al. (2002), and Egede and Zheng (2003) all reported a higher risk for the development of the disorder in females. The research is less clear regarding gender differences for female children and adolescents.

Type 1 DM is an autoimmune disease in which the immune system destroys the insulin-producing beta cells of the pancreas that regulate blood glucose. The condition has an acute onset and it is difficult to pinpoint when the symptoms begin in children and adolescents. Children with type 1 DM are at risk for long-term complications, including damage to kidneys, eyes, nerves, the cardiovascular system, blood vessels, and gums and teeth. The onset of the condition can occur at any age, but most often occurs in children and young adults.

Symptoms of type 1 DM typically develop over a short period of time and include increased thirst and urination, constant hunger, weight loss, and blurred vision. Frequently, children present with vomiting, a sign of diabetic ketoacidosis, and are mistakenly diagnosed as having gastroenteritis. DM can usually be differentiated from a gastrological infection by the frequent urination that accompanies continued vomiting in comparison to decreased urination due to dehydration when the vomiting is caused by a gastrological illness.

A combination of genetic and environmental factors increases the risk for type 1 DM. Autoimmune diseases, including celiac disease and autoimmune thyroiditis, are also associated with type 1 DM. Gender differences occur in children, adolescents, and young adults with type 1 DM. Ostman et al. (2008) evaluated all medical patients in Sweden from 1983 to 2002 and found that there was a clear predominance of newly diagnosed type 1 DM in males of all ages.

Type 2 DM occurs mainly in those who are overweight. In the past, type 2 DM was identified primarily in overweight adults over 40 years old. However, with the increase of obesity and inactivity in children and adolescents, the disorder has dramatically increased in younger individuals. According to the Kelly et al. (2006), the increased incidence of type 2 DM is a "first consequence" of the obesity epidemic among young people.

The first stage in the development is often insulin resistance, which causes an inadequate response to insulin and results in the need for increasing amounts of insulin to control blood glucose. At first, the pancreas responds by producing more insulin. After several years, insulin production decreases and DM develops.

Type 2 DM is more common in certain ethnic and racial groups, including African Americans, Hispanic Americans, American Indians, and some Asian and Pacific Islanders.

Symptoms of type 2 DM may be similar to type 1 DM symptoms. In addition, symptoms often develop slowly and insidiously in children and adolescents. A child may report feeling very tired, thirsty, or nauseated. A child may have to urinate often. Other symptoms may include weight loss, blurred vision, frequent infections, and/or slow healing of sores or wounds. However, some children may display no symptoms at all when diagnosed. Still other children may present with a vaginal yeast infection or burning during urination due to a yeast infection. Physical signs of DM include acanthosis nigricans, where the skin around the neck or in the armpits appears to be dark, thick, and feels velvety. Furthermore, high blood pressure and dyslipdemia are also associated with insulin resistance.

Type 2 DM has a number of risk factors, particularly being overweight and having a family member who has type 2 DM. Other risk factors include being a member of a high risk ethnic or racial group, having signs of insulin resistance, experiencing puberty, and being older than 10 years old. Children and adolescents with type 2 DM are also at risk for long-term complications of DM, including hypertension and lipid abnormalities.

GDM is a form of the disorder that is diagnosed in about 7% of all pregnancies, approximately 200,000 per year. GDM is more common among obese women, those with a family history of DM and certain ethnic and racial groups. The children of women with GDM have an increased risk of developing obesity and DM compared to other children.

A "hybrid" or "mixed" form of DM also exists. Some children have elements of both type 1 and type 2 DM, which may not be surprising because more children are overweight than ever before. Children with "hybrid" DM are likely to display both insulin resistance that is associated with type 2 DM and antibodies against the pancreatic islet cells that are associated with autoimmunity and type 2 DM. The signs and symptoms tend to be similar to other forms of the disorder.

Another rare form of the disease is maturity-onset DM, which is caused by a single gene defect that results in faulty insulin secretion. This form of the disorder is defined by its early onset, usually prior to age 25 (Nobre et al. 2002), absence of ketosis and autosomal dominant inheritance. Maturity-onset DM has been estimated to account for 2–5% of all DM cases and often goes unrecognized.

Finally, DM can occur in children and adolescents with other diseases, such as cystic fibrosis, as well as in those children who need glucocortoid medications. More recently, Ludvigsson (2006) discovered that children with celiac disease had a much greater risk of acquiring type 1 DM, compared with children without celiac disease. They also found that the age at which celiac disease was discovered did not affect whether children got DM later. Overall, secondary DM may account for 1–5% of all cases of the disorder. Diabetic neuropathy develops in 15–20% of those with type 1 DM and in a similar or higher percentage of those with type 2 DM. Although overt diabetic neuropathy or kidney failure is very uncommon in childhood or adolescence, diabetic kidney disease in susceptible patients begins soon after the onset of the disease and may accelerate during adolescence, leading to microalbuminuria or incipient diabetic neuropathy (Bogdanovic, 2008).

Identification

Children and adolescents may present with ketoacidosis as the first indication of diabetes, while others may present with modest fasting hyperglycemia that quickly changes to severe hyperglycemia and/or ketoacidosis in the presence of infection or other stress (Acton et al., 2002). Most children and adolescents diagnosed with type 2 DM are obese or overweight, insulin resistant, and have a family history of DM. They may also have physical signs of insulin resistance such as acanthosis nigricans. The American Academy of Pediatrics and the American Diabetes Association have developed testing criteria and risk factors (American Diabetes Association, 2005). Testing criteria include an assessment for being overweight (defined as BMI greater than the 85th percentile or weight greater than 120% of ideal for height) and at least two risk factors such as family history in first or second degree relative; American Indian, African-American, Hispanic, Asian American, or Pacific Islander heritage; signs of insulin resistance or conditions associated with insulin resistance such as hypertension, dyslipidemia, acanthosis nigricans, polycystic ovarian syndrome.

Behavioral and Emotional Issues

Several researchers have demonstrated that youth with DM are more likely to have emotional or behavioral problems than youth who do not have the disease (Anderson et al., 2001). Garrison (2005) evaluated 4,508 children from 5 to 12 years old and 3,094 adolescents from 13 to 18 years who had DM. Having an emotional or behavioral disorder did not result in increased hospitalizations for children, but did result in increased hospitalizations for adolescents. In particular, having an internalizing disorder, such as depression or anxiety, was associated with increased hospitalizations. Katon et al. (2004) analyzed the relationship between behavioral and clinical factors associated with depression among individuals with DM and cited the prevalence of depression and anxiety as well.

Several longitudinal studies of adolescents have indicated that depression in teenage years was associated with a higher risk of developing obesity in adolescence and early adulthood (Goodman and Whitaker, 2002; Richardson et al., 2003), resulting in an increased risk for the development of type 2 DM. Furthermore, depression earlier in life has also been shown in prospective studies to increase the risk of type 2 DM twofold (Eaton et al., 1996; Kawakami et al., 1999). Depression has been reported to decrease adherence to diet for diabetics (Ciechanowski et al., 2000). However, Dantzer et al. (2003) recently reviewed the literature on anxiety and depression in adolescents with diabetes and related that more information was necessary to understand the etiology and impact of anxiety and depression in young diabetics. They agreed that anxiety and depression appeared to be important in determining adaptation to the disease.

Wasserman and Trifonova (2006) reviewed the research on psychosocial factors in type 1 DM. They concluded that the stress-inducing nature of the disorder was associated with the development of anxiety and depression, and that in turn, there may be a negative influence on the DM and self-care. Furthermore, the authors examined the impact on health-related quality of life and noted that early diagnosis of emotional and behavioral disturbances in young diabetic patients is essential.

Although it has been repeatedly reported that smoking and increased insulin resistance are associated (Facchini et al., 1992; Ronnemaa et al., 1996), reports have shown higher rates of smoking in individuals with depression as compared to those without depression (Glassman et al., 1990). In a longitudinal study of adolescents, researchers discovered that depression increased susceptibility to peer pressure to start smoking (Patton et al., 1998, 1999). Katon et al. (2004) concluded that there was an association of both major and minor depression with higher BMI and smoking and that there may be bidirectional effects between obesity and depression. Furthermore, they posited that the association between depression and smoking is particularly problematic among those with diabetes. Although diabetic guidelines strongly recommend that patients with diabetes stop smoking, Anda et al. (1990) reported that smokers with depression were 40% less likely to quit than non-depressed smokers. In addition, smokers with a history of depression were found to be more likely to develop a major depressive episode when they tried to quit smoking (Dierker et al., 2002).

A number of researchers have focused on the psychological adjustment of children and adolescents with DM. Sultana et al. (2007) found that the self-esteem of diabetic children and adolescents was significantly lower than controls. In addition, the diabetes group was more defensive. In another study, Frank et al. (1998) found that the diabetic children's emotional and behavioral functioning was not related to their medical diagnosis, but noted that their parent's distress and depression were relevant factors in the child's functioning. Damiao and Pinto (2007) examined the experience of adolescents with type 1 DM and found that resilient adolescents were capable of healing their wounds, being in charge of their lives and living a full life.

Most of the research on children and adolescents with DM has focused on quality of life. Grootenhuis et al. (2007) investigated the prevalence of quality of life (QOL) problems in children with different chronic diseases, including DM. In comparison to healthy children, only a small number of differences were found. Naughton et al. (2008) examined 2,245 children aged 8–22 years old in the Search for Diabetes in Youth study and evaluated the demographic and management variables of youths with both type 1 and type 2 DM. The authors concluded that health-related quality of life (HRQOL) was lower for those with type 2 DM than those with type 1 DM. In addition, HRQOL was better for those with type 2 DM who had to inject insulin at least three times per day rather than take oral medication or no medication.

Furthermore, having two or more emergency room visits in the past 6 months was also associated with worse HRQOL. Finally, the study indicated that HRQOL was lower for girls in comparison to boys. In another recent study (deWitt et al., 2008), the researchers evaluated the effects of monitoring and discussion of HRQOL on adolescents. Mean scores on the Child Health Questionnaire (CHQ) subscales of psychosocial health, behavior, mental health, and family activities improved in those in the intervention group, who had the opportunity to discuss their disease during consultations. The authors concluded that monitoring and discussion of HRQOL in adolescents with DM have positive effects on psychosocial well-being, except for those in poorest control of their DM. Pecaud et al. (2007) reported that those with diabetes showed delayed psychosocial maturation, while Debono and Cachia (2007) noted the effects of impaired psychological well-being and poor perception of QOL in diabetics.

Cognitive Issues

A decline in cognitive function has been reported in children and adolescents with type 1 DM (Brands et al., 2005; Ferguson et al., 2003; Jacobson et al., 2007; Northam et al., 1999; Rovet et al., 1987; Schoenle et al., 2002; and Veldhuis et al., 2005). Typically the effects on cognition are mild and are influenced by the age of onset, hyperglycemia, and hypoglycemic episodes.

Reports using relatively new brain imaging techniques have also shown brain changes in adults and children that appear to be influenced by metabolic abnormalities present in DM (Musen, 2008). Furthermore, early detections of brain changes may be early indicators of subsequent cognitive abnormalities.

A number of researchers (Hershey et al., 2003; Hyllienmark et al., 2005; Prescott et al., 1990; Rovet & Ehrlich, 1999) have examined the role of hypoglycemia on intelligence in children with DM and found a relationship between cognition and diabetes. However, Perantie et al. (2008) evaluated the role of hypoglycemia and hyperglycemia in producing cognitive impairment and found that hypoglycemia and hyperglycemia have qualitatively different effects on cognitive function in type 1 DM. The authors also related that those with type 1 DM had lower verbal intelligence than sibling controls and that verbal intelligence was reduced with increased exposure to hyperglycemia but not to hypoglycemia. In addition, they reported that spatial intelligence and delayed recall were reduced only with repeated hypoglycemia, particularly when the hypoglycemic episodes occurred before the age of 5 years old.

Brismar et al. (2007) conducted a cross-sectional study of type 1 DM patients. They found that early age of DM onset and long duration of the disease were the strongest predictors of low scores in psychomotor speed, memory, processing speed, attention, working memory, verbal ability, general intelligence, executive function, and a low global score. They also reported that the number of hypoglycemic events had no defined effect on cognitive functioning.

Treatment

The basic components of treatment for children and adolescents with type 1 DM are insulin administration, blood glucose testing, nutrition management, hypoglycemic avoidance, and physical activity. Management of type 2 DM also involves nutrition management, blood glucose testing, and increased physical activity. Oral medication and/or insulin therapy may also be utilized in type 2 DM, if blood glucose levels cannot be maintained without medication and/or insulin.

Glucose monitoring in children and adolescents has been widely researched and has been shown to be a significant problem for many young diabetics. Gonder-Frederick et al. (2008) found that both children and their parents showed poor ability to recognize either high or low blood glucose levels. Rabbone et al. (2008) also evaluated glycemic control in newly diagnosed diabetic children and found that indwelling catheter therapy was helpful for selected continuous insulin infusion patients. Weinzimer et al. (2005) suggest that diabetic management in young patients should include regular and careful monitoring for glycemic control and the presence of hypoglycemia. They reported that a continuous glucose monitoring system can significantly help improve glycemic control. Buckingham et al. (2007) reported that incorporating real-time continuous monitoring into the daily treatment of children with type 1 DM was feasible. Shalitin and Phillip (2007) also argued that the use of continuous subcutaneous insulin infusion therapy was useful in maintaining blood glucose levels as close to normal as possible. As a result, the risk of hypoglycemic episodes was reduced as were micro and macrovascular complications. QOL was also improved. However, Steck et al. (2007) related that the achievement of optimal glycemic control in children is complicated by their variability in eating habits and activity levels.

Danne and Becker (2007) agreed that glycemic control was important in order to prevent or delay long-term complications in pediatric patients and the use of insulin was often instrumental. However, they expressed concern about the attainment of target glycemic levels without increased risk of hypoglycemia, as well as hormone-driven fluctuations in insulin requirements and the psychological and social impacts of weight gain and puberty.

Miles and Acerini (2008) reviewed the use of newer analog preparations for clinical use with children and adolescents with type 1 DM. They reported that clinical trials with pediatric patients suggest significant benefits in terms of reduced frequency of nocturnal hypoglycemia, better postprandial blood glucose control, and improved quality of life when compared with traditional insulins. In addition, there is evidence that patients may also benefit from reduced risk of excessive weight, particularly during adolescence. However, the authors raised possible concerns, including increased mitogenic potential and risk of tumor development. Rodrigues et al. (2007) evaluated the use of pramlintide, a synthetic analog of amylin, and concluded that pramlintide bolus may result in an increase in the risk of immediate postprandial hypoglycemia.

Diet and nutrition have also been studied. Recent recommendations by the American Diabetes Association suggest that children with type 1 DM should follow the recommendations for age, sex, and body type of the general population. For obese and overweight children with DM, weight-control strategies should be utilized. Nutritional education and nutritional counseling have also been advocated and it has been suggested that nutritional intervention begins at the onset of diagnosis. Maffeis and Pinelli (2008) have posited that behavioral intervention strategies to help parents improve mealtimes could be helpful in teaching diabetic children to learn to follow a structured eating schedule. For adolescents, they have suggested focusing on insulin misuse and eating disorders for weight control. Chien et al. (2007) evaluated a group of adolescents and found that 36.8% did not use any meal plan and had difficulty following prescribed regimens.

The effects of exercise on diabetic children have also been examined (American Diabetes Association, 2006). Regular physical exercise has been one of the cornerstones of diabetes therapy for many years. The benefits of regular physical exercise include an increased sense of well-being, improved blood pressure, improved QOL, and improved weight and BMI. For diabetic patients, there has been demonstrated to be decreased risk of complications from the disease and mortality. Recently, Rachmiel et al. (2007) reviewed the literature related to physical activity and diabetes in youth and reported that there are both physiological and metabolic benefits from regular exercise. According to the Juvenile Diabetes Research Foundation International, exercise makes insulin work more effectively because it takes less insulin to balance the carbohydrates consumed. As a result, children who exercise more may find that taking in their typical doses of insulin prior to eating a typical amount of food may result in decreased blood sugar levels. Furthermore, the Diabetes Research in Children Network (2007) evaluated children and teens with type 1 DM, specifically the impact of aerobic exercise. For most of the children in the study, blood glucose levels dropped about 25%. About one-third of the participants became hypoglycemic either during or right after exercise, but only one child had an increase in blood glucose concentrations. The authors also commented that the type of exercise, how long the exercise is done, and the time of the day all had roles in how exercise affects glucose levels in children.

A number of researchers have also cited the importance of the child's family in their care. Newbould et al. (2008) conducted semi-structured interviews with 69 children aged 8–15 and their parents. Their interviews highlighted the importance of a young person's family in their care and the need for health professionals to partner with the children as well as with their parents. Newbould et al. (2007) also examined the experiences and concerns of youngsters and their parents regarding the management of medication. Parents expressed concern regarding the level of support and awareness related to their children, while children expressed concern regarding access to and use of their medication at school and the potential impact on their medical management. In another study, Dashiff et al. (2008) synthesized findings from empirical studies about communication and interaction between parents and adolescents with DM. The authors concluded that maternal support, conflict, control, involvement, and emotional expression were all linked to DM outcomes with adolescents. Mattosinho and Silva (2007) studied adolescents with type 1 DM and their families through interviews and field observation in a qualitative study. They suggested that different practices in health vary from family to family.

Educational programs for diabetic children and adolescents have also been utilized. Although most education has focused on nutrition, Viklund et al. (2007) placed diabetic adolescents in a group educational program, "the schooner programme," and assessed participants' attitudes. Participants reported more positive attitudes toward diabetes and self-care, as well as more frequent contact with others with DM, as well as more frequent monitoring of blood glucose. The authors concluded that the group had a positive impact on attitudes toward their disorder.

Although many diabetic children and adolescents become involved in psychotherapy, there have been few studies on the efficacy of counseling on DM. Ellis et al. (2007) assessed whether therapist treatment fidelity was a predictor of treatment outcome in a trial of multi-systemic therapy with 10- to 16-year-old children with poorly controlled DM. Results suggested that conducting complex behavioral interventions with a high degree of fidelity can improve treatment outcomes among children with DM.

The use of cognitive-behavioral approaches may be helpful for children with DM and other chronic diseases. In their literature review, Barlow and Ellard (2004) reported that cognitive behavioral methods may positively impact metabolic control in children with DM.

A number of alternative and complementary therapies have been used for diabetic patients. Some individuals with DM use complementary and alternative therapies (CAM) to treat DM, despite the lack of research (National Diabetes Information Clearinghouse, 2008). Although some CAM approaches may be effective, others may be ineffective or even harmful. CAM includes acupuncture, biofeedback, guided imagery, chromium, ginseng, magnesium, and vanadium.

The benefit of added chromium has been debated and studied for several years. Although some research has reported that chromium supplementation may improve diabetic control and help insulin improve its action, no recommendations for supplementation yet exist. Some research has shown that American ginseng has glucose lowering effects, but researchers have also shown that the amount of glucose lowering compound in ginseng plants varies widely. Magnesium has been widely studied and evidence suggests that a deficiency of magnesium may contribute to certain diabetic complications. Research has also found that magnesium may worsen blood glucose control in type 2 DM. Furthermore, people with higher intakes of magnesium through the consumption of whole grains, nuts, and leafy green vegetables have a decreased risk of type 2 DM. Early studies on vanadium showed that vanadium normalized blood glucose levels in animals with DM. When people were given vanadium, they developed a modest increase in insulin sensitivity and were able to decrease insulin requirements. Investigations with children and adolescents have not been conducted, however.

Dannemann et al. (2008) noted that most studies on the use of CAM have focused on adults. They concluded that parents do not typically question the use of insulin. The most common types of CAM included homeopathy, vitamins and minerals, modified diet, aloe vera, and cinnamon. Those who used CAM had a higher family income and greater parent education, as well as a stronger interest in self-care. Zipitis and Akobeng (2008) evaluated whether vitamin D supplementation in infancy reduces the risk of type 1 DM and posited that vitamin D may offer protection against the development of type 1 DM.

Case Study

The following case discusses a youth with type 2 DM. Samantha is a 9-year-old Hispanic female, who resides with her parents and three older siblings in a middle class urban family. She weighed over 9 pounds at birth and weighed 115 pounds when only 7 years old. The family practitioner expressed concern at each yearly check-up and attempted to refer the family to a nutritionist. However, the child's mother did not follow through with a nutritionist, feeling that Samantha was just a "good eater." It should be noted that all family members were overweight, but no other member was grossly obese.

Samantha did not attend preschool, but attended kindergarten at a Catholic school in the neighborhood. In first grade, she began to be teased by the other children due to her weight and was often called "fatty." She had few friends at school and began to be isolated in second grade. Near the end of second grade, she told her mother that she hated herself and wished that she had never been born. When her mother related this information to the family doctor, she was referred to a child psychologist. After a diagnostic interview with the parents and Samantha, the psychologist convinced the family to follow through with a nutritionist. Around the same time, Samantha was diagnosed with type 2 DM. Significantly, Samantha's paternal grandmother and two paternal aunts had been treated for DM for years.

Samantha and her family regularly met with the nutritionist and made significant changes in meals at the home for the entire family. As a result, Samantha lost 15 pounds. In addition, Samantha began to exercise, again with family support. She also continued with therapy and decreased her isolation, resulting in a decrease in depression and an increase in self-esteem.

References

Acton, K.J., Burrows, N.R., Moore, K., et al. (2002). Trends in diabetes prevalence among American Indian and Alaska Native children, adolescents, and young adults. Am J Public Health, 92 (9), 1485–1490.

American Diabetes Association. (2005). Clinical practice recommendations: standards of medical care in diabetes. Diab Care, 28 (S1), 4–36.

American Diabetes Association. (2006). Effects of exercise on glucose levels in children with type 1 diabetes. Diab Care, 29, 20–25.

Anda, R., Williamson, D., Escobedo, L. et al. (1990). Depression and dynamics of smoking. JAMA, 264, 1541–1543.

Anderson, R.J., Freeland, K.E., Clouse, R.E. et al. (2001). The prevalence of comorbid depression in adults with diabetes: a meta-analysis. Diab Care, 24, 1069–1078.

Auslander, W.F., Thompson, S., Dreitzer, D. et al. (1997). Disparity in glycemic control and adherence between African-American and Caucasian youths with diabetes. Diab Care, 20 (10), 1569–1575.

Barlow, J.H., Ellard, D.R. (2004). Psycho-educational interventions for children with chronic disease, parents, and siblings: an overview of the research evidence base. Child Care Health Dev, 30 (6), 637–645.

Blazer, D.G., Moody-Ayers, S., Craft-Morgan, J. et al. (2002). Depression in diabetes and obesity. J Psychsom Res, 53, 913–916.

Bogdanovic, R. (2008). Diabetic nephropathy in children and adolescents. Pediatr Nephro, 23 (4), 507–525.

Brands, A.M., Biessels, G.J., deHaaan, E.H. et al. (2005). The effects of type 1 diabetes on cognitive performance: a meta-analysis. Diab Care, 28, 726–735.

Brismar, T., Maurex, L., Cooray, G. et al. (2007). Predictors of cognitive impairment in type 1 diabetes. Psychoneuroendocrinology, 32 (8–10), 1041–1051.

Buckingham, B., Caswell, K., Wilson, D.M. (2007). Real-time continuous glucose monitoring. Curr Opin Endocrinol Diabetes Obese, 14 (4), 288–295.

Centers for Disease Control & Prevention. (2005). National diabetes fact sheet, United States, 2005. Atlanta, GA: U.S. Department of Health & Human Services. Centers for Disease Control & Prevention.

Chien, S.C., Larson, E., Nakamura, N. et al. (2007). Self-care problems of adolescents with type 1 diabetes in southern Taiwan. J Pedatr Nurs, 22 (5), 404–409.

Ciechanowski, P., Katon, W., Russo, J. (2000). Depression and diabetes: impact of depressive symptoms on adherence, function and costs. Arch Intern Med, 60, 3278–3285.

Damiao, E.B., Pinto, C.M. (2007). "Being transformed by illness": adolescents' diabetes experience. Rev Lat Am Enfermagem, 15 (4), 568–574.

Danne, T., Becker, D. (2007). Paediatric diabetes: achieving practical, effective insulin therapy in type 1 and type 2 diabetes. Acta Paediatr, 96 (11), 1560–1570.

Dannemann, K., Hecker, W., Haberland, H. et al. (2008). Use of complementary and alternative medicine in children with type 1 diabetes mellitus—prevalence, patterns of use and cost. Pediatr Diab, 9 (3), 228–235.

Dantzer, C., Swendsen, J., Maurice-Tison, S. et al. (2003). Anxiety and depression in juvenile diabetes: a critical review. Clin Psychol Rev, 23 (6), 787–800.

Dashiff, C., Hardeman, T., McClain, R. (2008). Parent-adolescent communication and diabetes: an integrative review. J Adv Nurs, 62 (2), 140–162.

Debono, M., Cachia, E. (2007). The impact of diabetes on psychological well being and quality of life. Psychol Health Med, 12 (5), 545–555.

Delameter, A.M., Shaw, K.H., Applegate, E.B. et al. (1999). Risk for metabolic control problems in minority youth with diabetes. Diab Care, 22 (5), 700–705.

deWitt, M., Delemarre-van de Waal, H.A., Bokma, J.A. et al. (2008). Monitoring and discussing health-related quality of life in adolescents with type 1 diabetes improve psychosocial well-being: a randomized controlled trial. Diab Care, 31 (8), 1521–1526.

Diabetes Research in Children Network. (2007). Continuous glucose monitoring in children with type 1 diabetes. J Pediatr, 151 (4), 388–393.

Dierker, L., Avnenevoli, S., Stolar, M. et al. (2002). Smoking and depression: an examination of mechanisms of comorbidity. Am J Psychiatry, 159, 947–953.

Eaton, W., Armenian, H., Gallo, J. et al. (1996). Depression and risk for onset of type 2 diabetes: a prospective population-based study. Diab Care, 19, 1097–1102.

Egede, L., Zheng, D. (2003), Independent factors associated with major depressive disorder in a national sample of individuals with diabetes. Diab Care, 26, 104–111.

Egede, L., Zheng, D., Simpson, K. (2002). Comorbid depression is associated with increased health care use and expenditures in individuals with diabetes. Diab Care, 25, 464–470.

Ehehalt, S., Blumenstock, G., Willasch, A.M. et al. (2008). Continuous rise in incidence of childhood type 1 diabetes in Germany. Diabet Med, 25 (6), 755–757.

Ellis, D.A., Naar-King, S., Templin, T. et al. (2007). Improving health outcomes among youth with poorly controlled type 1 diabetes: the role of treatment fidelity in a randomized clinical trial of multisystemic therapy. J Fam Psychol, 21 (3), 363–371.

Facchini, F.S., Hollenbeck, C.B., Jeppesen, J. et al. (1992). Insulin resistance and cigarette smoking. Lancet, 339, 1619–1620.

Fagot-Campagna, A., Pettitt, D.J., Engelgau, M.M. (2000). Type 2 diabetes among North American children and adolescents: an epidemiologic review and a public health perspective. J Pediatr, 136 (5), 664–672.

Ferguson, S.C., Blane, A., Perros, P. et al. (2003). Cognitive ability and brain structure in type 1 diabetes: relation to microangiopathy and preceding severe hypoglycemia. Diabetes, 52, 149–156.

Frank, R., Hagglund, K.J., Schopp, L.H. et al. (1998). Diabetes and family contributors to adaptation in juvenile rheumatoid arthritis and juvenile diabetes. Arthritis Care Res, 11 (3), 166–176

Gallegos-Macias, A.R., Macias, S.R., Kaufman, E. et al. (2003). Relationship between glycemic control, ethnicity and socioeconomic status in Hispanic and non-Hispanic youths with type 1 diabetes mellitus. Pediatr Diab, 4 (1), 19–23.

Garrison, M.M. (2005). The impact of psychiatric comorbidities on readmissions for diabetes in youth. Diab Care, 28, 2150–2154.

Glassman, A., Helzer, J., Covey, L. et al. (1990). Smoking, smoking cessation and major depression. JAMA, 264, 1546–1549.

Goodman, E., Whitaker, R. (2002). A prospective study of the role of depression in the development and persistence of adult obesity. Pediatrics, 110, 497–504.

Gonder-Frederick, L., Zrebiec, J., Bauchowitz, A. et al. (2008). Detection of hypoglycemia by children with type 1 diabetes 6 to 11 years of age and their parents: a field study. Pediatrics, 121 (3), 489–495.

Grootenhuis, M.A., Koopman, H.M., Verips, E.G.H. et al. (2007). Health-related quality of life problems of children aged 8–11 years with a chronic disease. Dev Neurorehabil, 10 (1), 27–33.

Harjutsalo, V., Sjoberg, L., Tuomileheto, J. (2008). Time trends in the incidence of type 1 diabetes in Finnish children: a cohort study. Lancet, 371 (9626), 1777–1782.

Hershey, T., Lillie, R., Sadler, M. et al. (2003). Severe hypoglycemia and long-term spatial memory in children with type 1 diabetes mellitus: a retrospective study. J Int Neuropsychol, 9, 740–750.

Hyllienmark, L., Maltez, J., Dandenell, A. et al. (2005). EEG abnormalities with and without relation to severe hypoglycemia in adolescents with type 1 diabetes. Diabetologia, 48, 412–419.

Jacobson, A.M., Musen, G., Ryan, C.M. et al. (2007). Long-term effect of diabetes and its treatment on cognitive function. New Eng J Med, 356, 1842–1852.

Karvonen, M., Viik-Kajander, M., Moltchanova, E. et al. (2000). Incidence of childhood type 1 diabetes worldwide. Diab Care, 23 (10), 1516–1526.

Katon, W.J., Simon, R.G., Russo, J. (2004). Quality of depression care in a population-based sample of patients with diabetes and major depression. Med Care, 42 (12), 1222–1229.

Kaufman, F.R. (2002). Type 2 diabetes mellitus in children and youth: a new epidemic. J Pediatr Endocrinol, 15 (S2), 737–744.

Kawakami, N., Takatsuka, N., Shimizu, H. et al. (1999). Depressive symptoms and occurrence of type 2 diabetes among Japanese men. Diab Care, 22, 1071–1076.

Kelly, J., Rodriguez, B., Ruiz, R., et al. (2006, March 7). National Diabetes Education Program: A new partner for CCPH (a joint initiative of CDC & NIH). Bethesda, MD: National Diabetes Information Clearinghouse (NDIC).

Libman, I., Songer, T., LaPorte, R. (1993). How many people in the US have IDDM? Diab Care, 16 (5), 841–842.

Ludvigsson, J.F. (2006). Celiac disease and risk of subsequent type 1 diabetes: a general population cohort study of children and adolescents. Diab Care, 29, 2483–2488.

Maffeis, C., Pinelli, L. (2008). Teaching children with diabetes about adequate dietary choices. Br J Nutr, 99 (S1), 33–39.

Mattosinho, M.M., Silva, D.M. (2007). Therapeutic itinerary of the family and adolescent with type 1 mellitus diabetes. Rev Lat Am Enfermagem, 15 (6), 1113–1119.

Miles, H.L., Acerini, C.L. (2008). Insulin analog preparations and their use in children and adolescents with type 1 diabetes mellitus. Paediatr Drugs, 10 (3), 163–176.
Musen, G. (2008). Cognition and brain imaging in type 1 diabetes. Curr Diab Rep, 8 (2), 132–137.
National Diabetes Information Clearinghouse. (2008). Complementary and alternative medical therapies for diabetes. ndic@info.niddk.nih.gov
Naughton, M.J., Ruggiero, A.M., Lawrence, J.M. et al. (2008). Health-related quality of life of children and adolescents with type 1 or type 2 diabetes mellitus. Arch Pediatr Adolesc Med, 162 (7), 649–657.
Newbould, J., Francis, S.A., Smith, F. (2007). Young people's experience of managing asthma and diabetes at school. Arch Dis Child, 92 (12), 1077–1081.
Newbould, J., Smith, F., Francis, S.A. (2008). 'I'm fine doing it on my own': partnerships between young people and their parents in the management of medication for asthma and diabetes. J Child Health Care, 12 (2), 116–128.
Nobre, E.L., Lopes, L.O., Miranda, A. et al. (2002). Mature onset diabetes of the young. Acta Med Port, 15 (6), 435–439.
Northam, E.A., Anderson, P.J., Werther, G.A. et al. (1999). Predictors of change in the neuropsychological profiles of children with type 1 diabetes 2 years after disease onset. Diab Care, 22, 1438–1444.
Ogden, C.L., Flegal, K.M., Carroll, M.D. et al. (2002). Prevalence and trends in overweight among US children and adolescents. JAMA, 288 (14), 1728–1732.
Ostman, J., Lonnberg, G., Arnqvist, H.J. et al. (2008). Gender differences and temporal variation in the incidence of type 1 diabetes. J Intern Med, 263 (4), 386–394.
Patton, G., Carlin, J., Coffey, C. et al. (1998). Depression, anxiety, and smoking initiation: a prospective study over 3 years. Am J Public Health, 88, 1518–1522.
Patton, G.C., Selzer, R., Coffey, C., et al. (1999). Onset of eating disorders: population based cohort over 3 years. BMJ, 318, 765–768.
Pecaud, D., Crawford, S., Stephure, D.K. et al. (2007). Effect of type 1 diabetes on psychosocial maturation in young adults. J Adolescent Health, 40 (1), 29–35.
Perantie, D.C., Lim, A., Wu, J. et al. (2008). Effects of prior hypoglycemia and hyperglycemia on cognition in children with type 1 diabetes mellitus. Pediatr Diab, 9 (2), 87–95.
Prescott, J.H., Richardson, J.T., Gillespie, C.R. (1990). Cognitive function in diabetes mellitus: the effects of duration of illness and glycemic control. Br J Clin Psychol, 29 (Pt 2)L, 167–175.
Rabbone, I., Bobbio, A., Di Gianni, V. et al. (2008). Intensive insulin therapy in preschool-aged diabetic children: from multiple daily injections to continuous subcutaneous insulin infusion through indwelling catheters. J Endocrinol Inves, 31 (3), 193–195.
Rachmiel, M., Buccino, J., Daneman, D. (2007). Exercise and type 1 diabetes mellitus in youth: review and recommendations. Pediatr Endocrinol Rev, 5 (2), 656–665.
Richardson, L., David, R., Poulton, R. et al. (2003). A longitudinal evaluation of adolescent depression and adult obesity. Arch Pediatr Adolesc Med, 157, 739–745.
Rodrigues, L.M., Mason, K.J., Hammond, M.W. et al. (2007). The role of prandial pramlintide in the treatment of adolescents with type 1 diabetes. Pediatr Res, 62 (6), 746–749.
Ronnemaa, T., Ronnemaa, E.M., Puukkla, P. et al. (1996). Smoking is independently associated with high plasma insulin levels in nondiabetic men. Diab Care, 19, 1229–1232.
Rovet, J.F., Ehrlich, R.M. (1999). The effect of hypoglycemic seizures on cognitive function in children with diabetes: a 7-year prospective study. J Pediatr, 134, 503–506.
Rovet, J.F., Ehrlich, R.M., Hoppe, M. (1987). Intellectual deficits associated with early onset of insulin-dependent diabetes mellitus in children. Diab Care, 10, 510–515.
Schoenle, E.J., Schoenle, D., Molinari, L. et al. (2002). Impaired intellectual development in children with type 1 diabetes: association with HbA(1c), age at diagnosis and sex. Diabetologia, 45, 108–114.
Shalitin, S., Phillip, M. (2007). The role of new technologies in treating children and adolescents with type 1 diabetes mellitus. Pediatr Diab, 8 (S6), 72–79.

Steck, A.K., Klingensmith, G.J., Fiallo-Scharer, R. (2007). Recent advances in insulin treatment of children. Pediatr Diab, 8 (S-6), 49–56.
Sultana, S., Oommen, A., Shanmugham, V. (2007). Psychological adjustment in juvenile diabetics. J Indian Acad Appl Psychol, 33 (1), 39–46.
Veldhuis, J.D., Roemmich, J.N., Richmond, E.J. et al. (2005). Endocrine control of body composition in infancy, childhood and puberty. Endocr Rev, 26, 114–146.
Viklund, G.E., Rudberg, S., Wikblad, K.F. (2007). Teenagers with diabetes: self-management education and training on a big schooner. Int J Nurs Prac, 13 (6), 385–392.
Wasserman, L.I., Trifonova, E.A. (2006). Diabetes mellitus as a model of psychosomatic and somatopsychic interrelationships. Spanish J Psychol, 9 (1), 75–85.
Weinzimer, S.A., Doyle, E.A., Tamborlane, W.V. (2005). Disease management in the young diabetic patient: glucose monitoring, coping skills and treatment strategies. Clin Pediatr, 44 (5), 393–403.
Zipitis, C.S., Akobeng, A.K. (2008). Vitamin D supplementation in early childhood and risk of type 1 diabetes: a systematic review and meta-analysis. Arch Dis Child, 93 (6), 512–517.

Chapter 12
Juvenile Arthritis

Juvenile arthritis (JA) is any type of arthritis or an arthritis-related condition that develops in children or teenagers who are under 18 (Lawrence et al., 1998; Arthritis Foundation Website). About 294,000 children are affected by JA and rheumatologic conditions (Sacks et al., 2007). These children typically have pain, swelling, tenderness, and stiffness of joints, causing limited range of motion, joint contracture, which occurs when holding a painful joint in a flexed position for a long time, damage to joint cartilage and bone, causing joint deformity and limited joint use, and altered growth of bone and joints, causing short stature.

Juvenile idiopathic arthritis (JIA), also known as juvenile rheumatoid arthritis (JRA), or juvenile chronic arthritis (JCA), is the most common form of arthritis in children and is a chronic inflammatory disease of the joints (Cassidy and Petty, 1995; Janz et al., 1993). Although JIA is often a mild condition that causes few problems over time, the disorder can produce severe complications.

According to a number of researchers (Cassidy and Petty, 1995), JIA affects between 60,000 and 200,000 children and adolescents in the USA. Approximately 5% of children diagnosed with JIA have recurrent episodes of arthritis as adults and about 10% begin adulthood with severe functional disabilities (Robinson, 1998). Of children diagnosed with JIA, 60–80% do not suffer permanent joint damage (Milota et al., 1991). Death occurs in 2–4% of children with JIA worldwide. In the USA, the majority of deaths associated with JIA have occurred in children with a type of JIA known as systemic JIAA. Infections play a major role in these deaths (Cassidy and Petty, 1995).

JIA is a heterogeneous group of autoimmune conditions characterized by increased inflammation response in a child's immune system (Aslan et al., 2011; Berkun and Padeh, 2010; Ellis et al., 2009). The condition occurs mainly with peripheral arthritis and various endogenous and exogenous antigens are thought to contribute to the etiology of the disease in a genetically susceptible host.

Researchers believe that the child's immunological predisposition and environmental conditions help to cause the disorder (Aslan et al., 2011). Of the environmental factors, infections are considered to be the most significant etiological factor. In addition, investigators consider stress, trauma, and the psychosocial milieu as very significant in the etiology of the condition (Aslan et al., 2011;

M.L. Goldstein, S. Morewitz, *Chronic Disorders in Children and Adolescents*,
DOI 10.1007/978-1-4419-9764-7_12, © Springer Science+Business Media, LLC 2011

Berkun and Padeh, 2010). Maternal smoking and meteorological factors are possible etiological factors (Berkun and Padeh, 2010; Ellis et al., 2009).

Ellis et al. (2009) suggest that breastfeeding may affect risk for acquiring JIA. They recommend further research into the possible role of vitamin D, exposure to the sun, and infections in early life (also known as the hygiene hypothesis) as possible risk factors for JIA.

Although the link between infections and adult chronic arthritis is well established, the association between infections and JIA is not clearly delineated (Aslan et al., 2011). An investigation by Aslan et al. (2011) concluded that *Mycoplasma pneumoniae* and *Campylobacter jejuni* were common in patients with primer and recurrent JIA. The researchers recommend performing a pre-diagnosis of microorganisms, adding specific antimicrobial treatments to regular JIA treatments, and conducting molecular-based serial case studies.

Using a sample of 60 JIA patients during an active disease time period, Altun et al. (2004) did not find any relationship between *Chlamydophila pneumoniae* infection and JIA. However, the researchers recommend more research to confirm their findings.

The most common features of JIA are joint inflammation, joint contracture (stiff, bent joint), joint damage, and/or alteration or change in growth. Other symptoms may include joint stiffness following rest or decreased activity level; this condition is often referred to as morning stiffness or gelling. In addition, the condition may cause weakness in muscles and other soft tissues around involved joints. JIA typically impacts each child differently, and individuals may be affected variably by any particular symptom. Signs and symptoms differ from child to child and even from day to day for a given child.

JIA consists of three major types: oligoarticular, polyarticular, and systemic JIA. In oligoarticular (or pauciarticular) JIA, four or fewer joints are affected. Usually, large joints, such as knees, ankles, or elbows, are involved. Other joints, including spine, wrists, and even small toe or finger joints can also be affected, but these are less common.

Oligoarticular JIA often affects a particular joint on one side of the body rather than both sides of the body simultaneously. Approximately 40% of all children with JRA have this form of arthritis. According to the Arthritis Foundation (2008), there are two different types of oligoarticular JIA. The first type typically impacts girls under age 7 and is associated with the development of eye inflammation (either chronic iridocyclitis or uveitis) in about one-third of these children. The second type typically affects boys, who are usually 8 or older and involves the lower spine, hips, knees, ankles, and tendons. At times, the places at which tendons and ligaments attach to bones are also inflamed. These children often develop eye problems, typically acute uveitis, which results in redness and pain in the eyes. Furthermore, this form of arthritis may be the initial sign of another arthritis-related condition, including one of the spondyloarthropathies. This group of diseases typically affects the spine, tendons, and eyes and is associated with a specific genetic factor (hla-b27). Estimates of blindness range from 15 to 30% in children with JIA and chronic uveitis.

Saurenmann et al. (2007) evaluated the prevalence, risk factors, and outcomes of uveitis in patients with JIA. Based on an inception cohort of all 1,081 patients diagnosed with JIA at a tertiary care center, the investigators discovered that 142 of the 1,081 patients (13.1%) had acquired uveitis after an average follow-up period of 6.9 years. Young age at diagnosis, female gender, antinuclear antibody positivity, and the subtype of JIA were risk factors for uveitis. Risk factors varied depending on the patient's JIA subtype. Fifty-three of the 142 patients with uveitis acquired uveitis complications. Only 16 of the 175 affected eyes (9.1%) in 14 of 108 had best corrected visual acuity less than 20/0. Synechiae or cataract was related to abnormal vision.

Among 75 patients with uveitis related to JIA, Woreta et al. (2007) showed that ocular complications were documented in 67% of the eyes affected by JIA-related uveitis. Ocular complications were more likely to occur if patients had a greater than or equal to 1+ anterior chamber flare, a positive antinuclear antibody, and a shorter duration between arthritis diagnosis and uveitis. In involved eyes, the occurrence of 20/50 or worse and 20/200 or worse visual acuities were 36 and 34%, respectively. Measurements of 20/50 or worse and 20/200 or worse visual acuities were associated with greater than or equal to 1+ anterior chamber flare and having had previous intraocular surgery. Moreover, 20/200 or worse visual acuity was related to posterior synechiae.

Polyarticular JIA is a second form of JIA. This type affects five or more joints and impacts girls more often than boys. The disorder usually affects the small joints of the hands and fingers and can also affect weight-bearing joints as well as the jaw and neck. Polyarticular JIA often affects the same joints on both sides of the body. In addition, children with this type may display a number of other symptoms, including low-grade fever, nodules on parts of the body that receive pressure from objects, and a positive blood test for rheumatoid factor (RF). Less frequently, children with polyarticular JIA may exhibit inflammation of internal organs and/or anemia.

Children with polyarticular JIA may develop damage to some of their joints. Slower growth may occur in the jaw due to arthritis in the temporomandibular joint, resulting in jaw pain and discomfort when chewing. Neck stiffness and difficulty turning the head side to side may also occur. The risk of developing chronic uveitis is also increased, particularly in young girls. Approximately 40% of all children with JRA have this form of arthritis.

The third major form of JIA is systemic-onset JIA. This disorder is the least common type of JIA and appears to equally affect males and females. In addition, this disease appears to equally impact different ethnic groups. Recently, Shishov et al. (2007) related that in children with systemic JIA, Hispanics did not have longer duration of systemic features than non-Hispanics. This type is associated with high fevers, a rash, as well as internal inflammation in some children. The systemic symptoms of the disease may disappear completely after the first few months of the illness, but the joint-related symptoms may continue for a longer period of time. According to the Arthritis Foundation, about one-half of the children with systemic JRA see a disappearance of the illness within 1 year after onset. However, a return of the illness or a flare-up can occur without warning or after the onset of a viral infection such as chicken pox.

The most common symptoms of systemic JIA are high spiking fever of 103 degrees or higher, a joint pain, and inflammation and a rash that appears on the chest, thighs, and, at times, on other parts of the child's body. Other possible features of systemic onset JIA include pericarditis, pleuritis, anemia, and high white blood cells and platelets, as well as enlarged lymph nodes, liver, or spleen. Approximately 20% of all children with JIA have been identified with this form of arthritis.

Long-term problems are similar to polyarticular JIA. However, uveitis is relatively uncommon. Recently, Frosch and Roth (2008) reported that investigations have focused on mediators of the innate immune system in those with systemic JIA and found that IL-1beta, IL-6, IL-18, and phagocyte-specific S100 proteins were correlated with disease activity and secondary complications.

Identification

JIA has no formal laboratory assessments. Typically, laboratory studies utilized for adults show negative results in children with JIA. More commonly, identification of JIA involves examination of individual joints and overall functional status, including the length of morning stiffness and degree of fatigue. Because strength, mobility, and dexterity frequently change as the disease progresses, assessment by occupational and physical therapists is needed. This evaluation involves observation of posture in sitting and standing and alignment and gait, according to Harper et al. (2000).

Diagnosis usually involves a complete health history to determine the duration of symptoms, to assess family history of arthritis, and to rule out other possible causes. In addition, a physical examination to look for joint inflammation, rashes, nodules, signs of internal organ inflammation and/or eye problems that may suggest the presence of JIA is essential. Laboratory tests to rule out other diseases, x-rays, or other specialized x-ray procedures of joints, bones, and organs and tests of joint, blood, and tissue fluids to check for infections or inflammation are also typical of screening. However, radiological studies are often able to identify only advanced articular destruction in children.

Child health questionnaires can be used to measure the health status of children with JIA. Based on a sample of 116 Norwegian children with JIA of less than 2.5 years duration and 116 matched controls, Selvaag et al. (2003) evaluated the determinants and responsiveness of the Norwegian version of the Child Health Questionnaire (CHQ). The investigators found that the CHQ discriminated between children with early JIA and matched controls. Children with early JIA had worse physical health and slightly reduced psychosocial well-being than the matched controls. The child's pain, morning stiffness, the Child Health Assessment Questionnaire disability index, the erythrocyte sedimentation rate, the child's overall well-being, and the physician's global evaluation of disease activity were the strongest predictors of the CHQ physical summary measure.

Cognitive Functioning

In contrast to other systemic diseases in childhood, recent research has demonstrated that children with juvenile arthritis do not experience cognitive impairment. Anthony and Schanberg (2007) concluded that children with JIA are not likely to be at risk for cognitive impairments; they found average IQ scores among children with JIA. Feldmann et al. (2005) reported that children and adolescents with systemic JRA performed within normal limits on IQ tests and in memory, learning, attention, and fine motor abilities.

Koutantji et al. (1999) investigated the effects of chronic pain on processing and recall in a group of children with chronic arthritis. They reported that children in pain exhibited specific patterns of cognitive processing of pain information while they presented with normal depression and anxiety levels.

Psychosocial Functioning and Quality of Life

Pain associated with JIA is common and despite the use of biologic agents, pain continues to impair daily functioning and quality of life (QOL) (Kimura and Walco, 2007). Several researchers have investigated the impact of chronic pain in children and adolescents with JIA. Margetic et al. (2005) reported that pain perception was significantly correlated with depression scores for children with JIA. Hoff and her colleagues (2006) indicated that depressive symptoms play a role in longitudinal depressive symptoms of children with JIA. Varni et al. (1996) found that higher perceived pain intensity was associated with depressive and anxious symptoms, as well as lower self-esteem and increased behavior problems. Sandstrom and Schanberg (2004) reported that pain, peer rejection, and problematic social behavior were all associated with depressive symptoms in children with arthritis and that children with JIA were vulnerable for increased risk for internalizing problems. Palermo and Kiska (2005) evaluated the relationship between pain, QOL, and subjectively reported sleep disturbances in adolescents with arthritis. They noted that depressive symptoms were associated with increased sleep problems, which in turn, contributed to increased pain. Hommel et al. (2006) examined learned helplessness in children and adolescents with JIA and found that feedback contributed to poorer or greater internalization of success for problem solving.

In another study, Merlijn et al. (2003) examined a number of psychosocial factors related to the onset, exacerbation, and maintenance of chronic pain in adolescents. They found that adolescents with chronic pain are more vulnerable to neuroticism, negative fear of failure, and less expectation of social acceptance. Schanberg et al. (2000) stated that this population showed variability in daily mood, frequency of stressful daily events, and daily symptoms across days. Sallfors et al. (2004) also reported that children suffering from JA oscillated between hope and despair and that their subjective experiences were based on dependency on treatment, experiences of disturbed order in daily life, significant others, and environmental factors.

Pirra and Pullukat (2006) reviewed the literature on chronic pain in children and related that in many instances environmental factors are likely to have a significant role. Balague et al. (1994), Forre and Smerdel (2002), Jamison and Walker (1992), Merlijn et al. (2003), Morley (2004), Schanberg et al. (2001), and Snelling (1990) have all noted environmental factors in their research.

Schanberg et al. (2001) suggested that family environment and parental pain history may be related to how children with JIA cope with the disease. They found that parents with greater severity of current pain and pain in the past month had a greater likelihood of having children who reported higher levels of pain and worse health status. In addition, parents who reported that pain disrupted their life had a greater chance of having children reporting higher levels of current pain.

Anthony and Schanberg (2007) indicated that children with JIA displayed age-appropriate social competence, social behaviors, and nonverbal social skills. However, children who had their arthritis longer tended to have more problematic social behaviors. This included loneliness and lower frustration tolerance. Barlow et al. (1999) noted that children's greatest concerns were social acceptance and peer belonging. Reiter-Purtill et al. (2003) reported that children with active or severe JIA may be at risk for difficulties with social acceptance. Nash et al. (1998) indicated that adolescents with JIA were at risk for substance abuse. Almost 31% reported alcohol use.

A number of studies have also evaluated the impact of JIA on QOL. April et al. (2006) examined the perceptions about QOL among children with JIA as well as their parent's perceptions. There appeared to be agreement between the children and their parents. However, disease severity was strongly correlated with QOL in both groups.

Investigators have also explored the extent to which parental coping is associated with QOL in children with JIA. Based on a cohort of 182 parents caring for a child with JIA, Cavallo et al. (2009) showed that parents who experienced more severe psychosocial difficulties were more likely to employ coping techniques associated with understanding the medical condition of their child.

Sawyer et al. (2005) found a significant negative relationship between children's QOL and their experience of pain. Riddle et al. (2006) concluded that both the physical and pain domains of QOL were impacted by arthritis. The authors also reported that quality of life improved most in those children treated with steroids, despite the adverse side effects.

Connelly (2005) reported that a child with JA had lower hope when the parent reported more dissatisfaction with family functioning. Hope was not related to child or parent ratings of QOL. Reid et al. (2005) noted that parent–child interactions were generally not related to disability, but parent–child patterns influenced children's adaptation to pain during experimental tasks. Turkel and Pao (2007) concluded that increased survival could not be assumed to be associated with increased QOL and problems in psychosocial functioning may be the result of the chronic illness or by the treatment.

Children with JIA may experience a number of different emotions, including sadness, anger, and anxiety. Furthermore, children may blame their parents for the illness, engage in self-pity, or become angry due to restrictions on activities. They may also resent other children who do not have the disease, including siblings.

Parental response to a child with JIA is often a significant variable in the child's emotional reaction to the disease, as well as the child's pain tolerance. Aasland et al. (1998) indicated that adolescents with JIA reported more overprotection from parents than adolescents in the general population. Anthony (2005) reported that parental perceptions of child vulnerability are an important influence on adjustment of young children with JA. In addition, parental stress most significantly predicted symptoms of depression in the child. Wagner et al. (2003) found that parental stress was associated with increased depressive symptoms among children and adolescents with rheumatic disease. Similarly, Manuel (2001) related that higher levels of psychosocial stress among mothers increased psychological symptoms.

Sallfors and Hallberg (2003) conducted a qualitative study of parents living with a child with JA and discussed the role of parental stress. A core category labeled "parental vigilance" and two related categories labeled "emotional challenges" and "continual adjustment" were identified. According to Barlow et al. (1998), JA can affect parents by increasing their feelings of guilt, anxiety, anger, frustration, helplessness, powerlessness, and isolation.

Using a sample of 70 patients with JIA and their caregivers, Bruns et al. (2008) showed that caregiver burden was more associated with psychosocial difficulties than the physical condition of the JIA patients. Rossato et al. (2007) examined the impact on family members caring for a child with JA and identified motivational factors for these families, including the desire to see the child without pain and desiring the child to live a normal life.

Sibling response is also critical. Children may over-identify with the sibling with special needs, treat their sibling differently, and/or have anger toward the child with JIA. Others want to involve themselves in the caretaking to the point that they give up their own activities, while others feel a pressure to achieve or make up for what their sibling cannot do or can no longer do. Some feel guilty, as if they caused the illness. Brewer and Angel (1992) have reported that siblings of children with JA have more difficulty in later life than the children with JA. The authors have speculated that this is due to the tremendous energy and time put toward the child with arthritis, while discounting the needs of the other siblings.

Weiss et al. (2001) studied the sibling relationship characteristics in youth with JIA and found that severity of illness was positively associated with perceived conflict with siblings.

Treatment

Currently, JIA has no curative treatments, and researchers have had difficulty assessing the effectiveness of different therapies (Emery, 2004). Despite the use of effective biologic agents, children and adolescents with JIA and other types of rheumatic disease continue to have pain that impairs their function and reduces their quality of life (Kimura and Walco, 2007). Multiple factors account for the etiology of pain in children and adolescents with these conditions and therapy alone often does not relieve their pain. No standard of care exists for managing pain in these patients.

However, early identification and treatment can improve outcomes. Treatment for patients with JIA can include medications, exercise, splints, eye care, nutrition, dental care, and surgery. In addition, massage, acupuncture, acupressure, as well as herbs and supplements have been utilized with JIA. Behavioral interventions have been conducted to increase calcium intake total body bone mineral content (Stark et al., 2006). Furthermore, a number of pain-reducing strategies may be employed, including cognitive-behavioral therapy, meditation, yoga, progressive muscle relaxation, guided imagery, biofeedback, and hypnotherapy. Although early aggressive therapy for adults with arthritis has superior outcomes, researchers have conducted minimal research on patients with JIA. Recently, the Childhood Arthritis and Rheumatology Alliance (CARRA) conducted a trial of early aggressive therapy with 96 children. The results at this time (Wallace et al., 2008) revealed that early aggressive therapy of juveniles with polyarticular arthritis appears to be feasible.

Based on a review of 34 controlled investigations, Hashkes and Laxer (2005) recommend individualizing drug treatment based on the child's JIA subtype. They reported that nonsteroidal anti-inflammatory drugs (NSAIDs) are efficacious for only a minority of patients with JIA. NSAIDs are mainly effective for patients with oliogoarthritis. Haines (2007) reported that only a small percentage of children with arthritis respond to NSAIDs, but almost all respond to corticosteroids. Yet, NSAIDs are often perceived as the first line of medication employed and are the mainstay of the initial therapy, according to the Arthritis Foundation (2008). NSAIDs must be taken for at least 3–4 weeks to assess whether they are assisting in the control of pain and inflammation. These medications come in both pill and liquid form and may be taken from one to four times per day. The most common NSAIDs include ibuprofen, aspirin, naproxen, indomethacin, tolementin, and choline magnesium trisalicylate. Side effects include headache, stomach pain, anemia, and nausea and vomiting. Less commonly, one may experience blood in the urine, difficulty with concentration, fluid retention, thinning and scarring of the skin, and rarely stomach ulcer.

Although aspirin was commonly used many years ago, it is rarely prescribed currently. Cassidy and Petty (1995) described aspirin as the most widely prescribed drug for children. It may be utilized to control joint pain and reduce fever, but the danger of toxic reactions and side effects have lessened its use.

Slow-acting anti-rheumatic drugs (SAARDs) or disease-modifying anti-rheumatic drugs (DMARDs) are often used in combination with NSAIDs. These drugs do not relieve pain or inflammation immediately, but tend to change the progress of the joint disease, such as joint erosions or cartilage and bone destruction. These particular drugs are more powerful medications, and as a result, those children taking them need more frequent lab tests to monitor possible side effects.

Hydroxychloroquine (Plaquenil) is one of the most widely used SAARDs. It is utilized to control joint pain and swelling and may take 3–6 months to work. While not helpful in all cases, it may be helpful alone or in combination with other drugs. Common side effects include skin rash, gastrointestinal problems, and rarely eye damage.

Another large group of medications in the treatment of JIA are the immune system medications. The most popular drug has been methotrexate (Rheumatrex), which has been helpful with not only arthritis but also systemic illness. Methotrexate (MTX) can help control uveitis in more severe cases as well.

MTX has been found efficacious in treating prolonged oligoarthritis, polyarthritis and has been shown to be less effective in treating systemic arthritis (Hashkes and Laxer, 2005). MTX is employed as a second-line drug in instances in which JIA is resistant to NSAIDs, intra-articular corticosteroid injections, and physiotherapy (Niehues and Lankisch, 2006).

MTX typically takes 4–8 weeks to work and can be taken in pill or liquid form or injection. Few side effects have been reported at low doses, but blood tests are usually ordered monthly at first, and then every 6–8 weeks after 6 months. Common side effects include aversion to the drug, moodiness, diarrhea, nausea, mouth sores, infections, low white blood count, lung irritation, and liver irritation (Niehues and Lankisch, 2006).

Prospective controlled trials have demonstrated the efficacy of MTX in treating children with JIA (Niehues and Lankisch, 2006). The medication has been shown to have slightly superior efficacy than leflunomide. Researchers have not provided data on when to start MTX in children with JIA and what should be the duration of treatment.

Sulfasalazine (Azulfadine) and leflunomide may be alternatives to MTX (Hashkes and Laxer, 2005). Sulfasalazine helps with joint pain, swelling, and stiffness. In controlled studies, sulfasalazine has been shown to be effective (Herlin, 2002). It typically takes 6–12 weeks to work. Children with systemic JIA may have more side effects with this medication. Common side effects include upset stomach, diarrhea, decreased appetite, headache, achiness, itching, dizziness, nausea, vomiting, rash, light sensitivity, liver abnormalities, and lowered blood count.

Anti-tumor necrosis factor drugs are very efficacious in treating polyarticular course JIA that is unresponsive to MTX (Hashkes and Laxer, 2005). However, anti-tumor necrosis factor medications are less effective in the treatment of systemic arthritis. Research has not provided support for the best treatment of systemic and enthesitis-associated arthritis.

Penicillanime (DePen and Cuprimine) are rarely used for JIA and take up to 6 months to work. Finally, gold compounds (Auranofin, Ridaura, Myochrysine, and Solganol) are used to reduce morning stiffness and control joint pain and swelling. These medications are infrequently used with JIA patients at the present time. When used, children may take daily oral pills or weekly injections for 5 or 6 months and then less often. These drugs take 3–6 months to work.

Azathioprine (Imuran) is an immune system-suppressing medication, but not commonly used in treating children with arthritis. Typically, the medication is employed with children who have failed or cannot take MTX. The medication takes approximately 3 months to work. Common side effects of the drug include loss of appetite, nausea, vomiting, cough, fever and chills, skin rash, unusual weakness or tiredness, unusual bleeding or bruising, and rarely sterility.

Cyclophosphamide (Cytoxan) is rarely used for JIA, but is often employed with children with systemic lupus erythematosus, an arthritis-related condition. The drug takes several months to work. Common side effects include loss of appetite, nausea, vomiting, dizziness, cough, fever and chills, blood in the urine, burning during urination, confusion or agitation, unusual weakness or tiredness, and an increased risk of cancer.

Cyclosporine (Sandimmune) assists with joint inflammation as well as the systemic symptoms of systemic JIA. The medication usually takes 1–2 months to work. Possible side effects include fluid retention, high blood pressure, kidney problems, bleeding, tender or enlarged gums, loss of appetite, and trembling or shaking hands.

A recent development has been the use of biologic agents, aimed at specific proteins to control a variety of diseases including JIA. These drugs are typically made of antibodies that block high levels of inflammatory proteins in those with arthritis. The most widely used and researched drug in this class of drugs is etanercept (Enbrel), which blocks the protein.

TNF was initially approved for use with children in 1999. Lovell et al. (2008) evaluated the safety and efficacy of up to 8 years of treatment with etanercept therapy in children with polyarticular juvenile arthritis and reported that there was acceptable safety and that improvements in the signs and symptoms of JIA were maintained for up to 8 years. Furthermore, etanercept was found to be effective with many children and adolescents who had failed to receive relief from MTX.

Other biologic agents include infliximab (Remicade) and intravenous immunoglobulin (IVIG). Studies are underway to assess the use of infliximab in treating polyarthritis JIA (Hashkes and Laxer, 2006). IVIG has been used to treat several childhood rheumatic diseases and is usually given intravenously once per month. IVIG is sometimes utilized as part of the treatment of systemic JIA.

TNFalpha antagonist therapy seems to be linked to different adverse events. Pontkaki et al. (2006) evaluated the side effects of anti-TNF alpha blockers for JIA, using a sample of 95 patients, who had a median age of 14 years and had been treated for a median duration of 12 months. Nineteen patients also received MTX therapy and 56 patients were treated with infliximab associated with MTX. The investigators found that patients developed severe headaches and thrombocytopenia associated with etanercept therapy. The onset of Crohn's disease in three patients probably was linked to etanercept therapy.

In their study, Pontkaki et al. (2006) found that reactions to infusions and the anti-dsDNA positivity were side effects of infliximab therapy. They discovered that behavioral changes and pain amplification syndrome were side effects probably related to both etanercept and infliximab. Treatment with biological agents was possibly related with the flare-up or new onset of chronic iridocyclitis and single cases of thyroidal cancer, hypoglossal nerve paralysis, and a severe cytomegalovirus pulmonary infection.

Researchers are evaluating corticosteroid-sparing drugs, including biologic modifiers, in treating JIA-related uveitis (Hashkes and Laxer, 2006).

Glucocorticoid drugs, including dexamethasone, methylprednisolone, cortef, prednisolone, and prednisone, are the most potent of the anti-inflammatory drugs and are used to treat a variety of rheumatic diseases when there has not been a sufficient response to other medications. At times, this class of drugs is employed for a few weeks until other slower acting medications become effective in controlling pain. However, these medications have numerous side effects, including high blood pressure, slowed growth rate, reduced resistance to infection, Cushing's syndrome, mood swings, increased appetite and weight gain, and increased risk of ulcers. Furthermore, these medications cannot be discontinued suddenly and need to be tapered. In addition, a child's own natural glucocorticoids may not be produced adequately after using these drugs for more than 1 month.

Although analgesics, including Tylenol, Panadol, and Ultram, do not relieve inflammation, they do provide pain relief for children with JA. Herbs and supplements have also been utilized and have a significant attraction to parents of those with JIA, according to the Arthritis Foundation (2008). However, research has been minimal and inadequate at this time.

In patients with JIA, inflammation and glucocorticoid treatment influence growth and bone maturation (Bechtold et al., 2009). Longitudinal findings reveal that in JIA patients, changes in total bone mineral density and bone geometry and reductions in muscle mass and force are associated with errant bone maturation. Growth hormone (GH) therapy may influence body composition in a positive way. Clinicians use GH treatment to treat growth retardation in JIA patients who are being treated with glucocorticoids. GH treatments are designed to make growth velocity normal, increase height, bone mineral density, and bone mass. In addition, GH therapy alters bone geometry. JIA patients receiving GH treatments experience increases in muscle mass and bone size despite being on glucocorticoid treatments. Researchers believe that increases in bone size improve bone stability and lowering the risk of fractures. In addition to experiencing increases in muscle mass, JIA patients during GH therapy have stabilized or slightly lowered fat mass.

To improve bone accretion in children with JIA, Stark et al. (2006) conducted a behavioral intervention to increase dietary calcium and total body bone mineral content using a sample of 49 children, aged 4–10 years, with JIA. The researchers demonstrated that the behavioral intervention was effective in increasing calcium intake and total body bone mineral content in children with JIA over a 1-year period.

New investigations are assessing the potential use of anti-interleukin (IL)-1 and anti-IL6 receptor antibody treatment for systemic JIA (Hashkes and Laxer, 2006). New drug investigations and the use of combination therapy, including aggressive induction treatment in the early course of the disease, should improve the results for patients with JIA.

In addition to medications in the treatment of JIA, surgery, soft tissue release, and splints have been employed. Splints help keep the joint in correct position and relieve pain. Furthermore, splints may assist in stretching a joint back to its normal position. Soft tissue release can improve the position of a joint which has been pulled out of line by a contracture, by cutting and repairing the tight tissues caused by the contracture, thus allowing the joint to return to a normal position. Joint replacement surgery is typically only employed with older children and adolescents who have completed their growth and who have badly damaged joints. This form of surgery may reduce pain and/or improve function.

Exercise has been touted as a valuable tool in the treatment of JIA. Therapeutic exercise can assist in restoring lost motion in a joint and make it simpler for children to perform the daily activities of life, including walking, writing, and eating. Furthermore, exercise may also help with morning stiffness. Brewer and Angel (1992) and Janz et al. (1993) both indicated that exercise was essential to children with JIA. Zebracki et al. (2007) also reported that massage and prayer improved psychological functioning in children with JA. More recently, Stephens et al. (2007) compared different exercise therapies. However, Takken et al. (2008) concluded that there was no statistically significant evidence that exercise therapy can improve functional ability, QOL, aerobic capacity, or pain. No detrimental effects of exercise therapy were found in any study reviewed by the authors. Furthermore, studies did not demonstrate that exercise exacerbated JA.

Although sports and recreational activities may not take the place of therapeutic exercise, these may enhance social skills, self-esteem, and confidence. However, contact sports are never recommended, due to the increased risk of injury.

A number of psychotherapeutic interventions have also been utilized with children with JIA. Hagglund et al. (1996) developed a family-based approach for children with this condition. Rapoff (1996) cited the importance of using behavioral contracting strategies to reinforce treatment adherence. Clay et al. (1999) developed a computer-based system, employing an interactive CD-ROM with relaxation skills and coping strategies for pain reduction for treating chronic pain in children and adolescents. Furthermore, cognitive-behavioral therapy (CBT) has been widely used to reduce pain, including relaxation techniques, activity pacing, pleasant activity scheduling, distraction strategies, cognitive restructuring, imagery techniques, hypnotherapy, problem solving, and goal setting.

Ding et al. (2008) investigated the psychological functioning of children with JA and its association with disease activity and disability. The authors found that poor psychological outcome was associated with more severe disability, but not with the level of disease activity.

References

Aasland, A., Novik, T.S., Flato, B., et al. (1998). A multimodal prospective assessment of outcome in families of children with early onset chronic arthritis. Fam Syst Health, 16 (3), 267–280.

Altun, S., Kasapcopur, O., Asian, M., et al. (2004). Is there any relationship between Chlamydophila pneumoniae infection and juvenile idiopathic arthritis? J Med Microbiol, 53 (Pt 8), 787–790.

Anthony, K. (2005). Parental perceptions of child vulnerability in parents of preschool-aged and young children with arthritis: relationships with child adjustment, functional status and health care use. Dissert Abstracts Int, Section B, 65 (7-B), 3696.

Anthony, K., Schanberg, L.E. (2007). Assessment and management of pain syndromes and arthritis in children and adolescents. Rheum Dis Clin North Am, 33 (3), 625–660.

April, K.T., Feldman, D.E., Platte, R.W., et al. (2006). Comparison between children with juvenile idiopathic arthritis and their parents concerning perceived quality of life. Qual Life Res, 15 (4), 655–661.

Arthritis Foundation (2008). Arthritis fact sheet. Retrieved February 21, 2010 from: http://www.arthritis.org/media/newsroom/media-kits/JuvenileArthritisFactSheet.pdf

Aslan, M., Kasapcopur, O., Yasar, H., et al. (2011). Do infections trigger juvenile idiopathic arthritis? Rheumatol Int, Feb;31(2), 215–20. Epub 2009 Dec 13.

Balague, F., Nordin, M., Skovron, M.I., et al. (1994). Low back pain among school children: a field survey. Spinal Disord, 7 (5), 374–379.

Barlow, J.H., et al. (1998). The experience of parenting in the context of juvenile chronic arthritis. Clin Child Psychol Psychiatry, 3 (3), 445–463.

Barlow, J.H., Shaw, K.L., Harrison, K. (1999). Consulting the experts: children's and parents' perceptions of psycho-educational interventions in the context of juvenile chronic arthritis. Health Educ Res, 14 (5), 597–610.

Bechtold, S., Dalla Pozza, R., Schwarz, H.P., et al. (2009). Effects of growth hormone treatment in juvenile idiopathic arthritis: bone and body composition. Horm Res, 72 (Suppl 1), 60–64.

Berkun, Y., Padeh, S. (2010). Environmental factors and the geopidiology of juvenile idiopathic arthritis. Autoimmun Rev, 9 (5), 319–324.

Brewer, E.J., Angel, K.C. (1992). Parenting a child with arthritis: a practical, empathetic guide to help your child live with arthritis. Los Angeles, CA: Lowell House.

Bruns, A., Hilario, M.O., Jennings, F., et al. (2008). Quality of life and impact of the disease on primary caregivers of juvenile idiopathic arthritis patients. Joint Bone Spine, 75 (2), 149–154.

Cassidy, J., Petty, R. (1995). Textbook of pediatric rheumatology (3rd ed.). Philadelphia, PA: W.B. Saunders.

Cavallo, S., Feldman, D.E., Swaine, B., et al. (2009, March 11). Is parental coping associated with quality of life in juvenile idiopathic arthritis? Pediatr Rheumatol Online J. 7, 7.

Clay, D.L., Harper, D.C., Varni, J.W. (1999). Use of emerging technologies to address barriers to treatment research in pediatric chronic pain. Paper presented at the Florida conference on Child Health Psychology, Gainesville, FL.

Connelly, T.W. (2005). Family functioning and hope in children with juvenile rheumatoid arthritis. Am J Matern Child Nurs, 30 (4), 245–250.

Ding, T., Hall, A., Jacobs, K., et al. (2008). Psychological functioning of children and adolescents with juvenile idiopathic arthritis is related to physical disability but not to disease status. Rheumatol, 47 (5), 660–664.

Ellis, J.A., Munro, J.E., Ponsonby, A.L. (2009). Possible environmental determinants of juvenile idiopathic arthritis. Rheumatology, 49 (3), 319–324.

Emery, H. (2004). Pediatric rheumatology: what does the future hold? Arch Phys Med Rehabil, 85 (8), 1382–1384.

Feldmann, R., Weglage, J., Roth, J., et al. (2005). Systemic juvenile rheumatoid arthritis: Cognitive function and social adjustment. Ann Neurol, 58 (4), 605–609.

Forre, O., Smerdel, A. (2002). Genetic epidemiology of juvenile idiopathic arthritis. Scand J Rheum, 31 (3), 123–128.

Frosch, M., Roth, J. (2008). New insights in systemic juvenile idiopathic arthritis – from pathophysiology to treatment. Rheumatology, 47 (2), 121–125.

Hagglund, K.J., Doyle, N.M., Clay, D.L., et al. (1996). A family retreat as a comprehensive intervention for children with arthritis and their families. Arthritis Care Res, 9 (1), 35–41.

Haines, K.A. (2007). Juvenile idiopathic arthritis: therapies in the 21st century. Bull NYU Hosp Jt Dis, 65 (3), 205–211.

Harper, R.P., Kevins, C.A., Talman, R., Spears, R., Hutchens, B., Carlson, D.S., McIntosh, J.E., Ballinger, L.L. (2000). Masticatory function in patients with juvenile rheumatoid arthritis. Pediatric Dent, 79 (9), 1704–1711.

Hashkes, P.J., Laxer, R.M. (2005). Medical treatment of juvenile idiopathic arthritis. J Am Med Assoc, 294 (13), 1671–1684.
Hashkes, P.J., Laxer, R.M. (2006). Update on the medical treatment of juvenile idiopathic arthritis. Curr Rheumatol Rep, 8 (6), 450–458.
Herlin, T. (2002). Juvenile idiopathic arthritis. Ugeskr Laeger, 164 (34), 3941–3946.
Hoff, A.L., Palermo, T.M., Schluchter, M., et al. (2006). Longitudinal relationships of depressive symptoms to pain intensity and further disability among children with disease-related pain. J Pediatr Psychol, 31 (10), 1046–1056.
Hommel, K.A., Chaney, J.M., Wagner, J.L., et al. (2006). Learned helplessness in children and adolescents with juvenile rheumatic disease. J Psychosomatic Res, 60 (1), 73–81.
Jamison, R.N., Walker, L.S. (1992). Illness behavior in children of chronic pain. Psych Med, 22 (4), 329–342.
Janz, J., Harrison, J., Caldwell, T. (1993). Children with special health needs in school: developing and individualized educational program and an individualized health care plan. Paper presented at the Annual Convention of the Council for Exceptional Children, San Antonio, TX.
Kimura, Y., Walco, G.A. (2007). Treatment of chronic pain in pediatric rheumatic disease. Nat Clin Pract Rheumatol, 4, 210–218.
Koutantji, M., Pearce, S.A., Oakley, D.A., et al. (1999). Children in pain: an investigation of selective memory for pain and psychological adjustment. Pain, 81 (3), 237–244.
Lawrence, R.C., Helmick, C.G., Arnett, F.C., et al. (1998). Estimates of the prevalence of arthritis and selected musculoskeletal disorders in the United States. Arthritis Rheum, 41 (5), 778–799.
Lovell, D.J., Rieff, A., Ilowite, N.T., et al. (2008). Safety and efficacy of up to eight years of continuous etanercept therapy in patients with juvenile rheumatoid arthritis. Arthritis Rheum, 58 (5), 1496–1504.
Manuel, J.C. (2001). Risk and resistance factors in the adaptation of mothers of children with juvenile rheumatoid arthritis. J Pediatr Psychol, 26 (4), 237–246.
Margetic, B., Aukst-Margetic, B., Bilic, E., et al. (2005). Depression, anxiety and pain in children with juvenile idiopathic arthritis. Europ Psychiatry, 20 (3), 274–276.
Merlijn, V., Hunfield, J., van der Wouden, J.C., et al. (2003). Psychosocial factors associated with chronic pain in adolescents. Pain, 101 (1–2), 33–43.
Milota, C., Goldberg, M., Goldberg, P., et al. (1991). Count me in: resource manual on disabilities. Minneapolis, MN: PACER Center Inc. Retrieved February 27, 2010 from: http://www.eric.ed.gov/ERICDocs/data/ericdocs2sql/content_storage_01/0000019b/80/3/98/8a.pdf.
Morley, S. (2004). What impact does childhood experience have on the development of chronic pain? In R.H. Dworkin, W.S. Breitbart (Eds.), Psychosocial aspects of pain. Seattle, WA: IASP Press, pp. 57–72.
Nash, A.A., Britto, M.T., Lovell, D.J., et al. (1998). Substance use among adolescents with juvenile rheumatoid arthritis. Arthritis Care Res, 11 (5), 391–396.
Niehues, T., Lankisch, P. (2006). Recommendations for the use of methotrexate in juvenile idiopathic arthritis. Paediatr Drugs, 8 (6), 347–356.
Palermo, T.M., Kiska, R. (2005). Subjective sleep disturbances in adolescents with chronic pain: relationship between functioning and quality of life. J Pain, 6 (3), 201–207.
Pirra, T., Pullukat, R. (2006). Are the children of chronic pain patients more likely to develop pain? Enfance, 58 (1), 20–25.
Pontkaki, I., Gerloni, V., Gattinara, M., et al. (2006). Side effects of anti-TNFalpha therapy in juvenile idiopathic arthritis. Rheumatismo, 58 (1), 31–38.
Rapoff, M.A. (1996). Adherence. In S.T. Wegener, B.L. Belza, E.P. Gall (Eds.), Clinical care in the rheumatic diseases. Atlanta, GA: American College of Rheumatology, pp. 137–140.
Reid, G.J., McGrath, P.J., Lang, B.A. (2005). Parent-child interactions among children with juvenile fibromyalgia, arthritis and healthy controls. Pain, 113 (1–2), 201–210.
Reiter-Purtill, J., Gerhardt, C.A., Vannatta, K., et al. (2003). A controlled longitudinal study of the social functioning of children with juvenile rheumatoid arthritis. J Pediatr Psychol, 28 (1), 17–28.

Riddle, R., Ryser, C.N., Morton, A.A., et al. (2006). The impact of health-related quality of life from non-steroidal anti-inflammatory drugs, methotrexate or steroids in treatment for juvenile idiopathic arthritis. J Pediatr Psychol, 31 (3), 262–271.

Robinson, E.L. (1998). Arthritis (juvenile rheumatoid). In Le.A. Phelps (Ed.), Health related disorders in children and adolescents: a guidebook for understanding and educating. Washington, DC: American Psychological Association, pp. 62–67.

Rossato, L.M., Angelo, M., Silva, C.A. (2007). Care delivery for the child to grow up despite the pain: the family's experience. Rev Lat Am Enfermagem, 15 (4), 556–562.

Sacks, J., Helmick, C., Yao-Hua, L., et al. (2007). Prevalence of and annual ambulatory health care visits for pediatric arthritis and other rheumatologic conditions in the US in 2001–2004. Arthritis Rheum, 57, 1439–1445.

Sallfors, C., Hallberg, L. (2003). A parental perspective on living with a chronically ill child: a qualitative study. Fam Syst Health, 21 (2), 193–204.

Sallfors, C., Hallberg, L., Fasth, A. (2004). Well-being in children with juvenile chronic arthritis. Clin Exp Rheumatol, 22, 125–130.

Sandstrom, M.J., Schanberg, L.E. (2004). Brief report: peer rejection, social behavior and psychological adjustment in children with juvenile rheumatic disease. J Pediatr Psychol, 29 (1), 29–34.

Saurenmann, R.K., Levin, A.V., Feldman, B.M., et al. (2007). Prevalence, risk factors, and outcome of uveitis in juvenile idiopathic arthritis: a long-term follow-up study. Arthritis Rheum, 56 (2), 647–657.

Sawyer, M.G., Carbone, J.A., Whitham, J.N., et al. (2005). The relationship between health-related quality of life, pain and coping strategies in juvenile arthritis: a one-year prospective study. Qual Life Res, 14 (6), 1585–1598.

Schanberg, L.E., Anthony, K.K., Gil, K.M., et al. (2001). Family pain history predicts child health status in children with chronic rheumatoid arthritis. Pediatrics, 108 (3), e47.

Schanberg, L.E., Sandstrom, M.J., Starr, K., et al. (2000). The relationship of daily mood and stressful events in juvenile rheumatic disease. Arthritis Rheum: Arthritis Care Res, 13 (1), 33–41.

Selvaag, A.M., Flato, B., Lien, G., et al. (2003). Measuring health status in early juvenile idiopathic arthritis: determinants and responsiveness of the child health questionnaire. J Rheum, 30 (7), 1602–1610.

Shishov, M., Hendrickson, M., Burgos-Vargas, R., et al. (2007). Systemic features and early prognostic factors in Hispanic and non-Hispanic children from the US and Mexico with systemic juvenile idiopathic arthritis. Clin Exp Rheumatol, 25 (6), 907–914.

Snelling, J. (1990). The role of the family in relation to chronic pain. J Adv Nurs, 15 (7), 771–776.

Stark, L.J., Davis, A.M., Janicke, D.M., et al. (2006). A randomized clinical trial of dietary calcium to improve bone accretion in children with juvenile rheumatoid arthritis. J Pediatr, 148 (4), 501–507.

Stephens, S., Singh-Grewal, D., Bar-Or, O., et al. (2007). Reliability of exercise testing and functional activity questionnaires in children with juvenile diabetes. Arthritis Rheum, 57 (8), 1446–1452.

Takken, T., van Brussel, M., Engelbert, R.H., et al. (2008). Exercise therapy in juvenile idiopathic arthritis. Cochrane Database Syst Rev, Apr 16 (2), CD005954.

Turkel, S., Pao, M. (2007). Late consequences of chronic pediatric illness. Psychiatr Clin North Am, 30 (4), 819–835.

Varni, J.W., Rapoff, M.A., Waldron, S.A., et al. (1996). Chronic pain and emotional distress in children and adolescents. J Dev Behav Pediatr, 17 (3), 154–161.

Wagner, J.L., Chaney, J., Hommel, K., et al. (2003). The influence of parental distress on child depressive symptoms in juvenile rheumatoid arthritis diseases: the moderating effect of illness intrusiveness. J Pediatr Psychol, 28 (7), 453–462.

Wallace, C.A., Lovell, D.J., Giannini, E.H., et al. (2008). Interim report of the trial of early aggressive therapy (TREAT) in JIA Study. Childhood Arthritis and Rheumatology Research Alliance (CARRA). Retrieved on February 22, 2010 from: http://www.arthritis.org/carra-2008.php#TREAT.

Weiss, K.A., Schiaffino, K.M., Illowite, N. (2001). Predictors of sibling relationship characteristics in youth with chronic arthritis. Children's Health Care, 30 (1), 66–67.

Woreta, F., Thorne, J.E., Jabs, D.A., et al. (2007). Risk factors for ocular complications and poor visual acuity at presentation among patients with uveitis associated with juvenile idiopathic arthritis. Am J Ophthalmol, 143 (4), 647–655.

Zebracki, K., Holzman, K., Bitter, K.J., et al. (2007). Use of complementary and alternative medicine and psychological functioning in Latino children with juvenile idiopathic arthritis or arthralgia. J Pediatr Psychol, 32 (8), 1006–1010.

Chapter 13
Infants, Children, and Adolescents Affected by HIV/AIDS

In 2007, about 2 million children under 15 years of age were living with HIV/AIDS around the world (UNAIDS, July 2008). Innovations in treatment have increased the life expectancy of children with HIV and enhanced their quality of life (QOL) (Burns et al., 2008). Sub-Saharan Africa has the greatest number of children under 15 with 1 million, followed by South/Southeast Asia with 140,000, and Latin America with 44,000. In North America, 4,400 children under 15 were living with HIV/AIDS in 2007. Minority children are disproportionately affected by the condition. New drug treatments and voluntary testing have helped to reduce the mortality rate.

HIV-1 is the most prevalent cause of HIV in North America, Europe, Asia, and Africa (http://www.webmd.com). HIV-2 has produced epidemics in West Africa. However, HIV-2 also has been documented in Europe. HIV-2 has a slower disease progression than HIV-1 and the former is less transmissible. Subtypes of HIV-1 differ by geographic area. In the USA, HIV-1 subtype B is the main type. In Africa and Asia, non-B subtypes are especially prevalent. The heterogeneity of subtypes in Europe has been caused by the high transmission rate from Africa to European countries. In addition, in the USA non-B subtype HIV-1 is increasing. Some viral load tests are not sensitive to HIV-1 non-B subtypes.

Among children with HIV, most acquire the virus from their mothers prior to or during birth or via breastfeeding (NIAID, July 2004). Twenty-five percent of pregnant HIV-infected women in the USA who were not getting AZT treatment have transmitted the virus to their babies. Children have been infected through transfusions with HIV-contaminated blood or blood products. In addition, HIV-infected adults have infected children by sexually or physically abusing them.

Mother-to-Child Transmission

Around the world, mother-to-child transmission (MTCT) causes more than an estimated 90% of HIV infections in infants and children (NIAID, July 2004). A majority of these MTCT infections take place in the latter period of pregnancy or during birth. Researchers do not understand exactly how HIV transmission occurs. However, researchers believe that HIV develops in two ways. First, transmission

M.L. Goldstein, S. Morewitz, *Chronic Disorders in Children and Adolescents*,
DOI 10.1007/978-1-4419-9764-7_13,

of the virus may occur when maternal blood enters the fetal circulation. Second, the infant may acquire HIV by mucosal exposure to the virus during labor and delivery. Researchers are not sure about the role of the placenta in MTCT, and this mechanism is under investigation.

Risk of MTCT is substantially greater for mothers who have advanced HIV disease, increased levels of HIV in their bloodstream, or fewer immune system cells, CD4+T cells. Maternal drug use, extensive inflammation of fetal membranes, or a long period between membrane rupture and delivery also significantly increase MTCT. Research has shown that MTCT was almost two times as likely when HIV-infected women gave birth more than 4 h after rupture of the fetal membranes, compared to women who delivered within 4 h of membrane rupture.

Nursing mothers with chronic HIV infection may transmit HIV to their infants through breastfeeding (NIAID, July 2004). Researchers have found that infants have an additional 10–14% risk of MTCT among women with chronic HIV disease. Researchers estimate that one-third to one-half of HIV infections in developing countries occur due to breastfeeding. Safe alternatives to breastfeeding should be used where they are available and financially feasible. However, in developing countries, where safe alternatives to breastfeeding are often not easily accessible, the benefits of breastfeeding in reducing illness and death caused by other infections outweigh the risk of MTCT. In poor countries, to reduce MTCT, the World Health Organization recommends exclusive breastfeeding for 6 months. Mothers should then rapidly wean their babies if replacement feeding is affordable (Harris et al., 2009).

An investigation in 1994 carried out by the Pediatrics AIDS Clinical Trials Group (PACTG) revealed that AZT therapy was effective in reducing the risk of MTCT among HIV-infected women who had very little or no previous antiretroviral (ARV) treatment and CD4+T cell counts above 200/mm^3 (Connor et al., 1994; NIAID, July 2004). Under these circumstances, AZT therapy reduced MTCT risk from 25 to 8%. AZT treatment in this investigation was started in the second or third trimester and was continued during labor. In addition, infants were treated with AZT for 6 weeks following birth. The therapy did not result in any serious side effects in the mothers or infants, and researchers are conducting an extended follow-up of the mothers and infants.

In another investigation, PACTG showed that MTCT for newborn infants could be reduced to 1.5% in HIV-infected women who were treated with ARV therapy and received medical and obstetrical care during pregnancy (NIAID, July 2004). ARV agents lower viral replication and can reduce MTCT by lowering plasma viral load in pregnant women or by providing prophylaxis treatment to their newborns after they have been exposed to HIV (Volmink et al., 2007; Kilewo et al., 2009). In wealthy countries, highly active ARV therapy (HAART) has lowered vertical transmission rates to about 1–2%.

Kilewo et al. (2009) recommends evaluating the effectiveness of prolonged maternal prophylaxis of HAART for preventing MTCT of HIV-1 in breastfeeding mothers who do not need HAART. This treatment strategy should be compared with using postnatal ARV prophylaxis for infants to determine relative cost-effectiveness and safety.

Among HIV-infected adults, combination therapies have been found to be effective (NIAID, July 2004). More research is needed to determine the safety and mechanisms of combination therapies.

Unfortunately, AZT therapy is not accessible in many countries because of the high costs and logistics of following this treatment (NIAID, July 2004). A short-course AZT treatment is much lower. However, this regimen is still too costly in many nations. HIV/AIDS research agencies and international organizations are investigating ways to develop innovative strategies for offering AZT treatments at lower cost by reducing drug prices for developing countries and forming collaborations with the pharmaceutical industry (Volmink et al., 2007). An investigation in 1999 showed that short-course treatment with nevirapine for a breastfeeding population reduced the risk of HIV-1 transmission during the first 14–16 weeks of life by almost 50% compared to AZT (Marseille et al., 1999). A follow-up report showed that these findings remained after 18 months. According to the National Institute of Allergy and Infectious Diseases (NIAID), these results indicate that inexpensive treatments can potentially provide a less expensive alternative for reducing MTCT in developing countries.

Researchers need to assess the effectiveness of HAART in preventing MTCT in terms of both HIV transmission and infant mortality. Homsy et al. (2010), in a study of women on HAART in rural Uganda who delivered one or more infants between March 1, 2003, and January 1, 2007, showed that infants who were breastfed for less than 6 months had a six times greater risk of dying. The infants' risk of mortality was independent of the mothers' CD4+T cell count, maternal marital status, or the mothers' death. The researchers suggest that HIV-infected pregnant women in poor developing countries should be evaluated for HAART eligibility and treated as quickly as possible. Moreover, mothers should be encouraged to breastfeed their infants for at least 6 months after birth.

Other research by the International Perinatal HIV Group has shown that elective caesarian section delivery can lower the risk of vertical transmission of HIV (Riley and Greene, 1999; NIAID, July 2004). However, this procedure is not risk free. An MTCT rate of 2% has been reported when AZT therapy is combined with elective caesarian delivery.

Since a substantial number of MTCT takes place around the time of birth, MTCT risk is based in part on the amount of HIV in the mother's blood (NIAID, July 2004). Drug treatment only around the time of birth may lower NTCT transmission. NIAID is investigating the effectiveness of this treatment approach. Moreover, NIAID is evaluating the efficacy of ARV drugs, microbicides, and other approaches to reduce MTCT risk.

Diagnosis

Clinicians frequently have problems in diagnosing HIV infection in very young children (NIAID, July 2004). Babies, who are infected with HIV, particularly in the first months of life, frequently seem normal. Testing for HIV is not helpful for newborn infants or young infants because all infants born to HIV-infected mothers have antibodies to HIV, which are created by the mother's immune system and cross the placenta to the infant's bloodstream before birth and last up to 18 months. The infants' antibodies represent the mother's but not the infant's HIV infection status.

Researchers have created very accurate blood tests in diagnosing HIV infection in children 6 months of age and younger (NIAID, July 2004). Investigators developed the polymerase chain reaction (PCR), which can find very small amounts of the HIV virus in an infant's blood. Researchers have created another technique that enables clinicians to culture a sample of an infant's blood and determine if it contains HIV. Approximately one-third of infants who develop HIV can be identified at birth by PCR assays or HIV culture procedures. These procedures identify 90% of infants with HIV by 2 months of age and 95% by 3 months of age. Another innovative technique to both RNA and DNA PCR testing relies on dried blood spot specimens. This procedure facilitates easy collection and storage of specimens in different field settings.

HIV Disease Progression and Signs and Symptoms

HIV-infected children tend to exhibit one of two patterns of illness (NIAID, July 2004). Approximately 20% acquire the infection in the first year of life and a majority of children die by age of 4. In the other 80% of HIV-infected children, their rate of disease progression is slower. In many of the children in this latter group, the onset of AIDS symptoms do not occur until the child is school age or an adolescent. According to a European registry of HIV-infected children, 50% with HIV acquired in the perinatal period were alive at age 9.

The NIAID's Women and Infant's Transmission Study (WITS) has demonstrated that risk for a fast rate of disease progression is associated with maternal conditions, such as level of vitamin A, CD4+T-cell counts during pregnancy, infant viral load, and CD4+T-cell counts in the infant's first months of life (NIAID, July 2004). Early aggressive treatments may help infants at risk for this rapid rate of disease progression.

Many HIV-infected children do not gain weight normally or experience normal growth (NIAID, July 2004). They often develop slowly in terms of reaching their milestones related to motor skills and mental development, such as crawling, walking, and talking (Van Rie et al., 2008; Baillieu and Potterton, 2008). With the progression of their HIV disease, many of them acquire neurological problems, such as problems in walking, difficulty in school, seizures, and other symptoms of the brain disorder, HIV encephalopathy.

Van Rie et al. (2008) evaluated the impact of HIV/AIDS on neurodevelopment of preschool-aged children based on a sample of 35 HI-infected, 35 HIV-affected (HIV-unaffected AIDS orphans and HIV-uninfected children whose mothers had AIDS), and 90 control children, aged 18–72 months living in Kinshasa, Democratic Republic of Congo. Sixty percent of the HIV-infected children exhibited substantial delays in cognitive functioning, 29% had major delays in motor skills, 85% had delays in language expression, and 77% showed delays in language comprehension. Compared to control children, HIV-infected children had higher rates of delays. HIV-infected children, aged 18–29 months, exhibited worse functioning. Ninety-one percent had substantial mental delays and 82% demonstrated major delays in motor skills, compared to 46 and 4% in HIV-infected children, aged 30–70 months. Compared to control children, HIV-affected children showed more delays in motor skills and language expression. The investigators concluded that the HIV pandemic's effects go beyond the direct impact of HIV on the central nervous system. Children orphaned by AIDS and HIV-negative children whose mothers had symptomatic AIDS suffered major neurodevelopment delays, although to a lesser extent and in fewer domains than children infected by HIV. The authors found that older HIV-infected children did better because of a survival effect; while only those children with less severe disease survived.

In an investigation of 40 HIV-positive, ARV-naïve children, aged 18–30 months, in Johannesburg, South Africa, Baillieu and Potterton (2008) found that the children were delayed in cognitive functioning by an average of 7.63 months and delayed in motor skill development by an average of 9.65 months. Almost 98% of the children in the sample performed their expected age-based level for motor and cognitive development. Eighty-five percent of the children exhibited gross motor delay and 82.5% had delays in global language. The investigators suggest that disease progression and structural damage to the brain may cause delays in cognitive functioning. They attribute delays in language to neurological disability, delays in cognitive performance, or deprivations related to the environment. The authors suggest that children who suffer delays in gross motor development may occur because of reduced strength or HIV encephalopathy.

HIV-infected children may exhibit delayed motor development because of HIV infection of the central nervous system and the impact of opportunistic infections (OIs) (Ferguson and Jelsma, 2009). In addition, delayed motor functioning may be due to the indirect effects of the children's social environments. In their investigation of motor delay among 51 HIV-infected children (of whom 34 were being treated with ARV therapy) in Cape Town, South Africa, Ferguson and Jelsma (2009) reported that 66.7% of the HIV-infected children exhibited substantial delays in motor development compared with 5.7% in control children. The researchers found an unexpected number of control children exhibited major delayed functioning. The authors recommend monitoring the developmental functioning of HIV-infected children and offering stimulation and therapy to these children. In addition, the researchers recommend stimulation and treatment for uninfected children who are at risk for developmental delays because of their socioeconomic status.

Children with HIV, like adults with the disease, suffer potentially lethal OIs (NIAID, July 2004). HIV is a common cause of hospitalization in HIV-infected children and adolescents. In a study of the acute causes of hospitalization among 301 adolescents in Harare, Zimbabwe, Ferrand et al. (2010) showed that 69% of the HIV-positive adolescents and 19% of the HIV-negative adolescents hospitalized were for infections, with tuberculosis and pneumonia being the most prevalent infections. Twenty-eight percent of the adolescents were hospitalized for heart, lung, or other chronic health problems. Adolescents hospitalized for HIV-related reasons had a higher mortality rate than those hospitalized for non-HIV-related reasons (22 vs. 7%). Advanced HIV disease, pubertal immaturity, and chronic disease were related to higher mortality rates.

In HIV-infected children and adults, the incidence of OIs varies. A parasitic disease, toxoplasmosis, is less frequently occurring among HIV-infected children than among HIV-infected adults (NIAID, July 2004). However, children with HIV have a higher incidence of major bacterial infections than adults with HIV. Preventing OIs reduces disease burden and mortality in HIV-infected children and adolescents. The use of immunizations and chemoprophylaxis should vary depending on the patient's CD+4 cell count (Simpkins et al., 2009).

The leading cause of death in HIV-infected children with AIDS is *Pneumocystis carinii* pneumonia (PCP) (Morrow et al., 2010; NIAID, July 2004). PCP can make breathing increasingly more difficult and frequently causes hospitalization. In children, PCP and cytomegalovirus (CMV) are generally primary infections, while these conditions occur because of the reactivation of latent infections in adults.

During infancy, co-infection with CMV may affect the progression of HIV-1 disease (Slyker et al., 2009). Based on a sample of Kenyan HIV-infected and HIV-exposed but uninfected infants, Slyker et al. (2009) demonstrated that during the first months of life, CMV DNA was detected often. In 90% of HIV-exposed but uninfected infants and 93% of HIV-infected infants CMV DNA was detected by 3 months of age. The investigators found that in the first 1–3 months after detecting the virus, CMV viral loads were highest and then were quickly reduced after 3 months. HIV-infected infants had higher CMV peak viral loads than HIV-exposed but uninfected infants. In HIV-infected infants, CMV DNA was detected in three of the seven surviving infants who were tested between 19 and 21 months after developing the CMV infection. The authors also showed that peak CMV viral loads were positively correlated with peak HIV-1 viral loads. They conclude that CMV co-infection is prevalent in HIV-infected infants in Kenya, and dysfunctional containment of CMV replication is related to HIV-1 infection.

In children with HIV, chronic lung disorders are prevalent (Zar, 2008). These chronic lung conditions include lymphocytic interstitial pneumonitis (LIP), chronic infections, immune reconstitution inflammatory syndrome (IRIS), bronchiectasis, cancers, and interstitial pneumonia. Recurrent or persistent pneumonia may cause chronic lung disorders as a result of bacterial, mycobacterial, viral, fungal, or mixed infections. In areas with high tuberculosis (TB) prevalence, *Mycobacterium tuberculosis* is a major cause of chronic lung disease. HAART reduces incident TB (Martinson et al., 2009). In developing nations, with the increased availability of highly active ARV therapy (HAART), children have experienced an increased incidence of IRIS because of mycobacterial or other infections (Zar, 2008). Children are diagnosed as having chronic lung disease on the basis of chronic symptoms and persistent X-ray changes. However, definitive diagnosis can be problematic because clinical and radiological data often are not specific.

Pitcher et al. (2010) evaluated chest radiographic features of LIP in HIV-infected children and showed that using the Centers for Disease Control and Prevention

(CDC) criteria allowed for diagnosis of at least 75% of children with LIP. They suggest including children with persistent focal pulmonary opacification that is superimposed on diffuse nodularity to enhance the sensitivity of the CDC criteria.

Differentiating LIP from military TB is problematic in HIV-infected children who live in areas with a high prevalence of TB (Zar, 2008). LIP is found more frequently in children with HIV than in adults with HIV (NIAID, July 2004). LIP, like PCP, can impair breathing and frequently leads to hospitalization.

Studies have evaluated the risk factors for bronchiectasis in HIV-1 infected children. Using a retrospective, case–control investigation of 43 HIV-1 infected children with bronchiectasis and 57 controls, Berman et al. (2007) found that HIV-1-infected children with bronchiectasis were more likely to have had recurrent pneumonia, substantial immunosuppression, and LIP than controls.

In HIV-infected children, a yeast infection, severe candidiasis, often occurs (NIAID, July 2004). For example, in an investigation of 65 HIV-infected children and 40 uninfected siblings in Brazil, Cerqueira et al. (2009) demonstrated that oral *Candida* spp. was more prevalent in HIV-infected children than in their uninfected siblings. Candidiasis produces persistent diaper rash and infections in the mouth and throat, making it hard to eat. They found that the lack of HAART and the presence of dentinal carious teeth increase the risk of colonization of *Candida* spp. among these children.

Based on a literature review, dos Santos Pinheiro et al. (2009) found that HAART has significantly reduced the prevalence and severity of oral disease in HIV-infected children. However, they reported that HAART has been linked to an increased rate of oral lesions related to human papillomavirus and has the potential to increase oral squamous cell carcinoma at a later time.

Compared to children without HIV, those with the disease experience the same infections of childhood more often and with greater severity (NIAID, July 2004). HIV-infected children can suffer problems, such as seizures, fever, pneumonia, recurring colds, diarrhea, and dehydration. Opportunistic pathogens cause diarrhea in children with HIV whose disease progresses (NIAID, July 2004). These conditions frequently lead to lengthy hospitalizations and problems in nutrition.

Based on a sample of HIV-infected and uninfected children under 2 years of age, van Eijk et al. (2010) showed that diarrhea was more prevalent in HIV-infected children than uninfected children. However, specific bacterial pathogens were not related to diarrhea. The investigators note that diarrhea reduction methods will help all children and especially HIV-positive children.

Musiime et al. (2009), using a sample of HIV-infected children and uninfected children younger than 5 years of age, showed that *Escherichia coli*, *Salmonella*, and *Shigella* species produce diarrhea in HIV-positive and HIV-negative children. The researchers also found that most of these pathogens were resistant to cotrimoxazole.

In developing countries, many children with HIV/AIDS also have intestinal parasitic infections (Barrett et al., 2008). These infections contribute to the disease burden of children already suffering from HIV/AIDS. *Cryptosporidium parvum* is an intracellular parasite that infects gastrointestinal epithelium and causes diarrhea that is potentially lethal in individuals with AIDS. Based on a 6-year study of the incidence of *C. parvum* enteric infection in a cohort of children with HIV/AIDS, Barboni et al. (2008) discovered that 13.7% of the children had cryptosporidiosis. In 23% of the patients, mild or moderate eosinophilia was documented other intestinal parasites were recorded in 11 children.

Using a sample of 95 HIV-infected children and 87 uninfected children in Thailand, Wanachiwanawin et al. (2002) found that 25.3% of the HIV-infected children and 14.9% of the uninfected children with diarrhea had intestinal microsporidiosis. The investigators also demonstrated that *C. parvum* is a prevalent co-infective parasite, and pneumonia was the most prevalent concurrent disease in children with intestinal microsporidiosis. The authors conclude that in HIV-infected children and HIV-uninfected children with diarrhea, intestinal microsporidiosis is a significant health problem.

HIV-infected children are at increased risk of suffering malnutrition. For example, Wanachiwanawin et al. (2002) found that in HIV-infected children, malnutrition was more prevalent than in uninfected children. HIV-infected children with malnutrition have higher mortality rates than HIV-uninfected children (Fergusson and Tomkins, 2009). Based on an analysis of 17 studies of HIV prevalence and mortality in children being treated for severe acute malnutrition (SAM) in sub-Sahara Africa, Fergusson and Tomkins (2009) discovered that 30.4% of HIV-infected children had a greater likelihood of dying than HIV-uninfected children (8.4%). The mortality of HIV-infected children with SAM did not differ based on whether they were treated in community-based therapeutic care programs or in an inpatient nutrition rehabilitation unit. The authors found that in sub-Saharan Africa, HIV is prevalent in children with SAM, and these children face a substantial risk of mortality.

Treatment

Although general treatment principles are the same, therapy for infants, children, and adolescents with HIV differs in a number of ways from treatment for adults with the disease (NIAID, July 2004). Clinicians treating infants, children, and adolescents must take into account age-associated factors such as CD4+T-cell counts and drug metabolism. Clinicians should follow special formulations and therapy regimens based on whether their patients are infants, children, or adolescents. Pediatric HIV/AIDS treatment, like the therapy for infected adults, involves using powerful combinations of ARV drugs to suppress viral replication.

The use of HAART has substantially altered the natural history of HIV infection and organ-specific diseases in children (Guillén et al., 2010). Based on an observational investigation of 366 vertically HIV-infected children followed from 1990 to 2006, Guillén et al. (2010) reported that from 1996 to 2006, the children in the sample had a progressive increase in CD4+T count and reduction in HIV viral load. The children exhibited a reduction in mortality rates, AIDS, OIs, and organ-specific conditions, such as wasting syndrome, thrombocytopenia, LIP, and HIV-related encephalopathy in the 1997–1999 and 2000–2006 time periods.

Morrow et al. (2010) have analyzed obstacles in reducing PCP incidence. In their study of PCP in South African children, the investigators note that underutilization of the MTCT prevention programs and failure to use trimethoprim–sulfamethoxazole prophylaxis impede progress in reducing PCP incidence.

Researchers are focusing on both the creation of new ARV agents and ways to most effectively use existing therapies in developing nations (NIAID, July 2004). The research efforts focus on the most effective initial treatments, the conditions under which ineffective treatments should be altered, and treatments for children with advanced HIV/AIDS. In addition, researchers are evaluating the long-term benefits of these ARV therapies and the potential adverse effects of these treatments.

Treatment of chronic lung disease in HIV-infected children includes treatment for specific infections, pulmonary clearance procedures, and corticosteroid therapy for children with LIP who are hypoxic or who have airway compression from tuberculous nodes and HAART (Zar, 2008). Adjustments in drug regimens need to be made for children who are receiving TB treatment and HAART so that drug interactions are reduced and drug efficacy is achieved. Prevention of chronic lung disorders includes immunization, chemoprophylaxis, and micronutrient supplements. Chronic lung disorders may be prevented through the early initiation of HAART.

Investigators have evaluated the effectiveness of intravitreous ganciclovir in the treatment of CMV in HIV-infected children. Using a sample of 45 HIV-infected children, Surachatkumtonekul et al. (2008) showed that 13% of the children, aged 2–12 years, had CMV retinitis. All of the CMV retinitis lesions consisted of retinal hemorrhage and exudates lesions and occurred in the posterior pole. Three children had bilateral CMV retinitis. Four children were injected with intravitreous ganciclovir and each patient received injections an average of 5.6 times. The investigators showed that CMV retinitis lesions improved in every eye. In four eyes, visual acuity remained stable. However, endophthalmitis occurred in one eye a few days after the intravitrous ganciclovir injection. The researchers conclude that CMV retinitis is prevalent, and intravitreous ganciclovir can be an effective treatment. However, the therapy may lead to complications. The authors recommend the use of this therapy in settings with limited resources.

HAART enhances the immune status of HIV-infected patients, enabling them to minimize the potentially fatal complications of diarrhea and co-infection with *C. parvum* (Barboni et al., 2008).

Family members of HIV-infected individuals may be at increased risk of acquiring enteric parasites by living in close contact with their HIV-infected family members. A study by Raccurt et al. (2006) revealed that enteric parasites were less prevalent in HIV-infected patients who were under medical treatment than in their uninfected family members. Detecting and treating intestinal parasites in family members living in close proximity to HIV-infected individuals and teaching the family members the need for personal hygiene can maintain the health of HIV/AIDS patients and their family members.

Children with HIV/AIDS who live in residential facilities that closely monitor their personal hygiene and environmental conditions may help to control their risk of opportunistic infections. In a study of 41 HIV-infected children who lived in 2 institutions in Jamaica, Barrett et al. (2008) demonstrated that no opportunistic intestinal parasites were documented in the patients. In the sample, non-opportunistic parasites were found, including *Giardia lamblia* (12.2%) and *Ascaris lumbricoides* (2.4%). The authors conclude that close monitoring of the children's personal hygiene and environmental conditions may significantly reduce their risk for intestinal parasites.

Adherence to Antiretroviral Treatment in HIV-Infected Children

Adherence to ARV therapy is difficult to follow because of the complexity and toxicity of the regimens (Mellins et al., 2004). Using a sample of 75 HIV-infected children aged 3–13 years and their primary caregivers, Mellins et al. (2004) evaluated the possible effects of child psychosocial issues and caregiver/family conditions on adherence to ARV treatment. They discovered that 40% of the primary caregivers and 56% of the children reported missed doses of AR drugs in the previous month. The authors discovered that poorer parent–child communication, increased caregiver stress, less disclosure about the child's HIV status, and lower quality of life (QOL) predicted non-adherence to ARV treatment. The investigators recommend addressing developmental, psychosocial, and family problems to enhance adherence to ARV therapy.

Brackis-Cott et al. (2003) evaluated the views of HIV health-care providers regarding children's adherence to ARV. In their qualitative study, the health-care practitioners believed that limited therapy options were the greatest obstacle to ARV treatment adherence. The medical providers noted that a majority of HIV-infected children must follow complicated regimens that become more complex over time, making it difficult to achieve adherence. Clinicians were able to identify effective communication practices, but were unable to implement these practices in a consistent fashion. The practitioners report that the families of their patients face a variety of problems, including low socioeconomic status, psychosocial difficulties, substance abuse, and disclosure problems. The medical providers indicate that adherence to ARV treatment is an ongoing issue that is directly influenced by family problems.

Transitioning the Health Care of HIV-Infected Adolescents from Pediatrics to Internal Medicine

With the increased survival rate of children with HIV, adolescents must successfully transition medical care from pediatrics to internal medicine. Using qualitative interviews with adolescents with HIV, parents, and pediatric HIV clinicians, Vijayan et al. (2009) evaluated obstacles to HIV care and difficulties in transitioning care from pediatrics to internal medicine. The interview findings revealed that the stigma of having HIV, poor adherence to ARV treatment, adolescent sexuality, and poorly integrated social environments were major obstacles to effective HIV treatment. In terms of obstacles to transitioning care, the interview data showed that the stigma of HIV caused families to have negative perceptions and experiences that reduced their interest in contacting new HIV clinicians. In addition, pediatric HIV clinicians were concerned that internal medicine providers would require that their adolescent patients demonstrate too much independence. The interview findings also revealed that adolescents, caregivers, and clinicians worked together in a family-like relationship and it would be difficult to break up this relationship. The authors recommend developing effective transitioning programs based on an understanding the factors that impede pediatric HIV care and transitioning care.

Psychosocial Functioning and Quality of Life

The transition of HIV from an acute, terminal illness to a subacute, chronic illness has major consequences for HIV-infected children and their families (Brown et al., 2000). As HIV-infected children and adolescents live longer, reaching developmental milestones and accessing educational and social services will take on greater significance than in the past.

As children with HIV reach adolescence, researchers are increasingly evaluating factors that affect their QOL. HIV directly affects children's neurological, cognitive, and psychological functioning, which can lead to impairment in family, social, and school functioning. In addition, the disease often impairs children's social support mechanisms, making it very difficult for them to reach their full social potential (Steele et al., 2007). HIV-infected children have an increased likelihood of experiencing the adverse effects of parental illness and death and stigma from having HIV. Moreover, children with HIV must follow a complex therapy regimen for the rest of their lives.

The severity of HIV disease and the type of ARV therapy may influence physical, cognitive, psychosocial, family, and school functioning and QOL in children and adolescents (Lee et al., 2006; Storm et al., 2005). Martin et al. (2006) analyzed cognitive functioning in 41 school-age children with vertically acquired HIV infection who were treated with HAART. They demonstrated that children with minimal to moderate computed tomography (CT) scan abnormalities had lower composite scores on cognitive functioning and five subtests, especially impaired executive functions compared to children with normal CT scans. Children who had CD4+ counts less than or equal to 500 had lower scores on subtests that measure processing speed. Viral load did not predict cognitive functioning. The investigators suggest that HIV-infected children who are receiving HAART continue to face the possibility of acquiring central nervous system problems. In addition, the authors recommend assessing the neuropsychological status of children who have CD+4 counts less than or equal to 500.

Based on cross-sectional data for 940 children, aged 5–18 years, from the Pediatrics AIDS Clinical Trials Group Late Outcomes Protocol 219, Storm et al.

(2005) demonstrated that higher CD+4 cell counts, higher height for age growth, and absence of AIDS at the start of the study predicted fewer social/school impairments and improved HIV symptom status. Almost 50% of the HIV-infected children had at least some impairment in physical functioning. Thirty-eight percent of the children suffered one or more physical symptoms that were at least moderately distressing. Children reported more frequent impairments in energy-demanding activities (46%) than in basic activities of daily living (32%). Twenty-three percent of the children in the sample had extreme scores on the Behavior Problems Index, which are similar to children with chronic diseases and children who are socially and economically disadvantaged. Fifty-eight percent of the children indicated that they had one or more disabilities in social/school functioning.

Using data from the Pediatrics AIDS Clinical Trial Group Protocol 219 C Team, Lee et al. (2006) showed that HIV infection predicted lower functioning in children, 6 months to 4 years of age, and in children, aged 5–11 years, HIV disease was associated with poor health perceptions, physical resilience, and worse physical and social functioning. However, uninfected children, aged 5–11 years, exhibited worse psychological functioning. Among HIV-infected children and adolescents, those who had not received ARV treatment had poorer health perceptions. Moreover, HIV-infected adolescents who were not treated with ARV therapy exhibited worse physical symptoms.

Based on a sample of infected and uninfected children, aged 6–11 years, Grover et al. (2007) discovered that 80.7% of primary caregivers of infected children reported that their child had behavior problems compared with 18.3% of the controls.

Uninfected adolescents of HIV-infected mothers also may be at increased risk for engaging in delinquent behaviors because of the stigma of having an HIV-infected mother. Murphy et al. (2006) evaluated the extent and impact of HIV-related stigma among 118 HIV-positive mothers and their uninfected children and adolescents to whom the mother's HIV status previously had been disclosed. Adolescents who had high levels of stigma because of their mother's HIV status had a greater probability of engaging in delinquent activities compared to those with low levels of HIV-associated stigma.

Mellins et al. (2009) evaluated the rates and types of psychiatric disorders in HIV+ youths and HIV-exposed, but uninfected youths. Based on a sample of 340 youths aged 9–16 years and their caregivers, the investigators discovered that anxiety disorders, including social phobia, separation anxiety, and panic disorder, were the most prevalent diagnoses in both groups. Twenty-five percent of the youths had a behavior disorder, e.g., attention deficit hyperactivity disorder (ADHD), oppositional defiant disorder, and conduct disorder, and ADHD was the most prevalent behavior problem. Youths who were HIV+ had a higher prevalence of ADHD. Mood disorder and substance-abuse disorder were prevalent in 7 and 4% of the youths, respectively. Caregiver type and HIV status predicted HIV status in children and their mental health conditions.

An earlier investigation by Mellins et al. (2003) compared children with perinatal-acquired HIV and uninfected children and did not find an association between either HIV status or prenatal drug exposure and behavioral problems (Mellins et al., 2003). The authors showed that demographic factors were the best predictors of increased behavior problems.

In a chart review of 85 school-age children with perinatally acquired HIV, Mialky et al. (2001) discovered that 40% had an undetectable viral load. Eighty-five percent of the children were in public school and 76.5% were in their age-appropriate grade level. Fifty-three percent had to have some special educational services during school.

The type of ARV therapy may influence functioning and QOL in children and adolescents. However, Storm et al. (2005) evaluated the use of protease inhibitor combination therapy (PI therapy) in treating children with perinatally acquired HIV. They discovered that the QOL among children who were treated with PI therapy did not differ significantly from the QOL of children who received non-PI therapy. The investigators did not find any direct negative impact of PI treatment on QOL except for a higher rate of diarrhea. The results suggest that the use of PI combination treatments to prevent or slow disease progression and increase CD4+ cell counts and height growth can enhance QOL in HIV-infected children.

Another study from the Pediatrics AIDS Clinical Trial Group Protocol 219C Team revealed that adolescents who were treated with PI plus nonnucleoside reverse transcriptase inhibitor-containing treatment had poorer physical symptoms than adolescents who were treated with PI therapy (Lee et al., 2006).

Families are confronted with difficult question about whether they should disclose to their children about their condition (Steele et al., 2007). In addition, families often must decide whether to disclose their condition to other family members and others.

Mialky et al. (2001), in their study of school-age children with perinatally acquired HIV, reported that 43% of the children had been told their HIV status and disclosure occurred at the mean age of 9 years. In 23% of the cases, school staff had been notified about the child's HIV diagnosis.

Children who are disclosed to about their HIV status may exhibit better psychosocial functioning. Disclosure to individuals outside the family also may facilitate positive psychosocial functioning. However, more research needs to be conducted to determine the long-term impact of disclosures on the QOL of children.

Based on a longitudinal investigation of 395 children, 5 years of age and older, with perinatally acquired HIV youth, from the Pediatrics AIDS Clinical Trials Group, Butler et al. (2009) did not find any significant differences between pre-disclosure and post-disclosure QOL. The authors recommend that at an appropriate time, HIV disclosure should be made.

Family and Community Difficulties

HIV-infected children will continue to be adversely impacted by non-HIV conditions, such as poverty, insufficient medical care, and inadequate social support (Brown et al., 2000). Children orphaned by HIV/AIDS face substantial impairment in family, psychosocial, educational, and economic functioning. An estimated 2.3 million children in South Africa will be orphaned by HIV/AIDS by 2020 (Cluver and Gardner, 2007). Researchers are analyzing risk and protective factors for the psychosocial well-being of these children. A qualitative investigation of orphaned children, caregivers of orphaned children, and social services professionals showed that risk and protective factors for psychosocial well-being of children orphaned by HIV/AIDS include bereavement, level of family functioning, poverty, level of social support, access to educational services, and perceived stigma (Cluver and Gardner, 2007).

HIV-associated stigma can adversely impact the psychosocial well-being of HIV-infected mothers. In Murphy et al.'s (2006) study, mothers who reported a high degree of HIV-related stigma were more likely to have lower levels of physical and psychosocial functioning. Mothers with higher levels of HIV-associated stigma also had a greater likelihood of having more symptoms of depression. Children's level of stigma did not predict their levels of depression.

According to the China Ministry of Health, in 2007, at least 100,000 children in China were orphaned by AIDS (Zhao et al., 2007). Between 2007 and 2012, the UNICEF China Office estimates that additional 150,000–250,000 children will be orphaned by the disease. Zhao et al. (2007) note that little is known about the psychosocial and demographic characteristics of these children, effective ways to reduce grief, and appropriate care arrangements for these orphans. Based on a review of secondary data, scientific reports, government and non-government reports, and media accounts, Zhao et al. (2007) concluded that Chinese children who are orphaned by AIDS have very stressful lives. They often experience psychosocial difficulties and are unable to meet their basic needs such as getting sufficient food, education, and medical services. The authors recommend that health promotion programs and research efforts should focus on improving the psychosocial well-being of these children, who are especially susceptible to the adverse impact of parental death.

Social Support

Effective social support can help HIV-infected children and adolescents better cope with the stresses and stigma of the disease. Social support is especially critical for children and adolescents living with HIV/AIDS because the disease often disrupts essential social support systems (Steele et al., 2007). Social support helps the affected children and adolescents deal with the stigma of the disease and different psychosocial, school, family, financial, and community problems associated with this disease. Social support helps HIV-infected children and adolescents cope with the adverse effects of HIV disclosure and promotes adherence to the complex ARV regimen.

Social support is also essential for children affected by HIV/AIDS. Social support helps children cope with the psychosocial trauma of being orphaned by parents who died of AIDS or who are living with the disease. Children and adolescents orphaned by AIDS vary in their psychosocial well-being. In a study of AIDS orphans in rural China, Zhao et al. (2010) showed that children who had a healthy surviving parent had higher levels of social support and less depressive symptoms, loneliness, and post-traumatic stress disorder symptoms than children who had a sick surviving parent.

In their review of the literature, King et al. (2009) showed that interventions designed for improving the psychosocial well-being of children affected by HIV/AIDS are based on anecdotal evidence, descriptive research, and situational analyses. As a result, current practices do not offer a basis for developing effective psychosocial interventions for children impacted by HIV/AIDS. The authors recommend more collaboration between program developers and researchers to develop evidence-based interventions.

Social support and psychosocial interventions are also needed for the caregivers of children and adolescents living with HIV (Hansell et al., 1998). Based on an investigation of 70 primary caregivers of children living with HIV/AIDS, Hansell et al. (1998) revealed that seronegative caregivers (foster parents and extended members of the family) of children with HIV/AIDS face substantial stress in caring for these children. In this study, seronegative caregivers who received monthly social support-enhancing interventions were aided by these social support activities.

Prevention of HIV/AIDS and Sexually Transmitted Infections in Children and Adolescents

In the USA and globally, adolescents are at increased risk of developing sennxually transmitted diseases (STDs) and HIV. Therefore, HIV and STD reduction interventions are essential. Researchers have evaluated the characteristics and efficacy of these interventions and have analyzed the risk factors and protective factors related to acquiring HIV and STDs.

In a review of adolescent sexual risk-reduction programs, Robin et al. (2004) found that most of the investigations used randomized controlled methods and relied on delayed follow-up procedures. Researchers employed a variety of outcome measures, including when sexual intercourse is initiated, use of contraceptives, and frequency of sexual intercourse. The number of sessions in these interventions ranged from 1 to 80. A majority of programs employed adult facilitators. The programs often were designed to build skills in sexual communication, making decisions, and solving problems. Arts and craft programs, school councils, and community service learning settings were used to deliver the program content.

HIV/AIDS intervention programs often involve the collaboration between researchers and community residents. For example, Baptiste et al. (2005) describe the Chicago HIV Prevention and Adolescent Mental Health Project (CHAMP), which consisted of a collaboration between researchers and low-income, inner city residents to design and implement HIV/AIDS prevention programs for African-American youth.

In a review of the literature on the efficacy of HIV sexual risk reduction interventions, Johnson et al. (2003) showed that intensive behavioral programs lowered sexual HIV risk. Programs were effective because they enhanced the acquisition of skills, improved communication of sexual issues, enhanced condom use, and reduced the onset of sexual activity or the number of sexual partners.

Jemmott et al. (2005) assessed the effectiveness of a skill-based HIV/STD intervention in lowering self-reported unprotected sex among Latino and African-American adolescents in the USA. The investigators demonstrated that a skill-based HIV/STD intervention (consisting of information and skill training in safe sex practices) lowered risky sexual behaviors and the rate of STDs among Latino and African-American adolescents.

Kirby et al. (2004) evaluated the impact of the "Safer Choices" intervention on sexual behaviors of different sub-groups of high school students. The "Safer Choices" intervention seeks to lower the rate of unprotected sex by delaying the start of sexual activity, lowering its frequency, or increasing use of condoms. The components of the intervention comprise school organization, intense training with staff development, peer resources, parent education, and linkages between community and school. The investigators showed that "Safer Choice" lowered one or more indicators of risky sexual behavior among all high school students in the study. The program was particularly successful in reducing sexual risk behaviors among males, Latina/Latino, and young people who participate in unprotected sex.

Using a sample of 715 African-American adolescent females seeking sexual health services in Atlanta, Georgia, DiClemente et al. (2009) found that the sexual risk-reduction intervention resulted in a lower rate of chlamydial infection or recurrent chlamydial infection. In addition, adolescent females in the intervention had an increased percentage of condom-protected sex acts in the 60 days before the follow-up evaluations.

Kirby et al. (2006) reviewed school-based sex education and HIV education interventions in developing countries and found that most of the interventions lowered risky sexual behaviors. The authors noted that before school-based interventions can be recommended, they require rigorous evaluations.

In another investigation, researchers conducted a process evaluation of a school-based HIV/AIDS intervention in South Africa (Mukoma et al., 2009). Based on a study of 13 schools in the intervention group and 13 in the control group, the investigators discovered that some teachers adhered more to the intervention protocol than other teachers. The teachers' adherence to the protocol was affected by various individual factors and organizational characteristics. Those teachers who followed the current outcome-oriented educational practices, teacher training, having teacher manuals with detailed instruction about the lessons and activities, regular monitoring and support for teachers, and student interest in the lessons enhanced implementation of the intervention. Obstacles to implementation included large classes, having too many program activities, teacher opposition and lack of experience in using the program methods, teacher turnover, and having students who gave a low priority to life orientation.

Other researchers have assessed how different factors may influence the risk of HIV/AIDS among children and adolescent. Researchers have analyzed how adolescents' knowledge, perception and attitudes toward sexually transmitted infections (STIs), HIV/AIDS, safer sex, and sex education can affect adolescents' risk for STIs and HIV/AIDS (Anwar et al., 2010; East et al., 2007; McManus and Dhar, 2008).

Anwar et al. (2010) evaluated school students' knowledge about STIs in Pulau Pinang, Malaysia. Using a sample of 1,139 students, aged 15–20 years, the investigators showed that 10.6% of the sample indicated that they had never heard about STIs even though about 12.6% of the sample reported having had sexual experience. The researchers recommend the development of interventions that emphasize the association between STIs and risk of HIV/AIDS.

Based on a review of the literature on condom use in heterosexual adolescents and young people, East et al. (2007) showed that lack of knowledge about the prevalence of STIs, ambiguity about the use of contraception and safer sex practices, and the obstacles facing young women in negotiating safer sex practices are obstacles to condom use.

Rice et al. (2007), using a sample of 183 newly homeless youth, showed that the presence of peers who went to school, had jobs, and had good relations with their families reduced HIV risk behaviors among these newly homeless youth. Having more friends at baseline who commit theft, had suffered a drug overdose, had been arrested, or were a gang member increased the homeless youths' HIV risk behaviors.

Peer norms regarding sexual activity may affect HIV/AIDs risk among children and adolescents. In an investigation of 339 mainly ethnic minority youths, aged 9–16 who were perinatally exposed to HIV (61% HIV+), Bauermeister et al. (2009) discovered that young people were more likely to report participating in sexual activity if they reported having a greater number of their peers believe that sexually active boys were popular or cool.

Other investigations have assessed the influence of family factors on HIV/AIDS risks among children and adolescents. Using a longitudinal study of sexual risk behavior among adolescents of HIV-positive and HIV-negative drug-abusing or drug-dependent fathers, Brook et al. (2010) discovered that greater perceived discrimination and victimization, impaired father–child relations, increased adolescent social dysfunction and substance use predicted sexual risk behaviors.

References

Anwar, M., Sulaiman, S.A., Ahmadi, K., et al. (2010, January 30). Awareness of school students on sexually transmitted infections (STIs) and their sexual behavior: a cross-sectional study conducted in Pulau Pinang, Malaysia. BMC Public Health, 10, 47.

Baillieu, N., Potterton, J. (2008). The extent of delay of language, motor, and cognitive development in HIV-positive infants. J Neurol Phys Ther, 32 (3), 118–121.

Baptiste, D.R., Paikoff, R.L., McKay, M.M., et al. (2005). Collaborating with an urban community to develop an HIV and AIDS prevention program for black youth and families. Behav Modif, 29 (2), 370–416.

Barboni, G., Candi, M., Inés Villacé, M. (2008). Intestinal cryptosporidiosis in HIV infected children. Medicina (B Aires), 68 (3), 213–218.

Barrett, D.M., Steel-Duncan, J., Christie, C.D. (2008, June). Absence of opportunistic parasitic infestations in children living with HIV/AIDS in children's homes in Jamaica: pilot investigations. West Indian Med J, 57 (3), 253–256.

Bauermeister, J.A., Elkington, K., Brackis-Cott, E., et al. (2009). Sexual behavior and perceived peer norms: comparing perinatally HIV-infected and HIV-infected youth. J Youth Adolesc, 38 (8), 1110–1122.

Berman, D.M., Mafut, D., Djokic, B., et al. (2007, October). Risk factors for the development of bronchiectasis in HIV-infected children. Pediatr Pulmonol, 42 (10), 871–875.

Brackis-Cott, E., Mellins, C.A., Abrams, E., et al. (2003). Pediatric HIV medication adherence: the views of medical providers from two primary care programs. J Pediatr Health Care, 17 (5), 252–260.

Brook, D.W., Brook, J.S., Rubenstone, E., et al. (2010). A longitudinal study of sexual risk behavior among the adolescent children of HIV-positive and HIV-negative drug-abusing fathers. J Adolesc Health, 46 (3), 224–231.

Brown, L.K., Lourie, K.J., Pao, M. (2000). Children and adolescents living with HIV and AIDS: a review. J Child Psychol Psychiatry, 41 (1), 81–96.

Burns, S., Hernandez-Reif, M., Jessee, P. (2008). A review of pediatric HIV effects on neurocognitive development. Issues Compr Pediatr Nurs, 31 (3), 107–121.

Butler, A.M., Williams, P.L., Howland, L.C., et al. (2009). Impact of disclosure of HIV infection on health-related quality of life among children and adolescents with HIV infection. Pediatrics, 123 (3), 935–943.

Cerqueira, D.F., Portela, M.B., Soares, R.M. (2009, July–August). Comparison of techniques to evaluate the quantification of Candida spp. in HIV-infected children. Gen Dent, 57 (4), 438–441.

Cluver, L., Gardner, F. (2007). Risk and protective factors for psychological well-being of children orphaned by AIDS in Cape Town: a qualitative study of children and caregivers' perspectives. AIDS Care, 19 (3), 318–325.

Connor, E.M., Sperling, R.S., Gelber, R., et al. (1994, November 3). Reduction of maternal-infant transmission of human immunodeficiency virus type 1 with zidovudine treatment. Pediatric AIDS Clinical Trials Group Protocol 076 Study Group. N Engl J Med, 331 (18), 1173–1180.

DiClemente, R.J., Wingood, G.M., Rose, E.S., et al. (2009). Efficacy of sexually transmitted disease/human immunodeficiency virus sexual risk-reduction intervention for African American adolescent females seeking sexual health services: a randomized controlled trial. Arch Pediatr Adolesc Med, 163 (12), 1112–1121.

dos Santos Pinheiro, R., França, T.T., Ribeiro, C.M. (2009, September). Oral manifestations in human immunodeficiency virus infected children in highly active antiretroviral therapy era. J Oral Pathol Med, 38 (8), 613–622.

East, L., Jackson, D., O'Brien, L., et al. (2007). Use of the male condom by heterosexual adolescents and young people: literature review. J Adv Nurs, 59 (2), 103–110.

Ferguson, G., Jelsma, J. (2009). The prevalence of motor delay among HIV infected children living in Cape Town, South Africa. Int J Rehabil Res, 32 (2), 108–114.

Fergusson, P., Tomkins, A. (2009). HIV prevalence and mortality among children undergoing treatment for severe acute malnutrition in sub-Saharan Africa: a systematic review and meta-analysis. Trans R Soc Trop Med Hyg, 103 (6), 541–548.

Ferrand, R.A., Bandason, T., Musvaire, P., et al. (2010, February 2). Causes of acute hospitalization in adolescence: Burden and spectrum of HIV-related morbidity in a country with an early-onset and severe HIV epidemic: a prospective survey. PLoS Med, 7 (2), e1000178.

Grover, G., Pensi, T., Banerjee, T. (2007). Behavioural disorders in 6-11-year-old, HIV-infected Indian children. Ann Trop Paediatr, 27 (3), 215–224.

Guillén, S., García San Miguel, L., Resino, S. (2010, April). Opportunistic infections and organ-specific diseases in HIV-1-infected children: a cohort study (1990–2006). HIV Med, 11 (4), 245–252.

Hansell, P.S., Hughes, C.B., Caliandro, G., et al. (1998). The effect of a social support boosting intervention on stress, coping, and social support in caregivers of children with HIV/AIDS. Nurs Res, 47 (2), 79–86.

Harris, J.R., Greene, S.K., Thomas, T.K., et al. (2009, October 15). Effect of a point-of-use water treatment and safe water storage intervention on diarrhea in infants of HIV-infected mothers. J Infect Dis, 200 (8), 1186–1193.

Homsy, J., Moore, D., Barasa, A., et al. (2010, January 1). Breastfeeding, mother-to-child HIV transmission, and mortality among infants born to HIV-Infected women on highly active antiretroviral therapy in rural Uganda. J Acquir Immune Defic Syndr, 53 (1), 28–35.

Jemmott, J.B., Jemmott, L.S., Braverman, P.K., et al. (2005). HIV/STD risk reduction interventions for African American and Latino adolescent girls at an adolescent medicine clinic: a randomized controlled trial. Arch Pediatr Adolesc Med, 159 (5), 440–449.

Johnson, B.T., Carey, M.P., Marsh, K.L., et al. (2003). Interventions to reduce sexual risk for the human immunodeficiency virus in adolescents, 1985–2000: a research synthesis. Arch Pediatr Adolesc Med, 157 (4), 381–388.

King, E., De Silva, M., Stein, A., etal. (2009, April 15). Interventions for improving the psychosocial well-being of children affected by HIV and AIDS. Cochrane Database Syst Rev, 2, CD006733.

Kilewo, C., Karlsson, K., Ngarina, M., et al. (2009, November 1). Prevention of mother-to-child transmission of HIV-1 through breastfeeding by treating mothers with triple antiretroviral therapy in Dar es Salaam, Tanzania: the Mitra Plus study. J Acquir Immune Defic Syndr, 52 (3), 406–416.

Kirby, D.B., Baumler, E., Coyle, K.K., et al. (2004). The "Safer Choices" intervention: its impact on the sexual behaviors of different subgroups of high school students. J Adolesc Health, 35 (6), 442–452.

Kirby, D., Obasi, A., Laris, B.A. (2006). The effectiveness of sex education and HIV education interventions in schools in developing countries. World Health Organ Tech Rep Ser, 938, 103–150.

Lee, G.M., Gortmaker, S.L., McIntosh, K., et al. (2006). Quality of life for children and adolescents: impact of HIV infection and antiretroviral treatment. Pediatrics, 117 (2), 273–283.

Marseille, E., Kahn, J.G., Mmiro, F., et al. (1999, September 4). Cost effectiveness of single-dose nevirapine regimen for mothers and babies to decrease vertical HIV-1 transmission in sub-Saharan Africa. Lancet, 354 (9181), 803–809.

Martin, S.C., Wolters, P.L., Toledo-Tamula, M.A., et al. (2006). Cognitive functioning in school-aged children with vertically acquired HIV infection being treated with highly active antiretroviral therapy (HAART). Dev Neuropsychol, 30 (2), 633–657.

Martinson, N.A., Moultrie, H., van Niekerk, R., et al. (2009). HAART and risk of tuberculosis in HIV-infected South African children: a multi-site retrospective cohort. Int J Tuberc Lung Dis, 13 (7), 862–867.

McManus, A., Dhar, L. (2008, July 23). Study of knowledge, perception and attitude of adolescent girls towards STIs/HIV, safer sex and sex education: (a cross sectional survey of urban adolescent school girls in South Delhi, India. BMC Womens Health, 8, 12.**

Mellins, C.A., Brackis-Cott, E., Dolezal, C., et al. (2004). The role of psychosocial and family factors in adherence to antiretroviral treatment in human immunodeficiency virus-infected children. Pediatr Infect Dis J, 23 (11), 1035–1041.

Mellins, C.A., Elkington, K.S., Bauermeister, J.A., et al. (2009). Sexual and drug use behavior in perinatally HIV-infected youth: mental health and family influences. J Am Acad Child Adolesc Psychiatry, 48 (8), 810–819.

Mellins, C.A., Smith, R., O'Driscoll, P., et al. (2003). High rates of behavioral problems in perinatally HIV-infected children are not linked to HIV disease. Pediatrics, 111 (2), 384–393.

Mialky, E., Vagnoni, J., Rutstein, R. (2001). School-age children with perinatally acquired HIV infection: medical and psychosocial issues in a Philadelphia cohort. AIDS Patient Care STDS, 15 (11), 575–579.

Morrow, B.M., Hsaio, N.Y., Zampoli, M., et al. (2010, June). Pneumocystis pneumonia in South African children with and without human immunodeficiency virus infection in the era of highly active antiretroviral therapy. Pediatr Infect Dis J, 29 (6), 535–539.

Mukoma, W., Flisher, A.J., Ahmed, N., et al. (2009). Process evaluation of a school-based HIV/AIDS intervention in South Africa. Scand J Public Health, 37 (Suppl 2), 37–47.

Murphy, D.A., Austin, E.L., Greenwell, L. (2006). Correlates of HIV-related stigma among HIV-positive mothers and their uninfected children. Women Health, 44 (3), 19–42.

Musiime, V., Kalyesubula, I., Kaddu-Mulindwa, D. (2009, May–June). Enteric bacterial pathogens in HIV-infected children with acute diarrhea in Mulago referral and teaching hospital, Kampala, Uganda. J Int Assoc Physicians AIDS Care (Chic), 8 (3), 185–190.

NIAID. (2004, July). HIV infections in infants and children. Retrieved from http://www.niaid.nih.gov/factsheets/hivchildren.htm

Pitcher, R.D., Beningfield, S.J., Zar, H.J. (2010, February). Chest radiographic features of lymphocytic interstitial pneumonitis in HIV-infected children. Clin Radiol, 65 (2), 150–154.

Raccurt, C.P., Pannier Stockman, C., Eyma, E. (2006, October). Enteric parasites and AIDS in Haiti: utility of detection and treatment of intestinal parasites in family members. Med Trop (Mars), 66 (5), 461–464.

Rice, E., Milburn, N.G., Rotheram-Borus, M.J. (2007). Pro-social and problematic social network influences on HIV/AIDS risk behaviours among newly homeless youth in Los Angeles. AIDS Care, 19 (5), 697–704.

Riley, L.E., Greene, M.F. (1999, April 1). Elective cesarean delivery to reduce the transmission of HIV. N Engl J Med, 340 (13), 1032–1033.

Robin, L., Dittus, P., Whitaker, D., et al. (2004). Behavioral interventions to reduce incidence of HIV, STD, and pregnancy among adolescents: a decade in review. J Adolesc Health, 34 (1), 3–26.

Simpkins, E.P., Siberry, G.K., Hutton, N. (2009, September). Thinking about HIV infection. Pediatr Rev, 30 (9), 337–348.

Slyker, J.A., Lohman-Payne, B.L., John-Stewart, G.C., et al. (2009, October 23). Acute cytomegalovirus infection in Kenyan HIV-infected infants. AIDS, 23 (16), 2173–2181.

Steele, R.G., Nelson, T.D., Cole, B.P. (2007). Psychosocial functioning of children with AIDS and HIV infection: review of the literature from a socioecological framework. J Dev Behav Pediatr, 28 (1), 58–69.

Storm, D.S., Boland, M.G., Gortmaker, S.L., et al. (2005). Protease inhibitor combination therapy, severity of illness, quality of life among children with perinatally acquired HIV-1 infection. Pediatrics, 115 (2), e173–e182.

Surachatkumtonekul, T., Chokephaibulkit, K., Vanprapar, N., et al. (2008). Treatment of cytomegalovirus (CMV) retinitis with intravitreous ganciclovir in HIV-infected children. J Med Assoc Thai, 91 (3), 331–337.

UNAIDS. (2008, July). 2008 Report on the global AIDS epidemic. Geneva, Switzerland: Joint United Nations Programme on HIV/AIDS.

van Eijk, A.M., Brooks, J.T., Adcock, P.M., et al. (2010, March). Diarrhea in children less than two years of age with known HIV status in Kisumu, Kenya. Int J Infect Dis, 14 (3), e220–225.

Van Rie, A., Mupuala, A., Dow, A. (2008). Impact of the HIV/AIDS epidemic on the neurodevelopment of preschool-aged children in Kinshasa, Democratic Republic of the Congo. Pediatrics, 122 (1), e123–e128.

Vijayan, T., Benin, A.L., Wagner, K., et al. (2009). We never thought this would happen: transitioning care of adolescents with perinatally acquired HIV infection from pediatrics to internal medicine. AIDS Care, 21 (10), 1222–1229.

Volmink, J., Siegfried, N.L., van der Merwe, L., et al. (2007, January 24). Antiretrovirals for reducing the risk of mother-to-child transmission of HIV infection. Cochrane Database Syst Rev, 1, CD003510.

Wanachiwanawin, D., Chokephaibulkit, K., Lertlaituan, P., et al. (2002). Intestinal microsporidiosis in HIV-infected children with diarrhea. Southeast Asian J Trop Med Public Health, Jun; 33 (2), 241–245.

Zar, H.J. (2008, January). Chronic lung disease in human immunodeficiency virus (HIV) infected children. Pediatr Pulmonol, 43 (1), 1–10.

Zhao, G., Li, X., Fang, X., et al. (2007). Care arrangements, grief and psychological problems among children orphaned by AIDS in China. AIDS Care, 19 (9), 1075–1082.

Zhao, Q., Li, X., Fang, X., et al. (2010, July–August). Difference in psychosocial well-being between paternal and maternal AIDS orphans in rural China. J Assoc Nurses AIDS Care, 21 (4), 335–344.

Index

M.L. Goldstein, S. Morewitz, *Chronic Disorders in Children and Adolescents*,
DOI 10.1007/978-1-4419-9764-7, © Springer Science+Business Media, LLC 2011

MIX
Papier aus verantwortungsvollen Quellen
Paper from responsible sources
FSC® C105338

If you have any concerns about our products,
you can contact us on
ProductSafety@springernature.com

In case Publisher is established outside the EU,
the EU authorized representative is:
Springer Nature Customer Service Center GmbH
Europaplatz 3, 69115 Heidelberg, Germany

Printed by Libri Plureos GmbH
in Hamburg, Germany